P9-CWE-121

Artificial Neural Networks in Cancer Diagnosis, Prognosis, and Patient Management

Biomedical Engineering Series

Edited by Michael R. Neuman

Published Titles

Electromagnetic Analysis and Design in Magnetic Resonancer Imaging, Jianming Jin

Endogenous and Exogenous Regulation and Control of Physiological Systems, Robert B. Northrop

Artificial Neural Networks in Cancer Diagnosis, Prognosis, and Treatment, Raouf N.G. Naguib and Gajanan V. Sherbet

Medical Image Registration, Joseph V. Hajnal, Derek Hill, and David J. Hawkes

Introduction to Dynamic Modeling of Neuro-Sensory Systems, Robert B. Northrop

Forthcoming Titles

Noninvasive Instrumentation and Measurement in Medical Diagnosis, Robert B. Northrop

Handbook of Neuroprosthetic Methods, Warren E. Finn and Peter G. LoPresti

The BIOMEDICAL ENGINEERING Series
Series Editor Michael Neuman

Artificial Neural Networks in Cancer Diagnosis, Prognosis, and Patient Management

Edited by
Raouf N.G. Naguib
Gajanan V. Sherbet

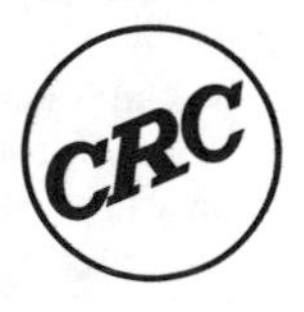

CRC Press
Boca Raton London New York Washington, D.C.

Library of Congress Cataloging-in-Publication Data

Artificial neural networks in cancer diagnosis, prognosis, and patient management / [edited by] Raouf N.G. Naguib and Gajanan V. Sherbet.
p. ; cm.— (Biomedical engineering series)
Includes bibliographical references and index.
ISBN 0-8493-9692-1 (alk. paper)
1. Cancer—Computer simulation. 2. Neural networks (Computer science) 3. Artificial intelligence—Medical applications. I. Naguib, Raouf N.G. II. Sherbet, G.V. (Gajanan V.) III. Biomedical engineering series (Boca Raton, Fla.)
[DNLM: 1. Neoplasms—diagnosis. 2. Diagnosis, Computer-Assisted. 3. Neoplasms—therapy. 4. Neural Networks (Computer). 5. Prognosis. QZ 241 A791 2001]
RC254.5 .A66 2001
616.99'4'00113—dc21 2001025509

Direct all inquiries to CRC Press LLC, 2000 N.W. Corporate Blvd., Boca Raton, Florida 33431.

International Standard Book Number 0-8493-9692-1
Library of Congress Card Number 2001025509
Printed in the United States of America 1 2 3 4 5 6 7 8 9 0
Printed on acid-free paper

குணம் நாடி குற்றம் நாடி அவற்றுள்
மிகைநாடி மிக்க கொளல்

"Weigh and closely scan both favourable and unfavourable features and the output will offer an option for action"

Thiru Valluvar
(Tamil Poet, Second Century, India)

Thirukkural, Chapter 51, Verse 504

PREFACE

The potential value of artificial neural networks (ANNs) as a predictor of malignancy has now been widely recognised. The concept of ANNs dates back to the early part of the 20th century; however, their latest resurrection started in earnest in the 1980s when they were applied to many problems in the areas of pattern recognition, control, and optimisation. Here we present a series of articles that emphasise the keen interest displayed by the scientific community in the application of neural networks in the management of human cancers, and also reflect the recent intense activity in this field. The neural systems use prognostic cancer markers as input neurons and provide an ideal means of combining the input signals so that the output neurons can provide a predictive basis on which to determine the course of patient management. In essence, the two characteristics that determine the reliability of neural networks are the discriminant analysis of the input variables and the correct classification of tumours with regard to the accuracy of the predictive output, whether in the form of diagnosis, its spread to regional lymph nodes, or patient survival. This versatility of the artificial neural networks is aptly encapsulated by the Tamil quotation.

One of the main objectives of this book is to ensure that the material reported in it emanates from a variety of institutions, in order that an objective and unbiased view of the different approaches undertaken by researchers in those institutions can be presented. Thus, the book contains chapters relating to different types of cancer. These have been written by leading international researchers in the field of artificial neural networks, as well as by leading experts in oncology, physicians, pathologists, and surgeons from Europe and North and South America.

The subject of artificial neural networks has been extensively treated in the literature and therefore the object of this book is not to present yet another monograph in this area. The aim, however, is to focus solely on their applicability in the field of oncology which, as witnessed by the growing number of publications, is rapidly developing into a major area of research in its own right. Chapter 1, therefore, presents a very brief introduction to ANNs whilst attempting to emphasise their direct relationship to the inherent problems in cancer diagnosis, prognosis, and patient management.

Breast cancer has been the focus of much research lately, especially with regard to the identification of molecular cancer markers. In Chapter 2, Angus et al. discuss some issues relating to prognosis in breast cancer patients. They highlight the clinical importance of molecular, cytological, and histological prognostic markers, including the proteins associated with metastatic potential. They also present an ANN analysis of the significance of the expression of the metastasis-associated *h-mts1* and *nm23* genes and their individual relationship to nodal spread of breast cancer. This is then followed in Chapter 3 by a discussion of the use of image cytometric measurements of DNA ploidy, the S-phase cell fraction and nuclear pleomorphism as prognostic aids. The practicalities and putative benefits of analysing these data using neural systems are then scrutinised.

The application of ANNs in lung cancer is the subject of Chapters 4 and 5. Chapter 4 is a contribution by Esteva and colleagues. The chapter presents the general issues involved in the prognostic analysis of patients with carcinoma of the lung, and assesses the accuracy of applying artificial neural networks to the prognosis of post-surgical outcome of lung cancer patients. Chapter 5 by Jefferson et al., on the other hand, focuses on the use of a genetic algorithm neural network for prognosis in surgically treated nonsmall cell lung cancer.

In Chapter 6, Speight and Hammond deal with the use of machine learning in screening for oral cancer. The chapter summarises the investigations into the application of ANNs in the selection of high-risk groups of patients, comparing their predictive performance with other machine learning techniques and evaluating the potential performance of machine learning for the detection of high-risk individuals. This chapter also discusses the merits of utilising machine learning for the prediction of risk of oral, and other cancers, as an adjunct to population screening.

The contribution by Wayman and Griffin in Chapter 7 describes the application of ANNs in the prediction of outcome for cancer of the oesophago-gastric junction. As the decision on whether a surgical procedure is necessary or not is made on the interpretation of pre-operative assessments of tumour stage and patient fitness, the correlation between pre- and post-operative findings is frequently poor. Thus, results relating to the application of ANNs to patients undergoing potentially curative resection of adenocarcinoma of the oesophago-gastric junction, both pre- and post-operatively, are reported in this chapter.

It is inevitable, as with any novel and fast growing area of research within a relatively tightly knit and closely collaborating community of researchers, that a degree of overlap will occur. This is particularly evident in the chapters on urological oncology, an area which has perhaps attracted a more concerted effort on the part of clinicians, engineers, and biomedical computing scientists. This is reflected in the number of chapters in this book that deal with this specific area of cancer from both a diagnosis and prognosis viewpoint.

Chapters 8 to 12 therefore represent a comprehensive treatment of this area of machine learning in urological oncology. Chapters 8 (Douglas and Moul) and 9 (Niederberger and Ridout) review the basic concepts of artificial neural networks and summarise their application in renal cell carcinoma (RCC), prostate, bladder, and testicular cancers. These reviews provide an insight into the difficult task of preoperative diagnosis of RCC, issues in prostate cancer diagnosis, outcome prediction, and patients' quality of life. These parameters are increasingly being regarded as important elements in the choice of treatment. The combined application of image analysis procedures and ANNs to identify bladder cells expressing the tumour antigen p300, as well as automated cytology-based interpretation in bladder cancer, are emphasised. Testicular cancer is reviewed, especially from the angle of pathologic stage I vs. stage II prediction in patients with clinical stage I nonseminomatous testicular cancer.

In Chapter 10, Stamey et al. give a detailed description of ProstAsure™, a neural-based technique to predict the risk of prostate cancer in men with a PSA $\leq$ 4.0 ng/ml, and predict tumour recurrence following radical prostatectomy. Hamdy reports, in Chapter 11, on the use of a neural network to predict prognosis and outcome in prostate cancer. Conventional input variables (age, stage, bone scan findings, grade, PSA, and type of treatment) are used in addition to data derived from the immunohistochemical staining performed on tissue specimens for the proto-oncogene bcl-2 and tumour suppressor gene p53. The presence of increased abnormal expression of these genes has been associated with disease progression in prostate cancer. Hamdy shows that ANNs can be used to assess the benefits, or otherwise, of such newer experimental tumour markers.

Finally, in the field of urological oncology, Chapter 12's authors Qureshi and Mellon present a study relating to the prediction of clinical outcome for patients with bladder cancer utilising prognostic markers identified at initial presentation. In this study, they seek to assess the ability of an ANN to predict the recurrence and stage progression in bladder cancer. This is carried out in a group of patients with newly diagnosed Ta/T1 bladder cancer, and 12-month cancer-specific survival in a group of patients with primary T2-T4 bladder cancer by using clinical, pathological and molecular prognostic indicators. In addition, the networks' predictions are compared with those of four consultant urologists supplied with the same data.

The final chapter is a contribution on skin cancer by Hintz-Madsen and his colleagues, where the authors describe a comprehensive study of the applications of ANNs in the diagnosis of melanoma. The accurate detection of this malignancy is heavily dependent upon the precise analysis of skin pigmentation, tumour shape, and colour.

There are several areas of neoplasia that have not been investigated by using the ANN tool. The editors hope this volume will not only emphasise the value of this tool in the study of this disease process but will provide a nucleus around which future work might be planned and executed.

Apart from minor cosmetic changes we have restrained from attempting to change either the structure or contents of each chapter. We sincerely felt that the views and technical contents presented by the authors should give an honest insight into the modes and practices of their efforts in this particularly sensitive, and perhaps contentious, area of research.

The experts who have contributed to this work have certainly made this book move from the possible to the achievable. We wish to thank them most sincerely. Without the time and effort they spent on their respective chapters, the objectives that we set for ourselves would not have been accomplished. Our research students have, over the years, been a tremendous source of inspiration. They have been instrumental in developing ideas and algorithms which, in many instances, seemed initially to be impractical. We are indebted to them for their efforts, original ideas, and many stimulating discussions. Our thanks also go to Sonia Clarke whose editing skills and careful attention to detail have made our task much easier than originally expected. We wish to thank Dr. M.S. Lakshmi for providing the Tamil quotation and its translation. Finally, we also wish to acknowledge the Cancer Research Campaign of the United Kingdom for supporting many aspects of this work.

R.N.G. Naguib, Ph.D.
G.V. Sherbet, DSc., FRCPath.
Editors

EDITORS

Raouf Naguib, Ph.D., is Professor of Biomedical Computing in the School of Mathematical and Information Sciences, Coventry University, England, where he also leads the Biomedical Computing Research Group. Prior to this appointment, he was a Lecturer at the University of Newcastle upon Tyne, England. Professor Naguib received the degrees of Ph.D., M.Sc. (with distinction), and D.I.C. from Imperial College of Science, Technology and Medicine, University of London, England, and the B.Sc. degree from Cairo University, Egypt. In 1995–1996 he was awarded the Fulbright Cancer Fellowship to pursue his research at the University of Hawaii in Mãnoa on the applications of artificial neural networks in breast cancer diagnosis and prognosis. Professor Naguib is a Chartered Engineer and a member of the Institution of Electrical Engineers (IEE), the Institute of Physics and Engineering in Medicine (IPEM), the American Association for Cancer Research (AACR), and a Senior Member of the Institute of Electrical and Electronics Engineers (IEEE). He is the representative of IEEE Engineering in Medicine and Biology Society (EMBS) to the European Society for Engineering and Medicine, and the IEEE-USA Committee on Communications and Information Policy. He is also a Special Area Editor for the IEEE Transactions on Information Technology in Biomedicine.

Professor Naguib has worked extensively on the applications of artificial neural networks in the field of clinical oncology. This work was also combined with studies on image processing, image cytometry and the stratification of significant conventional and experimental prognostic markers in a variety of cancers. His current interests lie in the applications of evolutionary computational models, fuzzy logic, genetic algorithms and parallel image processing methodologies to cancer diagnosis, prognosis and disease management. He also has a special interest in content-based image retrieval and human form perception for histopathological identification.

Professor Naguib has published more than 130 journal and conference papers and reports in many aspects of digital signal processing, image processing, artificial intelligence, evolutionary computation and biomedical engineering. He has also co-authored a book on digital filtering.

Gajanan Sherbet, DSc., FRCPath, is Professor at the Institute for Molecular Medicine, Huntington Beach, CA. He received the degrees of D.Sc. and M.Sc. from the University of London, and his Ph.D., M.Sc., and B.Sc. degrees from the University of Poona. Dr. Sherbet was Reader in Experimental Oncology and Deputy Director of the Cancer Research Unit in the Medical School of the University of Newcastle upon Tyne, England. Previous to this, Dr. Sherbet was a member of staff of the Chester Beatty Research Institute, Institute of Cancer Research, and University College Hospital Medical School in London. He has held prestigious fellowships such as the Beit Memorial and Williams Fellowship of the University of London. He held a career fellowship awarded by the North of England Cancer Research Campaign. For a brief period, he was a fellow of Harvard College, Cambridge, MA. Dr. Sherbet is Fellow of the Royal College of Pathologists (FRCPath), Royal Society of Chemistry (FRSC) and The Institute of Biology (FIBiol) of UK. He served as editor of Oncology, Experimental Cell Biology, and was senior editor of Pathobiology. Currently, Dr. Sherbet is a member of the editorial boards of Pathobiology and Anticancer Research.

Dr. Sherbet's major interest is in cancer metastasis. In recent years, he has been investigating the role of the calcium binding protein S100A4 in cell proliferation, cancer invasion, and metastasis. He recently demonstrated the potential value of S100A4 as a marker for assessing the progression of breast cancer. He is also studying the potential of artificial neural networks in the management of breast cancer, and has many publications in this field especially relating to the analysis of expression of cancer markers and image cytometric data of breast cancer by using artificial neural networks.

Dr. Sherbet has published numerous scientific papers in international journals. He was guest editor of *Retinoids*: *Their Physiological Function and Therapeutic Potential* (1997). He has written and edited several books on cancer; among them, *The Metastatic Spread of* Cancer (1987), *The Biology of Tumor Malignancy* (1982) and *The Biophysical Characterization of the Cell Surface* (1978). His book on *The Genetics of Cancer* (1997) was co-authored with Dr. M.S. Lakshmi. Dr. Sherbet's latest book on *Calcium Signalling in Cancer* (2001) was published by CRC Press.

CONTRIBUTORS

Brian Angus
Department of Pathology
Medical School, University of Newcastle
and
Royal Victoria Infirmary
Newcastle upon Tyne, UK

Stephen D. Barnhill
Horus Therapeutics, Inc.
Savannah, GA
and
Institute for the Advancement of Computer Assisted Medicine
Mercer University
Macon, GA, USA

Marta Bellotti
División Patologia Quirúrgica del Hospital de Clinicas "José de San Martin" de la Universidad de Buenos Aires
Buenos Aires, Argentina

Thomas H. Douglas
Urology Service, Department of Surgery
DeWitt Army Community Hospital
Fort Belvoir, VA
and
Centre for Prostate Disease Research
Department of Surgery
Uniformed Services University of the Health Sciences
Bethesda, MD, USA

Krzysztof T. Drzewiecki
Department of Plastic Surgery
National University Hospital
Copenhagen, Denmark

Hugo Esteva
Facultad de Medicina de la Universidad de Buenos Aires
and
División Patologia Quirúrgica del Hospital de Clinicas "José de San Martin" de la Universidad de Buenos Aires
Buenos Aires, Argentina

S. Michael Griffin
Northern Oesophago-Gastric Cancer Unit
Royal Victoria Infirmary
Newcastle upon Tyne, UK

Freddie C. Hamdy
University of Sheffield
and
Department of Urology
Royal Hallamshire Hospital Sheffield, UK

Peter Hammond
Department of Informatics
Eastman Dental Institute for Oral Health Care Sciences
University of London
London, UK

Lars Kai Hansen
CONNECT
Department of Mathematical Modelling
Technical University of Denmark
Lyngby, Denmark

Mads Hintz-Madsen
CONNECT
Department of Mathematical Modelling
Technical University of Denmark
Lyngby, Denmark

M.A. Horan
University Department of Geriatric Medicine
Hope Hospital
Salford, UK

M.F. Jefferson
University Department of Geriatric Medicine
Hope Hospital
Salford, UK

Jan Larsen
CONNECT
Department of Mathematical Modelling
Technical University of Denmark
Lyngby, Denmark

Thomas W.J. Lennard
Department of Surgery
Medical School
University of Newcastle
and
Royal Victoria Infirmary
Newcastle upon Tyne, UK

S.B. Lucas
University Department of Geriatric Medicine
Hope Hospital
Salford, UK

K. Rama Madyastha
Horus Therapeutics, Inc.
Savannah, GA
and
Institute for the Advancement of Computer Assisted Medicine
Mercer University
Macon, GA, USA

Alberto M. Marchevsky
UCLA School of Medicine
and
Division of Anatomic Pathology
Cedars Sinai Medical Centre
Los Angeles, CA, USA

J. Kilian Mellon
Department of Surgery Medical School
University of Newcastle
and
University Urology Unit
Freeman Hospital
Newcastle upon Tyne, UK

Judd W. Moul
Centre for Prostate Disease Research
Department of Surgery
Uniformed Services University of the Health Sciences
Bethesda, MD
and
Urology Service
Department of Surgery
Walter Reed Army Medical Centre
Washington, DC, USA

Raouf N.G. Naguib
BIOCORE
School of Mathematical and Information Sciences
Coventry University
Coventry, UK

Craig Niederberger
Department of Urology
University of Illinois at Chicago
Chicago, IL, USA

N. Pendleton
University Department of Geriatric Medicine
Hope Hospital
Salford, UK

Khaver N. Qureshi
Department of Urology
Royal Hallamshire Hospital
Sheffield, UK

Dustin Ridout
Department of Urology
University of Illinois at Chicago
Chicago, IL, USA

Gajanan V. Sherbet
Cancer Research Unit
University of Newcastle
Newcastle upon Tyne, UK
and
Institute for Molecular Medicine
Huntington Beach, CA, USA

Paul M. Speight
Department of Oral Pathology
Eastman Dental Institute for Oral Health Care Sciences
University of London
London, UK

Thomas A. Stamey
Department of Urology
School of Medicine
Stanford University
Stanford, CA, USA

John Wayman
Northern Oesophago-Gastric Cancer Unit
Royal Victoria Infirmary
Newcastle upon Tyne
and
West Cumberland Hospital
Whitehaven, UK

Cheryl M. Yemoto
Department of Urology
School of Medicine
Stanford University
Stanford, CA, USA

Hong Zhang
Horus Therapeutics, Inc.
Savannah, GA
and
Institute for the Advancement of Computer Assisted Medicine
Mercer University
Macon, GA, USA

Zhen Zhang
Department of Biometry and Epidemiology
Medical University of South Carolina
Charleston, SC
and
Institute for the Advancement of Computer Assisted Medicine
Mercer University
Macon, GA, USA

CONTENTS

Chapter 3

Artificial Neural Approach to Analysing the Prognostic Significance of DNA Ploidy and Cell Cycle Distribution of Breast Cancer Aspirate Cells **23**

R.N.G. Naguib and G.V. Sherbet

Chapter 4

Neural Networks for the Estimation of Prognosis in Lung Cancer **29**

H. Esteva, M. Bellotti, and A.M. Marchevsky

Chapter 5

The Use of a Genetic Algorithm Neural Network (GANN) for Prognosis in Surgically Treated Nonsmall Cell Lung Cancer (NSCLC) **39**

M.F. Jefferson, N. Pendleton, S.B. Lucas, and M.A. Horan

Chapter 6

The Use of Machine Learning in Screening for Oral Cancer **55**

P. M. Speight and P. Hammond

Chapter 7

Outcome Prediction of Oesophago-Gastric Cancer Using Neural Analysis of Pre- and Postoperative Parameters **73**

J. Wayman and S.M. Griffin

Chapter 8

Artifical Neural Networks in Urologic Oncology **93**

T.H. Douglas and J.W. Moul

Chapter 9

Neural Networks in Urologic Oncology **103**

C. Niederberger and D. Ridout

Chapter 10

Comparison of a Neural Network with High Sensitivity and Specificity of Free/Total Serum PSA for Diagnosing Prostate Cancer in Men with a PSA < 4.0 ng/mL **115**

T.A. Stamey, S.D. Barnhill, Z. Zhang, C.M. Yemoto, H. Zhang, and K.R. Madyastha

---

Chapter 11

Artificial Neural Networks and Prognosis in Prostate Cancer **125**

F.C. Hamdy

Chapter 12

Comparison between Urologists and Artificial Neural Networks in Bladder Cancer Outcome Prediction **133**

K.N. Qureshi and J.K. Mellon

Chapter 13

A Probabilistic Neural Network Framework for the Detection of Malignant Melanoma **141**

M. Hintz-Madsen, L.K. Hansen, J. Larsen, and K.T. Drzewiecki

Chapter 1

INTRODUCTION TO ARTIFICIAL NEURAL NETWORKS AND THEIR USE IN CANCER DIAGNOSIS, PROGNOSIS, AND PATIENT MANAGEMENT[§]

R.N.G. Naguib and G.V. Sherbet

I. PREAMBLE

The use of artificial neural networks (ANNs) in biological and medical research has vastly proliferated during the last few years. A recent MEDLINE search reveals more than 300 articles published in the last two years that have as a main identifier "neural network". Medical applications of ANNs have touched on a variety of areas such as anaesthesiology [1], radiology [2], cardiology [3,4], psychiatry [5], and neurology [6]. Our concern in this book, however, lies in their application in the field of cancer research, specifically concentrating on their potential uses in prognostic studies, survival analyses, and the prediction of outcome for patients afflicted with varying types and stages of cancer.

Although the process of cancer management may be somewhat deterministic, in that surgeons and pathologists can confidently ascertain the existence and extent of spread, such determination is usually reached through biopsies or axillary assessment at the expense of patient morbidity and health service resources. An automated, reliable, and noninvasive procedure would be greatly advantageous from the point of view of both patients and medical experts alike.

Similarly, reliable assessment of the progression of a tumour is essential for proper treatment. This has prompted researchers to search for prognostic factors, simple tests or measurements that could yield information about the biological features of the disease in relation to the state of its progression. Many such potential factors have been identified and studied, but none has been found to be completely reliable, and different factors may appear to contradict each other. As a result, clinicians are faced with increasing amounts of information about patients, but are finding it increasingly difficult to interpret this information in a useful way. Indeed, even elaborate survival analysis techniques based on univariate, multivariate, and proportional hazards paradigms have not so far culminated in a tangible advancement of prognostic assessment.

Neural network analysis has been shown to be particularly useful in those cases where the problem to be solved is ill defined, and development of an algorithmic solution is difficult.

[§] Many sections in this chapter have been extracted from our paper: Naguib R.N.G., Sherbet G.V., Artificial neural networks in cancer research, *Pathobiology*, 65, 129-139, 1997. The Publishers' agreement to reproduce this material is kindly appreciated.

0-8493-9692-1/01/$0.00+$1.50

This is exactly the situation with cancer data where a highly nonlinear, almost brain-like, approach is required to sift through the maze of available information.

II. ARTIFICIAL NEURAL NETWORKS

ANNs are parallel information-processing structures that attempt to emulate certain performance characteristics of the biological neural system.

The biological neuron has three types of components that are of particular interest in understanding the method of operation of its artificial counterpart. These are the dendrites, soma, and axon. Figure 1.1 illustrates a generic biological neuron [7]. Dendrites receive signals from other neurons via axons. These signals may originate as chemical, electrical, or temperature change and have to cross a synaptic gap by means of a chemical process. Incoming information is thus accumulated in the cell body, or soma. The soma then acts on the various input signals — usually through a simple summation process — and, when enough input is received, the cell fires, i.e., it transmits a signal over its output axon to other cells.

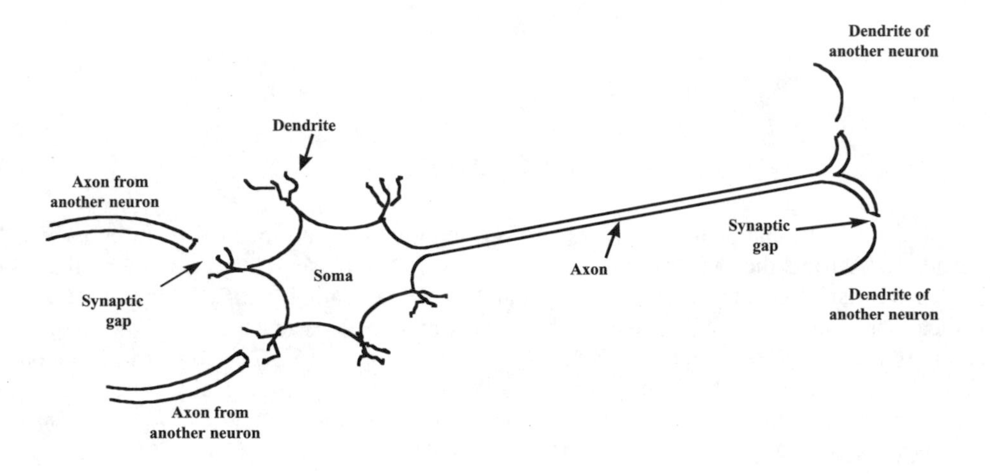

Figure 1.1 Schematic diagram of a generic biological neuron. A typical cell has three major regions: the cell body, which is also called the soma, the axon, and the dendrites. The axon is a long cylindrical connection that carries impulses from the neuron to the dendrites. The axon-dendrite contact area is called the synaptic gap. This is where the neuron introduces its signal to the neighbouring neuron. The receiving neuron either generates an impulse to its axon, or produces no response.

The mathematical model of an artificial neuron is shown in Figure 1.2. Here, the unit analogous to the soma is the processing element or node. Dendrites are represented by the different input values, which have to cross the synaptic gaps or weights. The output of the processing element is the result of applying a transfer function to its summation content. This transfer function may be a threshold function which only passes information if the combined activity only reaches a certain level, or it may be a continuous function of the combined input. In most practical neural network implementations such function is taken to be the sigmoid function (transfer function in Figure 1.2). It is clear that, since each connection has a corresponding weight, the signals on the input lines to a processing element are modified by these weights prior to being summed. Thus the summation function itself is a weighted summation.

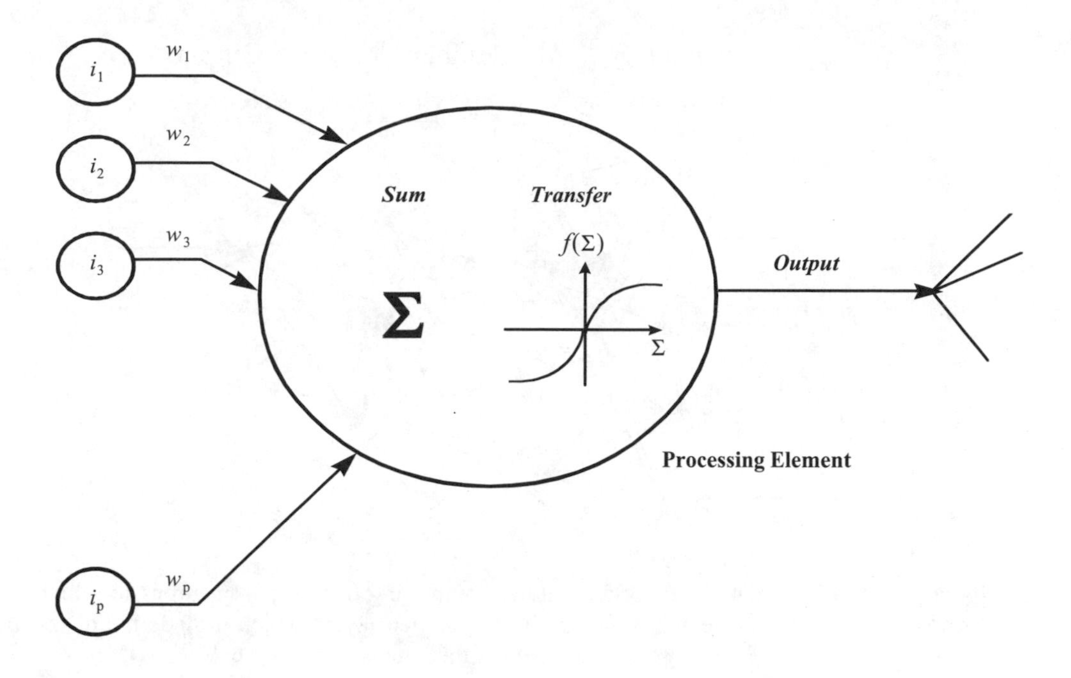

Figure 1.2 Mathematical model of an artificial neuron. The soma is represented by the processing elements. Inputs to the processing element represent the dendrites and the effects of the synaptic gap in the biological neuron are represented by the weights on the connections between inputs and processing element in the artificial model.

An artificial neural network consists of many processing elements joined together in the above manner. Processing elements are usually organised into groups called layers and, as such, a typical network consists of a sequence of layers successively connected by full or random connections. There are typically two layers with connection to the outside world: an input layer where data is presented to the network and an output layer which holds the response of the network to a given input. Layers distinct from the input and output buffers are called hidden layers. Such layers add to the learning nonlinearity required for the successful solution of complex problems. A feedforward fully interconnected artificial neural network is shown in Figure 1.3. In a feedforward network all signals pass from the input processing elements to the output processing elements (through intermediate or hidden units) without any connections back to the previous layers.

The application of such networks represents a major change in the traditional approach to problem solving. As is the case with the human brain, it is no longer necessary to know a formal mathematical model of the classification or recognition problem and then perform the test and recall phases based on this knowledge. Instead, if a comprehensive training set and a suitable network architecture are devised, then an error backpropagation algorithm can be used to adapt network parameters to obtain the input-output relationships required. The solution is obtained through experimentation and simulation rather than through rigorous and formal approach to the problem, as is the case with existing statistical methods currently applied in many cancer research studies.

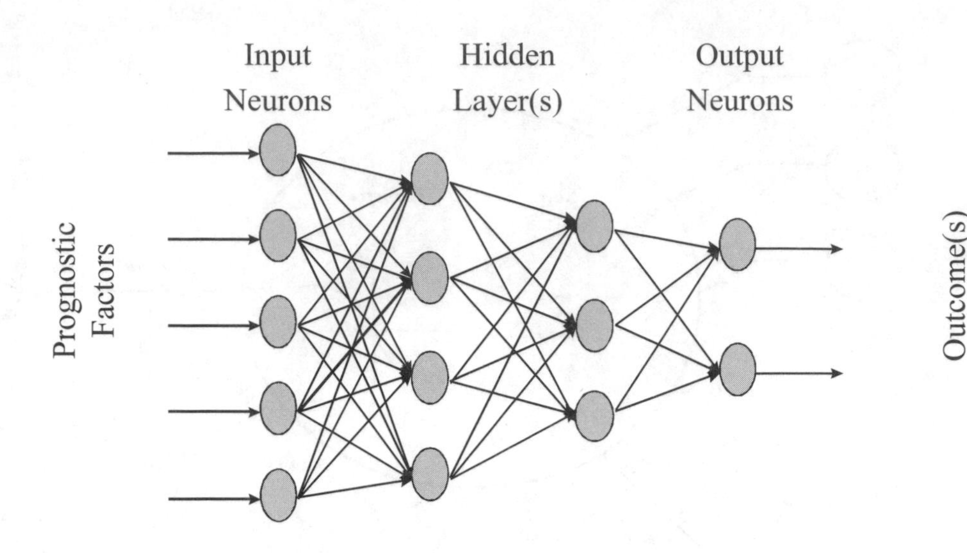

Figure 1.3 Artificial neural network structure, comprising of the input neurons to which the prognostic factors are presented, followed by the hidden layers which provide the necessary nonlinearity, and the output neurons which deliver the outcomes of the analysis.

The training procedure entails repeatedly presenting a collection of input-output pairs that represent the problem under consideration. The network is then able to study patterns or features within the data that will ultimately assist it in reaching the "correct" decision with respect to the desired output.

At each iteration, the network output is compared with the desired output and an error function is generated. When this error value exceeds a certain threshold, set by the designer and based upon the application at hand, the weights on the different interconnections within the network are reassessed and updated in readiness for the subsequent iteration. It is only when the error attains that threshold, or falls below it, that the network is said to have converged and is deemed to have "learnt" the interrelationships presented to it through the iterative process.

When presented with a new set of input data, the network should therefore be able to attain the correct corresponding decision based on its previous learning ability. In this sense, the network is capable of generalising, i.e., sensibly interpolating input patterns that are new to it [8]. This is undoubtedly one of the distinct strengths of neural systems.

The following is a very simplified summary of the task that an error backpropagation network needs to solve. Given a training data in the form of P vector pairs $\left(\mathbf{i}_p, \mathbf{d}_p\right)$, or the training set

$$\left\{ \left(\mathbf{i}_p, \mathbf{d}_p\right), \qquad p = 1, 2, \ldots P \right\} \tag{1}$$

where $\mathbf{i}$ and $\mathbf{d}$ are the input and desired output data vectors, respectively, then, for a given pattern p, the network maps $\mathbf{i}_p$ into an output vector $\mathbf{o}_p$ using a highly nonlinear operation, Γ, as follows

$$\mathbf{o}_p = \Gamma\left[\mathbf{W}\,\Gamma\left[\mathbf{V}\mathbf{i}_p\right]\right] \tag{2}$$

where **V** and **W** are the weight vector patterns pertaining to connections between the input and hidden and between the hidden and output layers, respectively.

The goal of the training is to produce $\mathbf{o}_p$ such that it replicates $\mathbf{d}_p$. The quality of approximation is determined by the error

$$E = \sum_{p=1}^{P} \left\| \mathbf{o}_p - \mathbf{d}_p \right\|^2 \tag{3}$$

Minimisation of the error in Equation (3) can be interpreted as a classical interpolation and estimation problem — given a set of input data, we seek parameters w and v that approximate the corresponding output data for a class of functions selected as in Equation (2).

Learning in artificial neural networks essentially assumes one of two paradigms: supervised or unsupervised.

Strictly speaking, the learning process described above is one type of supervised learning. At each instant when the input is applied, the desired response of the system is provided for comparison with the actual output.

In unsupervised learning, the desired response is not known *a priori*. Thus, explicit error information is unavailable to improve network behaviour. Since no information is available as to the correctness or incorrectness of the response, learning must somehow be accomplished based on observation of responses to inputs that yield marginal or no knowledge about them. The network is therefore training towards some optimum output where *optimum* is usually some clustering of the data.

In almost all applications of artificial neural networks in the field of cancer research, the target or desired output is explicitly provided. Almost invariably medical experts assist with the most likely diagnosis given a certain set of pathological information. Similarly, prognostic information is based on survival analysis procedures, and patient management is optimised through retrospective assessment of previous and long-term responses to treatment. Thus, in the vast majority of neural structures described in this book, supervised learning constitutes the basic mode of learning.

III. DISCUSSION

From the studies of neural application in cancer research addressed in this book, it is clear that ANNs have an impact on current cancer research from a number of different angles. Some of these are summarised below:

- From a prognostic viewpoint, it is clear that current statistical methods of survival analysis have not resulted in reliable conclusions as far as the individual patient's prognosis is concerned. Physicians can refer to information based on previous *group* studies and derive an extremely imprecise estimation of the likelihood of disease recurrence or progression. ANNs, on the other hand, provide the physician with much greater power to predict outcome on an individual basis.

- With the advent of National Health Service (NHS) screening programmes in the UK, an increasing number of patients afflicted with breast cancer are detected at an early stage when the lymph nodes are not involved. ANNs have the potential to classify patients accurately with respect to lymph node metastasis by including certain measures beyond the simple conventional ones. The result is a significant reduction in unnecessary patient morbidity and NHS resources. Therefore, accurate management of the disease could efficiently be achieved.

- Markers which are included in any one study are by no means exhaustive. As more factors and/or parameters are discovered and are deemed of value to the analysis, they can be easily integrated within the ANN, either replacing less important markers or in addition to existing ones. The data can then be reanalysed retrospectively or, indeed, prospectively, as the case may be. In short, the algorithms can be very easily updated to accommodate any relevant information that may have (or thought to have) a contributing value to the final outcome.

Although the contents of the following chapters in this book consider specific types of cancer, the methodology employed in relation to artificial neural analysis generally demonstrates clear and far-reaching implications on the early diagnosis of cancer and in the prediction of patient long-term outcome. However, we are not advocating the principle of an outright replacement of statistical methods but, having assessed the merits of their neural counterparts, to use those as complementary tools that enable clinicians and patients alike to reach a more accurate prediction with regard to the development of the disease. This should be augmented by having an ongoing critical comparison undertaken with the more traditional statistical techniques currently employed such as Cox's proportional hazards [9] and logistic regression [10], together with long-term prospective studies. Indeed, we firmly believe that it is through such prospective analyses that the position of ANNs as a viable diagnostic and prognostic tool will be established. This will also ultimately ascertain that the stigma associated with the neural approach – frequently referred to as a black box with unknown (and somewhat erratic) behaviour – will be unequivocally eliminated. Even under black box conditions, if the neural approach proves to offer a modest improvement over more established traditional statistical techniques, in prospective analyses, then its adoption, as a routine tool for clinical assessment of disease progression and patient outcome, cannot be discarded.

It is our hope that this book will help to contribute, even in a very small measure, to the future elucidation of the cancer dilemma. If intelligent biomedical computing techniques can assist in improving the quality of life of patients afflicted with this disease, then one battle will have been won. The war still goes on.

REFERENCES

1. **Narus S.P., Kück K., Westenskow D.R.,** Intelligent monitor for an anaesthesia breathing circuit, *Proc. Symp. Comp. Appl. Med. Care,* 96-100, 1995.
2. **Wu Y.C., Doi K., Giger M.L.,** Detection of lung nodules in digital chest radiographs using artificial neural networks: a pilot study, *J. Dig. Imag.*, 8,2, 88-94, 1995.
3. **Keem S., Meadows H., Kemp H.,** Hierarchical neural networks in quantitative coronary arteriography, *Proc. IEEE Int. Conf. on Artificial Neural Networks,* 459-464, 1995.
4. **Andrae M.H.,** Neural networks and early diagnosis of myocardial infarction, *The Lancet*, 347, 407-408, 1996.
5. **Dumitra A., Radulescu E., Lazarescu V.,** Improved classification of psychiatric mood disorders using a feedforward neural network, *Medinfo*, 8,1, 818-822, 1995.
6. **Moreno L., Piñero J.D., Sànchez J.L., Mañas J., Acosta L., Hamilton A.,** Brain maturation using neural classifier, *IEEE Trans. Biomed. Eng.*, 42,4, 428-432, 1995.
7. **Fausett L.,** *Fundamentals of Neural Networks — Architectures, Algorithms and Applications,* Prentice-Hall, Englewood Cliffs, NJ, 1994.

8. **Zurada J.M.,** *Introduction to Artificial Neural Systems,* West Publishing Company, 1992.
9. **Cox D.R.,** Regression models and life-tables, *J. Roy. Stat. Soc. [B]*, 34, 187-200, 1972.
10. **Erlichman C., Warde P., Gadalla T., Ciampi A., Baskerville T.,** RECAMP analysis of prognostic factors in patients with stage III breast cancer, *Breast Cancer Res. Treat.*, 16, 231-242, 1990.

Chapter 2

ANALYSIS OF MOLECULAR PROGNOSTIC FACTORS IN BREAST CANCER BY ARTIFICIAL NEURAL NETWORKS

B. Angus, T.W.J. Lennard, R.N.G. Naguib, and G.V. Sherbet

I. INTRODUCTION

The incidence of breast cancer is slowly increasing in most countries of the world, and the disease remains a significant cause of morbidity and mortality in populations. The financial consequences of the disease have a major impact on health economics and, because of the frequency of the condition, together with changes or variations in its management, there will be difficulties with resource planning, as well as differing outcomes amongst treated patients.

Recent observations have shown significant differences in outcome following treatment, which appear to be related to the centre where the patient is treated [1]. There may be a number of explanations for this, including facilities for specific adjuvant treatments at the base hospital, case load of the surgeon, case mix of referred patients and epidemiological factors in the population. One recurring theme in trying to explain these observations is that decisions relating to adjuvant treatments may not be consistent between centres or even within centres. This is hardly surprising given that breast cancer is anything but a homogeneous disease and there are many variables that affect prognosis and outcome. These include commonly available observations, such as tumour size, clinical stage, tumour type and grade, and the involvement or otherwise of the regional draining lymph nodes. Nodal involvement, in particular, has stood the test of time as being one of the most consistent predictors of outcome [2].

Clinicians have become used to using some or all of these parameters on which to base their recommendations for further treatments such as chemotherapy. Consistency in this area of decision-making is, however, far from transparent where, for example, some doctors recommend chemotherapy for grade 2 node negative tumours and others do not. Add in variables such as the age of the patient, coexistent disease, as well as perhaps some more detailed pathological data, for example, vascular or lymphatic invasion in the primary tumour with or without associated *in situ* carcinoma of varying grade, clearance of resection margins, total number of nodes involved and so on, and the clinician has a huge and bewildering number of interrelated factors to take into account. In specialised units, there may in addition be biological markers to take account of, including hormone receptor status, oncogene markers such as epidermal growth factor, c-*erb*B-2, PS2, *nm23,* and FGF [3]. Can we or

0-8493-9692-1/01/$0.00+$1.50

indeed the patient be sure that the advice from doctors in Newcastle will be the same as that in New York, Bristol, Paris, or Rome?

Attempts have been made to create reproducible, objective scoring systems to categorise patients according to risk, based on readily available pathological/morphological features within the primary tumour and nodes. The most familiar of these is the Nottingham prognostic index, a numerical score assigned to the patient, which can be used to estimate prognosis [4]. In longitudinal studies, this index has been shown to correlate well with survival curves of groups of patients [5] and it has the advantage of using readily available pathological criteria for its calculation. However, the parameters used to calculate the index are, by definition, limited and fixed and cannot be linked with other important variables which may influence outcome independently or in a correlated way. Use of multiple prognostic factors fitted into a proportional hazards model can overcome this difficulty, but large scale validation of this approach with long-term survival curves for different prognostic groups in a multicentre setting has not been possible.

The possibility of a reproducible multiparameter "intelligent" prognostic system is exciting and would provide a uniform yet personalised prediction of outcome, with reference to a large database of control patients. Artificial neural networks (ANNs) may provide that opportunity, allowing a set of variables relating to a patient and her tumour to be compared with a data set of known outcomes, while taking into account numerous nonlinear interrelationships between variables and the control data set. Prognostic variables that lend themselves to such an analysis and the background to their role in breast cancer follow.

II. PROGNOSTIC FACTORS IN BREAST CANCER

As discussed above, the outcome in breast cancer can be considerably influenced by patient management (treatment centre, time from presentation to surgery, timing of surgery relative to the menstrual cycle, specific chemotherapy regime employed, etc.). In determination of management of the individual patient, the physician would ideally wish to have available a reliable estimate of prognosis in order that therapy can be tailored to the patient's needs — those patients with a poor outlook receiving more aggressive regimes, and those with a good prognosis spared debilitating therapy.

Tumour associated prognostic factors can be viewed as belonging in two categories: firstly, established prognostic factors of known clinical predictive value, namely tumour stage, grade, and size and, secondly, factors which have been shown, at least in some studies, to be associated with outcome but which do not have proven independent value or value additional to other established factors. For example, tumour cell proliferation fraction has been shown in many studies to predict outcome in breast cancer but does not provide the clinician with a more accurate estimate of prognosis because the variable is accounted for within one of the established factors, tumour grade. The problem with prognostic factors as currently employed is their lack of predictive power; many patients with tumours deemed to be associated with a likely favourable outcome subsequently relapse and die. Here we briefly review prognostic factors, considering firstly those established factors in clinical use and then a number of biological factors, which have been shown to be associated with clinical behaviour.

A. ESTABLISHED PROGNOSTIC FACTORS IN CLINICAL USE: STAGE, GRADE, AND SIZE

Numerous studies have demonstrated the prognostic power of tumour stage (principally assessed as lymph node status), tumour size, and histological grade. Small tumours of low grade without evidence of lymph node spread are associated with an excellent outlook for the patient. Galea and colleagues have employed the three factors to develop the Nottingham Prognostic Index (NPI) [5] which uses a formula based on historic survival data to assign patients to low, intermediate, and high risk groups. The NPI has been validated in other studies [6,7] and provides an example of how prognostic factors can be combined in a clinically useful manner.

In the original description of the index, triple lymph node biopsy was employed to establish lymph node status (lower and apical axillary and internal mammary), but subsequent studies have shown that this can be replaced by the number of positive lymph nodes [7].

The NPI employs the most commonly used system for grading of tumours, namely that devised by Bloom and Richardson, as modified by Elston [4]. Tumours are assessed for degree of tubule formation, nuclear pleomorphism, and mitotic count from which is derived a score of 1 (good prognosis) to 3. In the assessment of tumour size the greatest of three dimensions assessed on the gross specimen is usually employed, but for smaller cancers, more accurate measurement is achieved using the histological section [8].

In the context of established prognostic factors, tumour histological type must be considered. Most invasive breast cancers are of invasive ductal (no special type) histological type. A small proportion of cases are, however, recognised as special cases, for example, tubular, lobular, cribriform, mucinous, and medullary carcinomas. Tubular, mucinous, and cribriform carcinomas are associated with a good prognosis [8]; they are of low histological grade, usually of small size and infrequently present with associated lymph node spread. Lobular carcinomas are almost always of Blooms grade II and behave according to the overall NPI score. Medullary carcinomas are of Blooms grade III, but some authors consider that they behave in a less aggressive manner than invasive ductal carcinomas of the same NPI score (or equivalent). The literature is not conclusive on this matter [9].

B. HORMONE RECEPTORS AND OESTROGEN REGULATED PROTEINS

It is now a routine in most laboratories to assess breast cancers for expression of oestrogen receptor protein (ER). This is done because of the predictive value of ER expression for response to endocrine therapy on relapse [10] and, to a lesser extent, because the enhanced survival in patients treated with adjuvant Tamoxifen is greater in patients with tumours expressing high levels of the protein [11]. However, a number of studies have also shown that ER is associated with superior prognosis [12]. Some investigators have shown that the prognostic value is confined to node positive patients [13] and the same group have shown that ER status does not provide additional predictive power when included in the multivariate analysis used to develop the Nottingham Prognosis Index, i.e., ER does not appear to be an independent prognostic marker [5]. Oestrogen receptor was originally identified and assayed in breast cancer using a radio-isotope competitive binding assay [10], but is now generally assessed by immunohistochemistry using monoclonal antibodies on paraffin embedded tissue [14,15].

Although ER was found to be predictive of response to endocrine therapy, around 50% of patients with ER positive tumours failed to respond to such treatment. It was considered that ER in these cases might be functionally inactive and a search was therefore made to identify proteins regulated or promoted by ER, which might indicate a functional ER apparatus. The first to be defined was progesterone receptor [16] and subsequently Cathepsin D [17,18] and pS2 [19-21] were identified. These molecules have been assessed regarding their potential prognostic value in breast cancer using immunohistochemistry. Progesterone receptor does appear to be of prognostic value, either alone or in combination with ER [22,23]; in some studies PgR has been shown to be superior to ER in predicting disease-free survival [24,25].

The role of Cathepsin D as a prognostic marker is controversial [26]. Using immunohistochemistry to detect the protein in tumour cell cytoplasm, Cathepsin D has been found to be associated with good [27] or poor [28] prognosis, or to be of no value [29-31]. A recent large study using a cytosolic assay of tumour lysates has shown, however, that Cathepsin D is a highly significant adverse prognostic factor in both node positive and node negative patients [32,33].

Expression of the oestrogen regulated protein pS2 has been shown to predict endocrine responsiveness in breast cancer. Early investigations showed no relationship between pS2 expression and prognosis [34], but a recent study assessing pS2 expression by Northern Blotting showed that pS2 was a significant prognostic variable [35].

C. MARKERS OF CELLULAR PROLIFERATION AND CELL CYCLE REGULATORS

Estimation of the mitotic index has an established place as a prognostic marker and is incorporated into the Bloom grading system described above. Mitoses are usually assessed as the number per 10 high power fields. Tissue fixation, intratumoral heterogeneity and sampling error all affect the reliability of measuring mitotic index [8]. Alternative and perhaps more accurate measures of tumour proliferative activity have thus been sought. These include assessment of S phase fraction by flow cytometry or BrDU labelling. The most widely employed method however is by immunostaining for the cell cycle associated antigen Ki 67, which has been shown to be superior to other markers such as PCNA and Ki S1 [36].

Cyclin D1 acts at the G1-S interface and indirectly promotes entry into S phase. The gene encoding the protein is amplified in around 20% of breast cancers. Contrary to expectations, immunostaining for cyclin D1 has been shown to correlate with ER expression and longer survival [37]. Clearly the role of cyclin D1 in breast cancer is complex and does not relate directly to cellular proliferation. Cyclin D1 (with other cyclins) acts in association with cyclin dependent kinases to inactivate the retinoblastoma (*rb*) gene protein (by phosphorylation) permitting activity of the E2F transcription factor family to promote S phase specific genes. Lack of *rb* protein or activity might therefore be predicted to be associated with cell cycle deregulation and poor outcome in breast cancer. However, although association between loss of *rb* expression and positive lymph node status, high tumour grade, and ER negativity have been shown, no relationship to outcome has been demonstrated.

D. p53 AND RELATED PROTEINS

Mutation of the p53 gene is a frequent event in many types of human cancer including breast carcinoma. Mutation impairs the ability of the cell to degrade the protein which thus accumulates and can be detected by immunohistochemistry. In a small proportion of cases, however, overexpression of p53 can occur in the absence of gene mutation [38]. Whilst the literature is not unanimous [39], most studies have shown that overexpression of p53 detected by immunohistochemistry is associated with markers of tumour aggressiveness, such as high grade and negative hormone receptor status, and also with poor outcome [40-47]. In view of the near universal involvement of p53 in human neoplasia, the potential prognostic significance of related proteins such as MDM2, which bind p53 and promote ubiquitin mediated degradation of the molecule, has been investigated. MDM2 is infrequently mutated but often overexpressed in breast cancer and in one study overexpression was shown to be associated with lymph node metastasis and poor outcome [48].

E. TYPE 1 GROWTH FACTOR RECEPTORS

The type 1 growth factor family comprises four known members viz. EGFR, c-*erb*B-2 (HER-2/neu), c-*erb*B-3 and c-*erb*B-4. The receptors function through tyrosine kinase activity induced by dimerisation which is ligand specific. Overexpression of EGFR was first shown to be of prognostic value by Sainsbury et al. using a radiolabelled ligand binding assay [49,50]. Subsequently a number of studies have confirmed this observation both by ligand binding assays and immunohistochemistry [51]. c-*erb*B-2 was first shown to be of prognostic value by Slamon et al. who demonstrated that amplification of the gene was associated with poor outcome [52]. It was subsequently shown that amplification was associated with overexpression of the protein detected by immunohistochemistry, and numerous studies have now shown that c-*erb*B-2 overexpression determined by IHC is associated with poor prognosis [53-56]. Little data has yet emerged regarding the prognostic significance of c-*erb*B-3 expression. Travis et al. found a weak association between expression and both larger tumour size and local recurrence of disease [57]. Knowlden et al. found an association between c-*erb*B-3 expression and positive ER status [58]. To date there have been no prognostic studies concluded with respect to the potential prognostic value of c-*erb*B-4.

III. PREDICTION OF NODAL METASTASIS BY NEURAL ANALYSIS

An increasing number of women with breast cancer are detected at an early stage of the disease when the lymph nodes are not involved. As explained above and in order to obviate the necessity to carry out axillary dissection, accurate surrogates for lymph node involvement need to be identified. Two studies by Naguib et al. examined the use of artificial neural networks to predict nodal involvement [59,60]. This neural approach was also extended to investigate its predictive applicability to the long-term prognosis of patients with breast cancer.

A number of established and experimental prognostic markers, which have been discussed in the previous section, were employed in these studies in an attempt to accurately determine patient outcome 72 months after first examination. The series included 81 unselected patients, presenting clinically, who had all undergone mastectomy for invasive breast carcinoma. A total of 12 markers were analysed for the prediction of lymph node metastasis while nodal status itself was used as an additional marker for the prognostic analysis (Table 2.1). In this latter case, the outcome related to whether a patient had relapsed within 72 months of diagnosis. In both cases, a number of marker combinations were analysed separately in an attempt to classify those most favourable marker interactions with respect to lymph node prediction and prognosis.

Patients were randomly divided into their training ($n = 50$) and testing ($n = 31$) sets and the simulation was developed using the NeuralWorks Professional II/Plus software (NeuralWare, Pittsburgh, PA, USA). Following surgery, of the 31 patients considered in the test set, 11 patients were identified as node positive and 20 as node negative. With respect to prognostic analysis, 8 women had suffered from relapse within the 72-month- period, while 23 were alive and well. It is against these figures that the accuracy of prediction of the neural network was assessed.

In the case of lymph node involvement, a total of 24 different combinations of measure were analysed, resulting in overall prediction accuracies ranging from 55% to 84%. The highest percentage of 84% relating to the correct prediction of axillary involvement was achieved in the test set by considering a combination of 9 of the 12 available markers. This represents an approximate improvement of 10% over the traditional approach, which considers the tumour grade and size only. The sensitivity and specificity were also shown to be 73% and 90%, respectively.

With regard to patient prognosis, again 84% classification accuracy was obtained using a subset of the markers, with a sensitivity of 50% and a specificity of 96%.

The above results, although relating to a relatively small sample of patients, nonetheless suggest that ANNs are capable of providing strong indicators for predicting lymph node involvement. There is no longer a need for axillary dissection with all its implications on patient morbidity and demands on clinical resources. Furthermore, the management of breast cancer and the planning of strategies for adjuvant treatments may also be facilitated through the use of neural networks for the long-term prognosis of patients.

Table 2.1 Prognostic markers used in the neural prediction of nodal metastasis (all biological markers determined by immunohistochemistry unless otherwise stated).

Marker No.	Description
Input neurons	
1	Grade – histological grade, modified Bloom and Richardson
2	Diameter – greatest diameter of tumour
3	ER(DCC) – oestrogen receptor, determined by the dextran coated charcoal method
4	ER – oestrogen receptor, frozen section
5	PgR – progesterone receptor, frozen section
6	ER/PgR – combined oestrogen and progesterone receptor, frozen section (cases scored positive if either receptor positive)
7	p53 protein – paraffin section, determined by monoclonal DO7B
8	*nm23* – antimetastatic gene protein, paraffin section, determined using NDPK-A antibody
9	*nm23* mRNA – fresh tumour tissue, messenger RNA determined by Northern Blotting
10	RB1 – retinoblastoma gene protein, frozen section, expression determined using monoclonal Mab1 (Triton), graded negative or positive
11	RB2 – retinoblastoma gene protein, frozen section, expression determined using monoclonal Mab1 (Triton), graded negative, weak or strong positive
12	RB3 – retinoblastoma gene protein, paraffin section, expression determined using monoclonal F284B31, graded negative or positive
Output neuron	
1	Nodal status

IV. PROTEINS ASSOCIATED WITH METASTATIC POTENTIAL

Among the notable putative genetic determinants are the *h-mts1* (also known as *CAPL and S100A4*) and *nm23* genes, which appear to influence the invasive and metastatic potential of tumours. The *h-mts1* and its murine homologue *18A2/mts1* encode a Ca^{2+}-binding protein belonging to the S-100 protein family [61]. The expression of these genes has been found to correlate strongly with the proliferative potential and invasive and metastatic behaviour of human cancer cell lines as well as murine tumour cell lines [61-70]. *nm23* is a putative metastasis suppressor gene whose expression has been found to correlate inversely with metastatic potential of some forms of human cancer. *nm23* was first identified in murine melanoma cell lines where it was found to be associated with low metastatic potential [71]. Subsequently it was shown that the protein possessed nonspecific nucleoside diphosphate kinase activity, and that in humans there were two forms of the protein: *nm23-*H_1 and *nm23-*H_2.

A. *h-mts1* AND NOT *nm23* EXPRESSION CORRELATES WITH NODAL SPREAD OF CANCER

A number of studies have shown that *nm23* expression is associated with less likelihood of nodal metastasis and superior survival in human breast cancer [72-74]. However, a more recent study assessing *nm23* by quantitative immunocytochemistry did not show association of *nm23* with survival [75]. Albertazzi and colleagues, including two authors (RNGN and GVS), showed that the levels of *nm23* did not correlate with nodal spread [76]. In the latter study, however, expression of the metastasis associated gene *h-mts1* did correlate with positive lymph node status. The study was carried out on a cohort of 47 women. Table 2.2 shows the data relating to 34 informative cases in relation to their *h-mts1* and *nm23* status. Of 19 patients with *h-mts1* positive carcinomas, 13 (68%) showed nodal metastasis. Compared with that, only 4 of 15 patients (27%) with *h-mts1* negative carcinomas were found to have nodal metastasis. This correlation of *h-mts1* positivity with the incidence of nodal metastasis was significant at $p < 0.05$ (using Fisher's exact test, where correlation was regarded as statistically significant when $p \leq 0.05$ in a two-tailed analysis), suggesting a significant parallelism between *h-mts1* expression and the presence of nodal metastasis.

Such a clear correlation was not encountered between *nm23* and nodal metastasis. Thus, although 8 of 10 patients with *nm23* negative tumours showed nodal spread, 15 of 24 patients whose tumours were *nm23* positive also had nodal metastasis. Therefore, in this series, *nm23* on its own did not appear to relate inversely to nodal metastasis.

There is now ample evidence that the products of these genes could have antagonistic actions. In the above-mentioned paper, Albertazzi et al. analysed whether their relative expression correlated with metastatic behaviour, and found that high expression of *h-mts1* relative to *nm23* seems to reflect far more accurately the state of nodal spread than does *h-mts1* alone. Such correlation of relative expression of the genes with metastatic spread was highly statistically significant at $p < 0.01$.

Table 2.2 Expression of *h-mts1* and *nm23* genes and their individual relationship to nodal spread of breast cancer.

Gene expression	Samples	N^+ (%)	N^- (%)	*p*
h-mts1 positive	19	13 (68.4)	6 (31.6)	
h-mts1 negative	15	4 (26.6)	11 (73.4)	< 0.05
nm23 positive	24	9 (37.5)	15 (62.5)	
nm23 negative	10	8 (80.0)	2 (20.0)	*n.s.*

Data from Albertazzi et al. *[76].*
N^+ *≡ node positive;* N^- *≡ node negative; n.s. ≡ not statistically significant.*

B. *h-mts1* EXPRESSION AND ER/PgR STATUS

Among other markers used by Albertazzi et al. is the ER/PgR status of breast cancer. ER/PgR positivity generally correlates inversely with epidermal growth factor receptor (EGFr) status, which has been regarded by some as an indicator of poor prognosis [50]. Furthermore, breast cancer cell lines that are high expressers of EGFr have been found to express *h-mts1* at a high level [70]. One may expect, therefore, that high *h-mts1* expression would correlate inversely with ER/PgR expression.

We measured ER/PgR expression and examined whether any correlation exists between these tumours [76]. The distribution of steroid receptor positivity was as follows: 12 tumours contained both ER and PgR, and 11 tumours contained only ER and one had only PgR, and 11 tumours were ER/PgR negative. Of the *h-mts1*-expressing tumours, 43% were ER/PgR positive. However, a majority of *h-mts1* negative tumours (13/17) were ER/PgR positive. This inverse correlation between ER/PgR positivity and *h-mts1* was statistically significant at $p = 0.0032$. No conclusions could be drawn from this as to any causal relation between expression of the gene and the regulation of ER/PgR. Nonetheless, it is significant that no correlation was seen between *nm23* expression and steroid receptor status.

V. ANALYSIS OF *h-mts1* AND *nm23* EXPRESSION BY ARTIFICIAL NEURAL NETWORKS

In view of the equivocal association of *nm23* with the metastatic potential of human cancer, we suggested that the relative expression of *h-mts1* and *nm23* might reflect tumour progression more accurately than either independently. As explained above, Albertazzi et al. have shown that high *h-mts1* expression is associated with metastatic spread to the regional lymph nodes. The expression of *nm23* on its own did not show a statistically significant inverse correlation with nodal spread. However, the expression status of the two genes taken together, correlated strongly with the occurrence of nodal metastases. Breast cancers with no detectable expression of *h-mts1* were found to be oestrogen and progesterone receptor positive. The clinical data together with the state of expression of steroid receptors and the expression levels of *h-mts1* and *nm23* genes were analysed using artificial neural networks for accuracy of prediction of nodal spread of the carcinomas. These analyses also support the conclusion that, overall, *h-mts1* expression appears to be associated with and indicative of more aggressive disease. Complemented with *nm23*, *h-mts1* could provide a powerful marker for predicting breast cancer prognosis.

In an attempt to predict nodal status, the ANN analysis carried out was based on Kohonen's self-organising maps and the back-propagation of errors. The system was again developed using the NeuralWorks Professional II/Plus software. The network was applied retrospectively to a cohort of 47 women.

Seven inputs were analysed by the ANN: the patient's age, the tumour size and grade, percentage ER- and PgR-expressing cells, and expression levels of *h-mts1* and *nm23*. Because nodal status was available for only 37 patients, the training set consisted of 17 randomly selected patients (7 node negative and 10 node positive). The validation set comprised the remaining 20 patients, of whom 10 were node negative and 10 were node positive.

Four separate analyses, detailed in Albertazzi et al., have allowed us to assess the relative predictive power of *h-mts1* and *nm23* expression, and from which the following observations could be inferred:

1. The combination of all markers clearly results in the best set of prediction statistics. This is an expected result, as each parameter, in its own right, makes a valuable contribution toward nodal status classification.

2. Omitting *h-mts1* results in the poorest statistics. This finding suggests that *h-mts1* is an important factor in the analysis, and its omission significantly reduces the prediction statistics: notably, sensitivity is reduced by 50%.

3. While the omission of *nm23* has a noticeable negative effect on the prediction statistics, this effect is not as pronounced as in case (2) above for *h-mts1*. This fact then suggests that *nm23* is an important factor that should not be neglected from the prediction analysis, but that its correlation with nodal involvement is perhaps not as prominent as that of *h-mts1*.

4. In our final analysis, we considered the use of *h-mts1* and *nm23* as sole inputs to the ANN. It is apparent from the results that genes do have an important effect on prediction statistics. In fact, the specificity parameter attained in this case is equal to that achieved by all seven parameters when analysed (90%), suggesting that the analysis of the various expression levels of both *h-mts1* and *nm23* is perhaps more effective in predicting node-negative status.

VI. CONCLUDING REMARKS

The patient and the clinician faced with a diagnosis of breast cancer have a huge amount of information to evaluate and upon which to base treatment decisions. Individual clinicians, patients and breast units will place different emphasis on prognostic markers, which potentially can produce differing recommendations on treatment proposals depending upon the personal biases and prejudices of the clinical team. An objective way of assessing prognosis, and thus future treatment strategies, would be a great advance in providing a uniform and standardised approach to the disease which importantly would subsequently permit reliable comparisons of treatment options in patient subgroups. This objectivity would not only hugely facilitate the clinical management of the patient but also would ensure that groupings of patients in clinical trials were genuinely similar. Artificial neural networks have the capability to provide objective assessment of multiple prognostic markers and guide the clinician and patient in the management of the individual case, as well as in ensuring homogeneous groups of patients who can be entered into meaningful, large, randomised, and controlled trials.

REFERENCES

1. **Sainsbury J.R.C., Rider L., Smith A., Macadam A.,** Does it matter where you live? Treatment variation for breast cancer in Yorkshire, *Br. J. Cancer,* 71, 1275-1278, 1995.
2. **Van der Ent F.W.C., Kengen R.A.M., Van der Pol H.A.G., Hoofwijk A.G.M.,** Sentinel node biopsy in 70 unselected patients with breast cancer: increased feasibility by using 10mCi radiocolloid in combination with a blue dye tracer, *Eur. J. Surg. Oncol.*, 25, 24-29, 1999.
3. **Hennessy C., Henry J.A., May F.E.B., Westley B.R., Angus B., Lennard T.W.J.,** Expression of the antimetastatic gene *nm23* in human breast cancer: an association with good prognosis, *J. Natl. Cancer Inst.,* 83, 281-285, 1991.
4. **Elston C.W., Ellis I.O.,** Pathological prognostic factors in breast cancer I: the value of histological grades in breast cancer — experience from a large study with long-term followup, *Histopathology,* 19, 403-410, 1991.
5. **Galea M.H., Blamey R.W., Elston C.E., Ellis I.O.,** The Nottingham Prognostic Index in primary breast cancer, *Breast Cancer Res. Treat.*, 22, 207-219, 1992.
6. **Collett K., Skjærven R., Mæhle B.O.,** The prognostic contribution of estrogen and progesterone receptor status to a modified version of the Nottingham Prognostic Index, *Breast Cancer Res. Treat.*, 48, 1-9, 1998.

7. **Balslev I., Axelsson C.K., Zedeler K., Rasmussen B.B., Carstensen B., Mouridsen H.T.,** The Nottingham Prognostic Index applied to 9,149 patients from the studies of the Danish Breast Cancer Co-operative Group (DBCG), *Breast Cancer Res. Treat.*, 32, 281-290, 1994.
8. **Page D.L., Jensen R.A., Simpson J.F.,** Routinely available indicators of prognosis in breast cancer, *Breast Cancer Res. Treat.,* 51, 195-208, 1998.
9. **Ridolfi R.L., Rozen P.P., Port A., Kinn D., Miké V.,** Medullary carcinoma of the breast — a clinicopathological study with 10-year followup, *Cancer,* 40, 1365-1385, 1997.
10. **Hawkins R.A., Roberts M.M., Forrest A.P.M.,** Oestrogen receptors and breast cancer: current status, *Br. J. Surg.,* 67, 153-169, 1980.
11. Tamoxifen and enhanced survival related to ER early breast cancer trialists collaborative group, systemic treatment of early breast cancer by hormonal, cytotoxic or immunotherapy, *Br. J. Surg.,* 78, 1-15, 1991.
12. **Rayter Z.,** Steroid receptors in breast cancer, *Br. J. Surg.,* 78, 528-535, 1991.
13. **Williams M.R., Todd J.H., Ellis I.O., et al.,** Estrogen receptors in primary and advanced breast cancer: An eight year review of 704 cases, *Br. J. Cancer,* 55, 67-73, 1987.
14. **Bevitt, D.J., Milton I.D., Piggot N., Henry L., Carter M.J., Toms G.L., Lennard T.W.J., Westley B., Angus B., Horne, C.H.W.,** New monoclonal antibodies to oestrogen and progesterone receptors effective for paraffin section immunohistochemistry, *J. Pathol.*, 183, 228-232, 1997.
15. **Saccani J.G., Johnston S.R.D., Salter J., et al.,** Comparison of new immuno-histochemical assay for oestrogen receptor in paraffin wax embedded breast carcinoma tissue with quantitative enzyme immunoassay, *J. Clin. Pathol.,* 47, 900-905, 1994.
16. **Horwitz K.B., McGuire W.L.,** Estrogen control of progesterone receptor in human breast cancer — correlation with nuclear processing of estrogen receptor, *J. Biol. Chem.,* 252, 2223-2228, 1978.
17. **Maudelonde T., Khalaf S., Garcia M., et al.,** Immunoenzymatic assay of Mr 52,000 cathepsin D in 182 breast cancer cytosols: low correlation with other prognostic parameters, *Cancer Res.,* 48, 462-466, 1988.
18. **Henry J.A., McCarthy A.L., Angus B., et al.,** Prognostic significance of the estrogen-regulated protein, cathepsin D, in breast cancer — an immunohistochemical study, *Cancer,* 65, 265-271, 1990.
19. **Luqmani Y.A., Ricketts D., Ryall G., Turnbull L., Law M., Coombes R.C.,** Prediction of response to endocrine therapy in breast cancer using immunocyto-chemical assays for pS2, oestrogen receptor and progesterone receptor, *Int. J. Cancer*, 54, 619-622, 1993.
20. **Henry J.A., Piggott N.H., Mallick U.K., et al.,** PNR-2/pS2 immunohistochemical staining in breast cancer: correlation with prognostic factors and endocrine response, *Br. J. Cancer,* 63, 615-622, 1991.
21. **Hurlimann J., Gebbard S., Gomez F.,** Oestrogen receptor, progesterone receptor, pS2, ERD5, HSP27 and cathepsin D in invasive ductal breast carcinomas, *Histopathology,* 23, 239-248, 1993.
22. **Mason B.H., Holdaway I.M., Mullins P.R., Yee L.H., Kay R.G.,** Progesterone and estrogen receptors as prognostic variables in breast cancer, *Cancer Res.,* 43, 2985-2990, 1983.
23. **Chevallier B., Heintzmann F., Mosseri V., et al.,** Prognostic value of estrogen and progesterone receptors in operable breast cancer — results of a univariate and multivariate analysis, *Cancer,* 62, 2517-2524, 1988.
24. **Clark G.M., McGuire W.I., Hubay C.A., Pearson O.H., Marshall J.S.,** Progesterone receptors as a prognostic factor in stage II breast cancer, *N. Engl. J. Med.,* 309, 1343-1347, 1983.
25. **Thorpe S.M., Rose C., Rasmussen B.B., et al.,** Prognostic value of steroid hormone receptors: multivariate analysis of systemically untreated patients with node negative primary breast cancer, *Cancer Res.,* 47, 6126-6133, 1987.

26. **Westley B.R., May F.E.B.,** Cathepsin D and breast cancer, *Eur. J. Cancer,* 32A, 15-24, 1996.
27. **Henry J.A., McCarthy J.L., Angus B., et al.,** Prognostic significance of the estrogen-regulated protein, cathepsin D, in breast cancer, *Cancer,* 65, 265-271, 1990.
28. **Winstanley J.H.R., Leinster S.J., Cooke T.G., Westley B.R., Platt-Higgins A.M., Rudland P.S.,** Prognostic significance of cathepsin-D in patients with breast cancer, *Br. J. Cancer,* 67, 767-772, 1993.
29. **Domagala W., Striker G., Szadowska A., Dukowicz A., Weber K., Osborn M.,** Cathepsin D in invasive ductal NOS breast carcinoma as defined by immunohistochemistry, *Am. J. Pathol.,* 141, 1003-1012, 1992.
30. **Têtu B., Brisson J., Côté C., Brisson S., Potvin D., Roberge N.,** Prognostic significance of cathepsin D expression in node-positive breast carcinoma: an immunohistochemical study, *Int. J. Cancer,* 55, 429-435, 1993.
31. **O'Donoghue A.E.M.A., Poller D.N., Bell J.A., et al.,** Cathepsin D in primary breast carcinoma: adverse prognosis is associated with expression of cathepsin D in stromal cells, *Breast Cancer Res. Treat.,* 33, 137-145, 1995.
32. **Foekens J.A., Look M.P., Bolt-de Vries J., Meijer-van Gelder M.E., van Putten W.L.J., Klijn J.G.M.,** Cathepsin-D in primary breast cancer: prognostic evaluation involving 2810 patients, *Br. J. Cancer,* 79, 300-307, 1999.
33. **Westley B.R., May F.E.B.,** Prognostic value of Cathepsin D in breast cancer, *Br. J. Cancer,* 79, 189-190, 1999.
34. **Henry J.A., Piggott N.H., Mallick U.K., Nicholson S., Farndon J.R., Westley B.R., May F.E.B.,** pNR-2/pS2 immunohistochemical staining in breast cancer: correlation with prognostic factors and endocrine response, *Br. J. Cancer,* 63, 615-622, 1991.
35. **Thompson A.M., Elton R.A., Hawkins R.A., Chetty U., Steel C.M.,** PS2 mRNA expression adds prognostic information to node status for 6-year survival in breast cancer, *Br. J. Cancer,* 77, 492-496, 1998.
36. **Pinder S.E., Wencyk P., Sibbering D.M., Bell J.A., Elston C.W., Nicholson R., Robertson J.F.R., Blamey R.W., Ellis I.O.,** Assessment of the new proliferation marker MIB1 in breast carcinoma using image analysis: associations with other prognostic factors and survival, *Br. J. Cancer,* 71, 146-149, 1995.
37. **Barnes D.M.,** Cyclin D1 in mammary carcinoma, *J. Pathol.,* 181, 267-269, 1997.
38. **O'Neill M., Campbell S.J., Save V., Thojmpson A.M., Hall P.A.,** An immunochemical analysis of mdm2 expression in human breast cancer and the identification of a growth-regulated cross-reacting species p170, *J. Pathol.,* 186, 254-261, 1998.
39. **Rosen P.P., Lesser M.L., Arroyo C.D., Cranor M., Borgen P., Norton L.,** p53 in node-negative breast carcinoma: an immunohistochemical study of epidemiologic risk factors, histologic features, and prognosis, *J. Clin. Oncol.*, 13, 821-830, 1995.
40. **Allred D.C., Clark G.M., Fuqua S.A.W.,** Overexpression of mutant p53 associated with increased proliferation and poor outcome in node negative breast cancer, *J. Natl. Cancer Inst.,* 85, 200-206, 1993.
41. **Silvestrini R., Benini E., Daidone M.G., Veneroni S., Boracchi P., Cappelletti V., Fronzo G.D., Veronesi U.,** p53 as an independent prognostic marker in lymph node-negative breast cancer patients, *J. Natl. Cancer Inst.,* 85, 965-970, 1993.
42. **Elledge R.M., Fuqua S.A.W., Clark G.M., Pujol P., Allred D.C., McGuire W.L.,** Prognostic significance of p53 gene alterations in node-negative breast cancer, *Breast Cancer Res. Treat.,* 26, 225-235, 1993.
43. **Stenmark-Askmalm M., Stål O., Sullivan S., Ferraud L., Sun X.-F., Carstensen J., Nordenskjöld B.,** Cellular accumulation of p53 protein: an independent prognostic factor in stage II breast cancer, *Eur. J. Cancer,* 30A, 175-180, 1994.

44. **Thor A.D., Moore D.H., Edgerton S.M., Kawasaki E.S., Reihsaus E., Lynch H.T., Marcus J.N., Schwartz L., Chen L.-C., Mayall B.H., Smith H.S.,** Accumulation of p53 tumor suppressor gene protein: An independent marker of prognosis in breast cancers, *J. Natl. Cancer Inst.,* 84, 846-854, 1992.
45. **Anderson T.I., Holm R., Nesland J.M., Heimdal K.R., Ottestad L., Børresen A.-L.,** Prognostic significance of *TP*53 alterations in breast carcinoma, *Br. J. Cancer,* 68, 540-548, 1993.
46. **Cattoretti G., Rilke F., Andreola S., D'Amato L., Delia D.,** p53 expression in breast cancer, *Int. J. Cancer,* 41, 178-183, 1988.
47. **Bosari S., Viale G.,** The clinical significance of p53 aberrations in human tumours, *Virchows Arch.,* 427, 229-241, 1995.
48. **Jiang M., Shao Z.M., Wu J., Lu J.S., Yu L.M., Yuan J.D., Han Q.X., Shen Z.Z., Fontanta J.A.,** P21/waf1/cip1 and mdm-2 expression in breast carcinoma patients as related to prognosis, *Int. J. Cancer,* 74, 529-534, 1997.
49. **Sainsbury J.R.C., Farndon J.R., Sherbet G.V., Harris A.L.,** Epidermal growth factor receptors and oestrogen receptors in human breast cancer, *The Lancet,* 1, 364-366, 1985.
50. **Sainsbury J.R.C., Farndon J.R., Needham G.K., Malcolm A.J., Harris A.L.,** Epidermal growth factor receptor status as predictor of early recurrence of and death from breast cancer, *The Lancet,* 1, 1398-1402, 1987.
51. **Klijn J.G.M., Berns P.M.J.J., Schmitz P.I.M., Foekens J.A.,** The clinical significance of epidermal growth factor receptor (EGF-R) in human breast cancer: a review on 5232 patients, *Endocr. Rev.*, 13, 3-17, 1992.
52. **Slamon D.J., Clark G.M., Wong S.G., Levin W.J., Ullrich A., McGuire W.L.,** Human breast cancer: Correlation of relapse and survival with amplification of the HER2/*neu* proto-oncogene in human breast and ovarian cancer, *Science,* 235, 177-182, 1987.
53. **Gusterson B.A., Gelber R.D., Goldhirsch A., Price K.N., et al.,** for the International (Ludwig) Breast Cancer Study Group, Prognostic importance of c-*erb*B-2 expression in breast cancer, *J. Clin. Oncol.*, 10, 1049-1056, 1992.
54. **Toikkanen S., Helin H., Isola, J., Joensuu H.,** Prognostic significance of HER-2 oncoprotein expression in breast cancer: a 30-year follow-up, *J. Clin. Oncol.*, 10, 1044-1048, 1992.
55. **Têtu B., Brisson J.,** Prognostic significance of HER-2/*neu* oncoprotein expression in node positive breast cancer, *Cancer,* 73, 2359-2365, 1994.
56. **Ravdin P.M., Chamness G.C.,** The c-*erb*B-2 proto-oncogene as a prognostic and predictive marker in breast cancer: a paradigm for the development of other macromolecular markers — a review, *Gene,* 159, 19-27, 1995.
57. **Travis A., Pinder S.E., Robertson J.F., Bell J.A., Wencyk P., Gullick W.J., Nicholson R.I., Poller D.N., Blamey R.W., Elston C.W., Ellis I.O.,** c-*erb*B-3 in human breast carcinoma: expression and relation to prognosis and established prognostic indicators, *Br. J. Cancer,* 74, 229-233, 1996.
58. **Knowlden J.M., Gee J.M., Seery L.T., Farrow L., Gullick W.J., Ellis I.O., Blamey R.W., Robertson J.F., Nicholson R.I.,** c-*erb*B-3 and c-*erb*B-4 expression is a feature of the endocrine responsive phenotype in clinical breast cancer, *Oncogene,* 17, 1949-1957, 1998.
59. **Naguib R.N.G., Adams A.E., Horne C.H.W., Angus B., Smith A.F., Sherbet G.V., Lennard T.W.J.,** The detection of nodal metastasis in breast cancer using neural network techniques, *Physiol. Meas.*, 17, 297-303, 1996.
60. **Naguib R.N.G., Adams A.E., Horne C.H.W., Angus B., Smith A.F., Sherbet G.V., Lennard T.W.J.,** Prediction of nodal metastasis and prognosis in breast cancer: a neural model, *Anticancer Res.*, 17, 2735-2742, 1997.

61. **Ebralidze A., Tulchinsky E., Grigorian M., Afanasyeva A., Senin V., Revsova E., Lukanidin E.,** Isolation and characterisation of a gene specifically expressed in metastatic cells and whose deduced gene product has a high degree of homology to Ca^{2+}-binding protein family, *Genes Develop.*, 3, 1086-1093, 1989.
62. **Ebralidze A., Florene V., Lukanidin E., Fostad O.,** The murine *mts1* gene is highly expressed in metastatic but not in non-metastatic human tumour cells, *Clin. Exp. Metastasis*, 8, suppl. 1, 35, 1990.
63. **Parker C., Whittaker P.A., Weeks R.J., Thody A.J., Sherbet G.V.,** Modulators of metastatic behaviour alter the expression of metastasis associated *mts1* and *nm23* genes in metastatic variants of the B16 murine melanoma, *Clin. Biotech.*, 3, 217-222, 1991.
64. **Parker C., Lakshmi M.S., Piura B., Sherbet G.V.,** Metastasis-associated *mts1* gene expression correlates with increased p53 detection in B16 murine melanoma, *DNA Cell Biol.,* 13, 343-351, 1994.
65. **Parker C, Whittaker P.A., Usmani M.S., Lakshmi M.S., Sherbet G.V.,** Induction of *18A2/mts1* gene expression and its effects on metastasis and cell cycle control, *DNA Cell Biol.*, 13, 1021-1028, 1994.
66. **Merzak A., Parker C., Koochekpour S., Sherbet G.V., Pilkington G.J.,** Overexpression of the *18A2/mts1* gene and down-regulation of the TIMP-2 gene in invasive human glioma cell lines *in vitro*, *Neuropathol. Appl. Neurobiol.*, 20, 614-619, 1994.
67. **Grigorian M.S., Tulchinsky E.M., Zain S., Ebralidze A.K., Kramerov D.A., Kriajevska M.V., Georgiev G.P., Lukanidin E.M.,** The *mts1* gene and control of tumour metastasis, *Gene*, 134, 229-238, 1993.
68. **Davies B.R., Davies M.P.A., Gibbs F.E.M., Barraclough R., Rudland P.S.,** Induction of the metastatic phenotype by transfection of a benign mammary epithelial cell line with the gene for p9Ka, a rat calcium-binding protein, but not with the oncogene EJ-*ras*-1, *Oncogene*, 8, 999-1008, 1993.
69. **Lakshmi M.S., Parker C., Sherbet G.V.,** Metastasis associated *mts1* and *nm23* genes affect tubulin polymerisation in B16 melanomas — a possible mechanism of their regulation of metastatic behaviour, *Anticancer Res.*, 13, 299-304, 1993.
70. **Sherbet G.V., Parker C., Usmani B.A., Lakshmi M.S.,** Epidermal growth factor receptor status correlates with cell proliferation-related *18A2/mts1* gene expression in human carcinoma cell lines, *Ann. NY Acad. Sci.*, 768, 272-276, 1995.
71. **Steeg P.S., Bevilacqua G., Kopper L., et al.,** Evidence for a novel gene associated with low tumour metastatic potential, *J. Natl. Cancer Inst,* 80, 200-204, 1988.
72. **Royds J.A., Stephenson T.J., Rees R.C., Shorthouse A.J., Silocks P.B.,** *nm23* protein expression in ductal *in situ* and invasive human breast carcinoma, *J. Natl. Cancer Inst.,* 85, 727-731, 1993.
73. **Hennessy C., Henry J.A., May F.E.B., Westley B.R., Angus B., Lennard T.W.J.,** Expression of the antimetastatic gene *nm23* in human breast cancer: an association with good prognosis, *J. Natl. Cancer Inst.*, 83, 281-285, 1991.
74. **Tokunaga Y., Urano T., Furakawa K., Kondo H., Kanematsu T., Shiku H.,** Reduced expression of $nm23\text{-}H_1$, but not of $nm23\text{-}H_2$, is concordant with the frequency of lymph node metastasis of breast cancer, *Int. J. Cancer,* 55, 66-71, 1993.
75. **Charpin C., Garcia S., Bonnier P., Martini F., Andrac L., Horschowski N., Lavaut M.-N., Allasia C.,** Prognostic significance of *nm23*/NDPK expression in breast carcinoma assessed on 10-year follow-up by automated and quantitative immunocytochemical assays, *J. Pathol.,* 184, 401-407, 1998.
76. **Albertazzi E., Cajone F., Leone B.E., Naguib R.N.G., Lakshmi M.S., Sherbet G.V.,** Expression of metastasis-associated genes *h-mts1* (S100A4) and *nm23* in carcinoma of breast is related to disease progression, *DNA Cell Biol.,* 17, 335-342, 1998.

Chapter 3

ARTIFICIAL NEURAL APPROACH TO ANALYSING THE PROGNOSTIC SIGNIFICANCE OF DNA PLOIDY AND CELL CYCLE DISTRIBUTION OF BREAST CANCER ASPIRATE CELLS

R.N.G. Naguib and G.V. Sherbet

I. INTRODUCTION

The evolution of cellular diversity, which is an inherent property of neoplastic progression, has been attributed to genetic instability. Genetic instability often manifests itself in neoplasms in the form of chromosomal and DNA aneuploidy, altered DNA repair properties, gene amplification, and deletion and point mutations. There is a general recognition that genetic instability often occurs in parallel with the generation and evolution of variant cell clones with enhanced invasive and metastatic properties. Hence DNA ploidy has assumed a position of some importance as a significant indicator of cancer progression and regarded putatively as a prognostic factor in several forms of human cancer.

DNA aneuploidy has been correlated with early recurrence of endometrial carcinomas, as well as with the degree of myometrial invasion by the tumour [1]. In contrast, diploid DNA has been correlated with less aggressive carcinomas of the pancreas, and higher DNA ploidy with decreased median survival [2,3]. Similar findings have also been reported in respect of colorectal cancer [4] and hepatocellular carcinoma [5]. The survival in patients with prostatic adenocarcinoma has also been correlated with DNA ploidy [6]. However, many investigators are reluctant to accept DNA ploidy as a prognostic marker [7-9].

II. BREAST CANCER FINE-NEEDLE ASPIRATES

The detection of tumour dissemination to the regional lymph nodes is of paramount importance in the management of the disease. Several surrogates for histological assessment of axillary lymph nodes are currently available [10], which are able to predict nodal metastasis with varying degrees of success. Azua et al. measured the DNA ploidy in fine-needle aspirates (FNAs) of breast cancer patients [11]. They found DNA quantification to be significantly related to survival times. In another study involving a large series of breast cancer, Gilchrist et al. found that DNA ploidy strongly correlated with lymph node metastasis and early death [12]. A highly significant relationship between DNA ploidy and the presence of tumour in the

0-8493-9692-1/01/$0.00+$1.50

axillary lymph nodes, sometimes with distal metastases, has been found in a small series of breast cancer [13].

DNA aneuploidy might be a consequence of cells entering the S-phase prematurely. The close association between aneuploidy and the size of the S-phase fraction (SPF) seems to suggest this. According to Wenger et al. aneuploidy tumours show a virtual doubling of the S-phase fraction [8]. However, Sherbet and Lakshmi found that DNA ploidy was totally unrelated to SPF. DNA ploidy is also associated with the expression of genes encoding growth factor and hormone receptor genes. Also the expression of cell proliferation-related genes such as p53 and metastasis-related genes such as the S100A4 has been found to correlate with DNA ploidy. Hence some credence should be given to the association of DNA ploidy with SPF [13]. The size of the S-phase fraction, together with DNA ploidy and other prognostic markers, generally appears to serve as a powerful predictor of early relapse, albeit with reservations as to its significance in certain tumour types [14].

III. ANALYSIS OF IMAGE CYTOMETRIC DATA USING ARTIFICIAL NEURAL NETWORKS

The divergence of opinion concerning the prognostic significance of these cellular features could be attributed to the degree of sophistication of statistical techniques employed and the difficulties associated with assigning weighting to individual cellular attributes or dissecting out specific features in order to assess their individual merits as prognostic factors. We demonstrated in previous studies that artificial neural networks (ANNs) are capable of predicting lymph node metastasis in breast cancer patients using measurements relating to the expression of specific markers [15,16]. We previously investigated FNA samples relating to benign conditions as well as carcinomas of the breast using image cytometry (ICM). We showed that cellular features such as DNA ploidy, size of the SPF, cell cycle distribution, and nuclear pleomorphism of breast cancer FNA cells could be analysed using ANNs and successfully used to predict subclinical metastatic disease [17]. In that study, DNA ploidy ranged from $2n$ to $12.5n$, the median being $4n$, with a few tumours being hypodiploid. The relative distribution of cells between the G_0G_1 and G_2M phases of the cell cycle, viz. the G_0G_1/G_2M ratio, which is regarded as an aspect of DNA aneuploidy, did not correspond with DNA aneuploidy. Only 25% of samples were aneuploid by this criterion, as compared with 82% that were hyperdiploid as indicated by DNA indices. Nonetheless, by neither criterion did DNA ploidy show any relationship to nodal status. The size of the SPF ranged from 2% to 36%, with a median value of 12%. The nuclear pleomorphism index (NPI) ranged from 0.58 to 1.0.

Neural analysis demonstrates that a high degree of accuracy can be attained for the prediction of nodal involvement, based on the four cellular parameters extracted by ICM techniques. Prediction of lymph node involvement reaches an overall prediction accuracy of 87%, with equally high sensitivity and specificity values (70% and 95%, respectively). We have also analysed the effect of individual parameters on the neural analysis. The omission of SPF results in an increased sensitivity, but all other parameters are of lower values when compared with those of the combined markers. Therefore, it could be concluded that the inclusion of SPF in the analysis results in a negative effect on sensitivity but appears to be a highly significant factor for predicting node-negative status.

DNA ploidy measured by nuclear DNA content does not appear to be a significant marker in the analysis, since its omission has no bearing whatsoever on the different statistics. However, when the G_0G_1/G_2M ratio is omitted, the results are worsened, indicating the positive effect that the ratio has on the neural outcome prediction and the importance of its inclusion in the analysis. A statistical analysis of DNA ploidy distribution by either criterion did not relate to nodal spread. This contrasts with the ANN analysis, which indicates a positive effect on neural-based prediction. The ratio G_0G_1/G_2M indeed reflects a facet of DNA aneuploidy. The presence of >10% of cells in the G_2M peak indicates a hyperdiploid state of a cell population [18,19]. This possibly provides a more reliable and stringent technique for the determination of aneuploidy than by using the criterion of DNA index. The use of specialised staining methods such as Feulgen rather than the haematoxylin could make the DNA indices more accurate. This may be reflected in the much smaller (25%) of samples being judged hyperdiploid by G_0G_1/G_2M ratio than by DNA index. Although cell cycle distribution, which is based on measurements of the integrated nuclear densities, is also subject to this source of error, this will not affect the intrinsic degree of aneuploidy because the calculation of the ratio G_0G_1/G_2M will have eliminated it.

The omission of the NPI in the analyses has mixed effects. Whereas specificity, positive predictive value and overall accuracy decrease, sensitivity, and negative predictive value increase significantly. This may be interpreted as suggesting that NPI may not faithfully reflect the degree of malignancy of a tumour, although nuclear pleomorphism has been traditionally viewed as such. However, the determination of NPI by the formula A/P^2 , where A and P are the nucleus area and perimeter, respectively, may only be a crude estimation of NPI, since these measurements could be refined by making them at higher resolutions. Nonetheless, the A/P^2 method provides a quantification of the feature at the specified resolution of the nuclei.

In a separate study, Mat-Sakim et al. have compared the results derived from the neural approach with those obtained using logistic regression [20]. Our study demonstrated that SPF was an independent prediction marker to identify node negative patient. This is in concordance with the findings of Muss et al. that SPF or DNA index is an independent prognostic factor for survival analysis [21]. Based on the χ^2 value, the ANN and logistic regression analyses resulted in identical results (ANN χ^2 test = 10.7989, p = 0.9992). When analysis is carried out using statistical methods, it is important to consider the significance level of the results obtained. Conventionally, the p value is related to hypothesis testing of the data. In the case of a neural approach, there is no formal method of assessing the significance of each individual variable or network. The choice of a p value of 0.05 for the inclusion of a variable may be too strict when a univariate analysis is used initially to identify significant variables for their further inclusion into a regression model. Using this cutoff value may fail to identify biologically important variables. Multivariate analysis is performed to indicate the possibility that a collection of variables, each of which is weakly associated with the outcome, can become important predictors of outcome when considered collectively. In this study however, univariate models seemed to give a better fit compared to multivariate models.

Ravdin et al. compared the performance of neural networks with statistical methods by obtaining a value of the χ^2 test [22]. This was a measure of goodness of fit of the test. Prediction using ANNs gave improved results. There the neural approach appears to be able to perform efficiently even with a small set of data.

IV. CONCLUSIONS

In summary, it can be seen that the artificial neural approach to analysing ICM data of breast tumour FNA can provide a sensitive and accurate way of predicting nodal involvement. It also provides an important insight into the predictive significance of the various metrics analysed.

The advantage of the ICM technique is its greater simplicity and that its application does not require special procedures other than those of cell staining routinely used in cytology laboratories. SPF can be determined with a degree of reliability, which depends upon the clarity of differentiation of the G_0G_1 and G_2M peaks of cell distribution. Cell identification and the assessment of premalignant lesions is easily achieved in image analysis [23]. The differentiation of benign cells from malignant ones is not a serious problem in breast cancer. Furthermore, image cytometry is able to measure features such as nuclear pleomorphism, which is regarded as an important indicator of malignancy. It is needless to say that the image analysis methodology requires a sophisticated image analysis system.

The data analysis described here can be applied wherever instrumentation is available, which can perform densitometric measurements of DNA staining of cells as aspirates or tissue sections. It may be noted, nonetheless, that determinations of DNA ploidy using ICM and conventional flow cytometry have shown significant concordance in several studies [24-27]. We therefore regard ICM data relating to breast cancer FNA cells as eminently suited for analysis using ANN techniques. Currently we are extending the study to include the evaluation of ICM data as a putative predictor of patient survival.

REFERENCES

1. **Giovagnoli M.R., Lukic A., Muraro R., Figlioini M., Pachi A., Vecchione A.,** Image cytometry for DNA analysis in endometrial carcinoma correlated with other prognostic parameters, *Int. J. Oncol.*, 7, 809-815, 1995.
2. **Linder J.S., Lindholm J., Falkmer U.S., Blasjo M., Sundelin P., Von Rosen A.,** Combined use of nuclear morphometry and DNA ploidy as prognostic indicators in non-resectable adenocarcinoma of the pancreas, *Int. J. Pancreatol.*, 18, 241-248, 1995.
3. **Southern J.F., Warshaw A.L., Lewandrowski K.B.,** DNA ploidy analysis of mucinous cystic tumours of the pancreas — correlation of aneuploidy with malignancy and poor prognosis, *Cancer*, 77, 58-62, 1996.
4. **Sampedro A., Urdiales G., Martinez-Nistal A., Riera J., Hardisson D.,** Prognostic value of DNA image cytometry in colorectal carcinoma, *Analy. Quant. Cytol. Histol.*, 18, 214-220, 1996.
5. **Bottger T., Seiffert J., Morschel M., Junginer T.,** The DNA content of the tumour cell — a new prognostic parameter for hepatocellular carcinoma, *Langenbecks Arch. Chirug.*, 381, 232-236, 1996.
6. **Azua J., Romeo P., Valle J., Azua J.,** DNA quantification as a prognostic factor in pancreatic adenocarcinoma, *Analy. Quant. Cytol. Histol.*, 18, 330-336, 1996.
7. **Hedley D.W., Clark G.M., Cornelisse C.J., Killander D., Merkel D.,** Consensus review of the clinical utility of DNA cytometry in carcinoma of the breast, *Breast Cancer Res. Treat.*, 28, 55-59, 1993.
8. **Wenger C.R., Beardslee S., Owens M.A., Pounds G., Oldaker T., Vendely P., Pandian M.R., Harrington D., Clark G.M., McGuire W.L.,** DNA ploidy, S-phase and steroid receptors in more than 127,000 breast cancer patients, *Breast Cancer Res. Treat.,* 28, 9-20, 1993.
9. **Camplejohn R.S., Ash C.M., Gillett C.E., Raikundalia B., Barnes D.M., Gregory W.M., Richards M.A., Millis R.R.,** The prognostic significance of DNA flow cytometry in breast cancer — results from 881 patients treated in a single center, *Br. J. Cancer*, 71, 140-145, 1995.
10. **Rutger E.J.T.,** Breast cancer questions for future trials, *Eur. J. Surg. Oncol.*, 21, 237-239, 1995.
11. **Azua J., Romeo P., Serrano M., Tello D.M., Azua J.,** Prognostic value from DNA quantification by static cytometry in breast cancer, *Analy. Quant. Cytol. Histol.*, 19, 80-86, 1997.
12. **Gilchrist K.W., Gray R., Vandrielkulker A.M.J., Mesker W.E., Ploem-Zaaijer J.J., Ploem J.S., Taylor S.G., Rormey D.C.,** High DNA content and prognosis in lymph node positive breast cancer — a case control study by the University of Leiden and ECOG, *Breast Cancer Res. Treat.*, 28, 1-8, 1993.
13. **Sherbet G.V., Lakshmi M.S.,** *The Genetics of Cancer,* Academic Press, London and New York, 1997.

14. **Berek J.S., Martinezmaza O., Hamilton T., Trope C., Kaern J., Baak J., Rustin G.J.S.,** Molecular and biological factors in the pathogenesis of ovarian cancer, *Annals Oncol.*, 4, 3-16, 1993.
15. **Naguib R.N.G., Adams A.E., Horne C.H.W., Angus B., Sherbet G.V., Lennard T.W.J.,** The detection of nodal metastasis in breast cancer using neural network techniques, *Physiol. Meas.*, 17, 297-303, 1996.
16. **Naguib R.N.G., Adams A.E., Horne C.H.W., Angus B., Smith A.F., Sherbet G.V., Lennard T.W.J.,** Prediction of nodal metastasis and prognosis in breast cancer — a neural model, *Anticancer Res.*, 17, 2735-2741, 1997.
17. **Naguib R.N.G., Mat-Sakim H.A., Lakshmi M.S., Wadehra V., Lennard T.W.J., Bhatavdekar J., Sherbet G.V.,** DNA ploidy and cell cycle distribution of breast cancer aspirate cells measured by image cytometry and analysed by artificial neural networks for their prognostic significance, *IEEE Trans. Info. Tech. Biomed.,* 3, 61-69, 1999.
18. **Scott N.A., Beatty Jr W.R., Weiland L.H., Cha S.S., Lieber M.M.,** Carcinoma of the anal canal and flow cytometric DNA analysis, *Br. J. Cancer*, 60, 56-58, 1989.
19. **Tribukait B., Gustafson H., Esposti P.L.,** The significance of ploidy and proliferation in the clinical and biological evaluation of bladder tumours — a study of 100 untreated cases, *Br. J. Urol.*, 54, 130, 1982.
20. **Mat-Sakim H.A., Naguib R.N.G., Lakshmi M.S., Wadehra V., Lennard T.W.J., Bhatavdekar J., Sherbet G.V.,** Analysis of image cytometry data of fine needle aspirated cells of breast cancer patients — a comparison between logistic regression and artificial neural networks, *Anticancer Res.,* 18, 2723-2726, 1998.
21. **Muss H.B., Kute T.E., Case L.D., Smith L.R., Booher C., Long R., Kammire L., Gregory B., Brockschmidt J.K.,** The relationship of flow cytometry to clinical and biological characteristics in women with node negative breast cancer, *Cancer,* 64, 1894-1900, 1989.
22. **Ravdin P.M., Clark G.M., Hilsenbeck S.G., Owens M.A., Vendely P., Pandian M.R., McGuire W.L.,** A demonstration that breast cancer recurrence can be predicted by neural network analysis, *Breast Cancer Res. Treat.*, 21, 47-53, 1992.
23. **Falkmer U.G.,** Methodological aspects of flow and image cytometric nuclear DNA assessments in prostatic adenocarcinoma, *Acta Oncologica*, 30, 201-203, 1991.
24. **Baretton G., Blasenbreu S., Vogt T., Lohrs U., Rau H., Schmidt M.,** DNA ploidy in carcinoma of the gall bladder — prognostic significance and comparison of flow and image cytometry on archival tumour material, *Pathol. Res. Practice*, 190, 584-592, 1994.
25. **Gandour-Edwards R.G., Donald P.J., Yu T.L.C., Howard R.R., Teplitz R.L.,** DNA content of head and neck squamous carcinoma by flow and image cytometry, *Arch. Otolaryng. Head Neck Surg.*, 120, 294-297, 1994.
26. **Papadopoulos I., Weichert-Jacobsen K., Nurnberg N., Sprenger E.,** Quantitative DNA analysis in renal cell carcinoma — comparison of flow and image cytometry, *Analy. Quant. Cytol. Histol.*, 17, 272-275, 1995.
27. **Epp R.A., Justice W.M., Garcia F.U., McGregor D.H., Giri S.P.G., Kimler B.F.,** Retrospective DNA ploidy analysis by image and flow cytometry in head and neck cancer, *Laryngoscope*, 106, 1306-1313, 1996.

Chapter 4

NEURAL NETWORKS FOR THE ESTIMATION OF PROGNOSIS IN LUNG CANCER

H. Esteva, M. Bellotti, and A.M. Marchevsky

I. INTRODUCTION

The assessment of prognosis has always been an important part of medical practice. When Greek physicians had only a few therapeutic strategies to offer, their capability for diagnosis, but mainly their skill to reach accurate prognosis, were the basis of professional prestige. Even though modern medicine has been continuously enhancing its efficiency for treatment, the science of prognosis has also included increasingly sophisticated aspects. Nowadays, prognosis means not only forming a general idea about the outcome of patients, but rather, the attainment of a sharper prediction of disease evolution in terms of clinical presentation, natural history of the illness, and response to therapy. Therapy itself can also vary in accordance with trends within different prognostic groups. The variety of data to be considered is similarly increasingly high. Lung cancer is an especially complex disease from that point of view. Several pathologic types and subtypes of biological behaviour of lung cancer, different evolution stages from the time of diagnosis, treatment, and individual responsiveness that cannot be precisely measured, need to be combined to make accurate individual prognostic statements.

II. CARCINOMA OF THE LUNG

Carcinoma of the lung is the generic name for malignant epithelial neoplasms of the lung. Its incidence has been steadily increasing during the 20th century until it recently became the major cause of death (in women as well as it was previously among men). The relationship between smoking and enhanced risk of lung cancer has been recognised since the 1950s.

The World Health Organisation (WHO) classifies lung cancer from a histopathological point of view as: (1) squamous cell carcinoma (well, moderately and poorly differentiated); (2) adenocarcinoma (not otherwise specified and bronchoalveolar); (3) adenosquamous carcinoma; (4) small cell undifferentiated carcinoma (classic, combined); (5) large cell undifferentiated carcinoma; and (6) giant cell carcinoma [1]. With general consensus, small cell undifferentiated carcinoma is considered separately from other primary bronchogenic carcinomas. Embryological origin and early systemic spread of this neuro-endocrine malignancy are different than those of other pulmonary neoplasms. Bronchogenic carcinomas

0-8493-9692-1/01/$0.00+$1.50

have broadly been divided into small cell and nonsmall cell bronchogenic carcinomas. This chapter is related to the latter category.

Nonsmall cell bronchogenic carcinomas include adenocarcinoma, squamous cell carcinoma (also called epidermoid carcinoma), and large cell undifferentiated carcinoma, as the more frequent types. Cell doubling time also decreases in that order. Adenocarcinoma has the longer doubling time and, therefore, a slower growing rhythm. The fact that most adenocarcinomas grow in the peripheral areas of the lung makes their growth largely asymptomatic. As a consequence, many of them have long silent subclinical periods, and distant metastases are frequently present at the time of diagnosis. On the other hand, it is the higher degree of cellular differentiation that they demonstrate that implies less sensitivity to radiotherapy and chemotherapy.

Squamous cell carcinoma usually grows inside the larger bronchi. This central location makes it an earlier symptomatic tumour. It is usually more sensitive to adjuvant radio- and chemotherapy. Large cell undifferentiated carcinoma is the most aggressive variety.

Since the first long-term successful excision of a lung cancer by Evarts Graham in 1933 [2], surgery has remained the sole therapeutic method that can cure patients with nonsmall cell carcinomas that are localised to the lung or adjacent regional lymph nodes, but it is only applicable to tumours that show local or regional spread. Even though it can be combined with adjuvant or neo-adjuvant therapy, prognosis is worst for extended lesions. Only very early lesions treated nonsurgically with endobronchial laser therapy or high dose endobronchial brachitherapy have recently shown significant 5-year survival rates [3]. Surgeons and pathologists have been developing clinicopathologic classifications in order to establish a common standard to estimate the progression of tumours. Successive efforts have led to the present TNM mode of classification for lung cancer [4]: four broad stages (Stage I – IV) have been defined according to size, localisation and local invasion of the tumour (T1-T4), different levels of lymphatic nodal involvement (N0-N3), and presence of metastasis (M0-M1). Surgical treatment is generally appropriate from Stage I to Stage IIIa. Chemotherapy and/or radiotherapy are the usual adjuvant or neo-adjuvant strategies that are adopted. TNM classification is useful as a prognostic and therapeutic guideline for patients with nonsmall cell carcinoma of the lung. It is basically an anatomical staging system that overlooks many other currently well-known biological factors that influence tumour development. In addition, the TNM system provides only a general idea about prognostic groups, and can hardly be translated into an individual prognostic determination of value.

In addition to tumour stage, cell differentiation also characterises progression of lung neoplasms, even between similar tumour types. It is usually evaluated by morphological cytohistological methods. In recent years, the development of special techniques such as flow cytometry, immunohistochemistry, *in situ* hybridisation, and molecular biology brought new possibilities for the more accurate classification of tumours.

As a consequence of better tolerated chemotherapeutic regimes, it has become increasingly important to develop new methods to identify patients with lung cancer who are at a high risk of distant metastasis or local recurrence. These patients may benefit from surgical treatment combined with cytotoxic drugs and/or radiotherapy used as neo-adjuvant or adjuvant agents [5].

In addition, evaluation of a large number of prognostic variables is needed to develop a comprehensive prognostic system for patients with lung cancer. This was the impetus behind our interest in the application of neural networks in the assessment of prognosis of nonsmall cell lung cancer.

III. MEDICAL APPLICATIONS OF ARTIFICIAL NEURAL NETWORKS

Medical applications of artificial neural networks are mostly based on their ability to handle classification problems: multiple examples are presented to the system together with the known output; the neural network is allowed to "learn" by adaptation using various paradigms [6-12]. Trained neural networks can then classify prospectively information from new patients. Such networks "learn" by finding subtle association between multiple elements of information that are not immediately apparent to a trained observer [12]. Theoretically, the larger the neural network the more powerful is its potential classification ability. Indeed, in comparison, the human brain has billions of neurons with innumerable connections that cannot be presently simulated even on the most powerful supercomputers.

Neural networks are best trained by using as large a dataset as possible, with numerous features of information and a large number of examples to learn from. They are different from multivariate statistical methods in that they are more flexible and can learn by "adaptation".

Classifications generated by artificial neural networks can be used in medicine to develop objective classifications of illnesses or to estimate prognosis [13-17]. For example, artificial neural networks have been applied in research studies for automatic tumour classification based on data collected through image analysis methods of histologic and cytologic slides, and are currently used in new computer-based automated systems for the interpretation of gynaecologic cytology smears. Such systems have effectively been recently approved by the Federal Drug Administration for quality assurance purposes in gynaecologic cytology [7]. They can also be used for the development of multivariate prognostic models of survival, of predicting local tumour recurrence and/or the possibility of lymph node metastasis, and for the selection of optimised groups of diagnostic tests. They can also be used to predict the response of patients to particular treatments and other questions that confront physicians on a daily basis [13-17].

IV. ARTIFICIAL NEURAL NETWORKS

A. ARCHITECTURE

Artificial neural networks consist of multiple processing elements or "neurons" organised in multiple layers [12,17]. Each neuron in a layer is connected to all neurons of the next layer. Information flows in one direction from one layer to another. Artificial neural networks can have complex architectures with multiple neuronal layers and recurrent flows of information. In general, the neurons of an artificial neural network are organised into an input layer, one or multiple hidden layers and an output layer.

The neurons of the input layer receive information about different features collected from patients (e.g., age, tumour size, molecular markers, etc.). The neurons in the hidden layers are used to create a variable number of numerical combinations, whereas those in the output layer generate a number that represents the "answer" provided by the system. For example, an artificial neural network system can be designed so that if the output is 1 it means the patient is dead, while if the output is 0 the patient is alive. The neurons "receive" a numerical input, process the information using a mathematical function, and "transmit" an output signal to another neuron. Various mathematical functions have been designed for the processing of information by artificial neurons, such as linear, step, ramp, sigmoid, Gaussian, or others. The numerical signal transmitted from one neuron to another is the connection "strength". Artificial neural networks represent their "knowledge" in a numerical matrix of these connection strengths.

B. TRAINING ARTIFICIAL NEURAL NETWORK SYSTEMS

The numerical data collected from patients is usually organised in a spreadsheet. Discrete data, such as presence or absence of a symptom (e.g., chest pain, pulmonary osteoarthropathy or others), can be represented numerically such as 1 (present) or 0 (absent). The data is divided during the design of a study into two random groups: training and testing sets. A proportion of the cases (usually 70-80%) is presented to the system for adaptive learning while the test cases are saved as "unknowns" to study the accuracy of the system. Input data is usually normalised to -1 to +1 by the artificial neural network software. The software may also customarily have a facility that allows investigators to label certain columns in the data as input and others as output (the known answers provided to the system during learning). The following simple steps can explain how artificial neural networks learn to estimate prognosis in lung cancer.

The network may initially be composed of only two layers (input and output). The input layer could consist of a few neurons (e.g., four neurons processing four prognostic features such as tumour size, presence of nodal metastases, DNA content, and a molecular marker). The output layer could consist of a single neuron that estimates prognosis. All values calculated by the output neuron as 0-0.49 are equivalent to "patient alive", while outputs ranging from 0.5-1 are equivalent to "patient dead".

Following definition of this simple network architecture, we proceed to study the data from a group of lung cancer patients, using only some of the patients for training. The data from each patient may be listed in a spreadsheet row (tumour size, presence of nodal metastases, DNA content, a molecular marker and known outcome for this patient). The neural network normalises all data to values ranging from 0-1 and processes each row at a time. During the first learning cycle, each input neuron reads the value of its corresponding prognostic feature and calculates a numerical output, using a mathematical function, that is presented to the output neuron as a "connection strength". The output neuron processes these four values, using another similar — or different — mathematical function, and calculates a value also ranging from 0-1. The artificial neural network compares this value with the correct answer (0-0.49 or 0.5-1) provided by the investigator. The training process is therefore "supervised".

Unsupervised training paradigms learn without the benefit of exposing the artificial neural network to the correct answers during the training process. The network repeats the learning cycle, but this time it modifies each connection strength using a mathematical function. The process is repeated multiple times until the artificial neural network estimates the best possible combination of connection strengths that will yield the fewest classification errors. At that stage, the artificial neural network is regarded as fully trained and is no longer modified. The data from each test patient are then presented to the trained system, and analysed in a single cycle. The results estimated by the artificial neural network can then be compared with the answers already known to the investigator. If the trained neural network is considered reliable, it can then be used to estimate prospectively the prognosis of other lung cancer patients. This simple example describes only two layers of neurons each composed of only a few processing elements. It is thus devoid of the nonlinearity feature that is an important trait of artificial neural networks. In reality, at least one hidden layer and a much larger number of possible combinations of connection strengths are needed to arrive at correct classifications.

C. ESTIMATING THE RELIABILITY OF ARTIFICIAL NEURAL NETWORKS

It is important to study the true predictive value of artificial neural networks, their so-called generalisation rate, before they can be used in clinical practice [15]. Trained artificial neural networks need to be tested in prospective studies analysing large numbers of patients to understand their reliability in "real life". Analysis of multivariate data with various statistical methods and neural network technology can yield spurious results due to multiple combinations of random events. It has been estimated theoretically that the number of training cases required to develop robust multivariate statistical classification methods that are able to generalise to large populations is approximately ten times the number of features in the model [18]. It is still controversial whether these theoretical considerations apply to artificial neural network technology; this requirement could pose daunting practical challenges.

V. PRACTICAL APPLICATION OF NEURAL NETWORKS IN THE PROGNOSIS OF LUNG CANCER PATIENTS

In order to practically evaluate the accuracy of artificial neural networks in the prognosis of postsurgical outcome of lung cancer patients, we have recently published a retrospective study of a known group of 67 patients who had been followed up for at least 5 years after treatment [14].

In our study, the input layer consisted of 12 neurons. Three of them represented information about tumour type (adenocarcinoma, squamous cell carcinoma or large cell undifferentiated carcinoma), the others consisted of information relating to DNA index, percentage of cells in the different mitotic phases (G_1, S, G_2 and %S + G_2M), MIB-1, p53 and IP (%PCNA + %MIB-1/2). The relative importance of each one of these parameters as a prognostic factor has been intensively investigated.

A. TUMOUR TYPE

Tumour type can have an important impact on surgical outcome. It is mainly linked to clinical presentation (central vs. peripheral tumours), which implies a different kind of operation (pneumonectomy or lobectomy) to obtain an oncologically safe excision. On the other hand, the biology of each type is different in terms of cell growing time and aggressiveness, as discussed below. In order to avoid the first factor, we only subjected our study to patients who underwent lobectomies (i.e., peripheral tumours) without adjuvant therapy. Differences could then be attributed to biological behaviour. Nevertheless, although the Kaplan-Meier curves showed some trend to a better survival for patients with squamous cell carcinoma, the difference was not statistically significant. Tumour type could not then be considered as an isolated prognostic factor in our population.

B. PLOIDY LEVELS

Nuclear DNA distribution patterns, or ploidy levels, of malignant cells deviate from normal. Minor numerical chromosomal aberration may be hardly detectable through conventional DNA-cytophotometric techniques. Flow cytometry is a rapid method that measures ploidy (DNA content) in the tumour cells. Ploidy can be a direct reflection of defects produced by chromosomic aberrations. These DNA measurements may thus result in distribution patterns that cannot be distinguished from those found in normal tissue or benign lesions, whereas major numerical changes in chromosomal complement unequivocally show histogram patterns clearly deviating from those found in normal cells.

The variable cytometry DNA pattern in aneuploid tumours may reflect a high degree of genomic instability, which in itself may lead to the generation of new phenotypes leading to a rapid progression of the disease. The histograms are classified as diploid and aneuploid. A histogram is considered diploid when the DNA index ranges between 0.90 to 1.20, and aneuploid when it is outside this range. The percentage of cells in the G_1, S, G_2, and G_2M phases of the mitotic cycle is also calculated from the histogram. In different studies of nonsmall cell lung cancer, it has been shown that the frequency of aneuploidy varies from 21 to 80% [19].

In our study, diploid histograms were obtained for 10 patients who were free of disease (FOD), and from 18 patients with recurrent tumour or tumour specimens who had died (REC/DEAD). Aneuploid histograms were found in 20 FOD and 29 REC/DEAD patients. There were no statistically significant differences. Thus, it was clear that flow cytometric data were not a prognostic factor by themselves in our study.

Nevertheless controversy still remains and, while some authors have shown that aneuploidy correlates with an unfavourable prognosis [19], or demonstrated through multivariate analysis that it is an independent predictor of survival [20], others could not show any prognostic significance [21].

Flow cytometry can also analyse the nonproliferating (G_0) cells or the proliferating (G_1-S-G_2/M) cells. The S-phase fraction had a mean 5.01% cells for diploid tumours and 10.84% for aneuploid tumours in our study. Its measurement had only a univariate statistically significant difference.

C. IMMUNOHISTOCHEMICAL PROLIFERATION MARKERS

Immunohistochemical proliferation markers are based on the fact that cycling cells can be detected by means of antibodies that target growth related proteins, such as the proliferating cell nuclear antigen (PCNA), the activating factor of polymerase and Ki-67 antigen. Ki-67 antigen is an IgG immunoglobulin that reacts with a nuclear antibody expressed in all human proliferating cells during the late G_1, S, M, and G_2 phases of cell cycle; it is absent in the G_0 phase [22,23]. Equivalently, the MIB-1 antigen represents cells in the earlier stages of the G_1 phase.

The antibodies anti-PCNA and monoclonal antibody PC10, a protein associated with cell proliferation, were compared with Ki-67. There were differences in the numbers of positive cells, which may reflect the longer half-life of PCNA protein. In our patients, the percentages of PCNA immunoreactivity ranged from 0 to 90% (mean 46%) and were statistically significant by univariate study of variance and by analysis through the Cox proportional hazards model.

On the other hand, percentages of MIB-1 immunoreactivity ranged from 0 to 70% and were not statistically significant by recurrence or survival rates. Percentages of MIB-1 immunoreactivity correlated with S-phase only in diploid cases [24].

The oncoprotein p53 is a suppressor gene functioning during the development and progression of tumours. It controls cell proliferation. The product of the p53 gene is a phosphoprotein of 53000 daltons, located at chromosome 17p13. It is indeed when there is DNA damage that it stops the cells from entering the S-phase until such damage is repaired. Disturbance of the p53 function may occur by somatic mutations. Mutations of p53 have been described in cigarette smokers with bronchial epithelial dysplasia. They probably play a role in early lung carcinoma and could be associated with poor prognosis in patients with nonsmall cells lung cancer [13, 25, 26].

Percentages of p53 immunoreactivity ranged from 0 to 95% (mean 46%) in our cases and were statistically significant by univariate analysis of variance and by analysis with the Cox proportional hazards model.

D. NEURAL PROCESSING

Data relating to our 67 patients were presented to the input layer of the neural network. After at least 5 years of follow-up, 30 patients were alive and free of disease (FOD) and 37 had recurrences or had succumbed to the disease (REC/DEAD). On the other hand, the predictive value of the tests explained above was poor when considered on an individual basis.

In addition to the above input neurons, the artificial neural network simulated in this study consisted of 12 neurons in a hidden layer and a single output neuron. The output neuron identified one of the two possible outcomes under investigation: FOD or REC/DEAD. If the calculated output was close to 1, the system estimated REC/DEAD; if it was close to 0, it estimated FOD. The system was trained with cases that were presented with known answers (supervised learning). It calculated an output value for each training case and compared it with the correct answer. In the following iteration the network adjusted the calculation using a learning rate defined by the user. The operation was repeated multiple times until the calculated output matched the correct answer. Training was completed using a sigmoidal transfer function, a learning rate of 1.0, and a training tolerance of 0.1. The latter is defined by the user and indicates to the neural network that, during training, values between 0.9 and 1 are correct classifications for REC/DEAD and outputs between 0 and 0.1 are correct classifications for FOD. Twenty such networks were simulated and deemed trained after 1883 to 2000 cycles. All cases, except for one, were used for training. The case left out was used as an "unknown" exemplar for testing purposes. Each of the 20 neural networks had a different randomly selected test case, using a jack-knife cross-validation method [13]. Testing was performed based on a tolerance of 0.4.

As a result, the 20 neural networks trained to completion (no errors) classified correctly the test cases in all instances.

VI. CONCLUSIONS

Lung cancer has been a fatal illness until the first surgical successful case in 1932. Since then, resectable cases began to have better prognostic survival than unresected ones. Soon however, it became evident that patients with anatomically similar lesions had different outcomes, depending on an increasing number of biological variables. Research in this area of oncology has resulted in the discovery and definition of many of these, and hopefully many more will be defined in the future. But in the meantime, no isolated test capable of providing the exact prognosis for an individual patient (the true goal of everyday medical practice) is available. The multiplicity of factors that characterise neoplasms requires a system capable to globalise and precisely evaluate all those factors in order to give an answer in terms of treatment and outcome for the individual patient. Artificial neural networks could be that tool. Usual statistical methods have been designed to compare population groups rather than individual patients; whereas neural networks can classify individuals.

Nonetheless, the neural approach can also be hindered by technical problems as we have discussed elsewhere [14]. In theory, a minimum of 10 to 20 cases per neuronal connection is necessary to validate a neural network reliably. In relation to the problem of patients with nonsmall cell lung cancer, the use of a model with 144 neuronal connections ($12 \times 12 \times 1$) implies the need to test 1440 to 2880 unknown cases before developing a system that could theoretically apply to *any* patient. This is an almost impossible task for a single institution, so it is probably necessary to train artificial neural networks with data from multiple centres to develop clinically useful prognostic systems. That could pose additional problems of adequacy of methods and standardisation from one institution to another.

Interestingly, physicians' accuracy for clinically establishing prognosis of nonsmall cell lung cancer patients has recently been tested [27]. Their clinical skills were compared to a series of prognostic factors analysed by the Cox statistical regression model and attained very similar performances.

It has been stated that physicians appear to use information that is not rigorously identified in the prognostic factor analysis process in order to reach their conclusions. This probably conforms with the essence of the medieval concept which considered that humans' capacity for spiritual knowledge is the combination of "*ratio plus intellectus*", defining "*intellectus*" as "*simplex intuitus*" [28]. In fact, "intuition" itself will always be a complex quality to be mathematically analysed. The use of artificial neural networks in the complex field of prognosis can be considered a genuine assay to inject an additional element of mathematical prowess into the art of medicine.

REFERENCES

1. **WHO (World Health Organization)**, The World Health Organisation histological typing of lung tumours, *Am. J. Clin. Pathol.*, 77, 123-136, 1982.
2. **Graham E.A., Singer J.J.,** Successful removal of an entire lung for carcinoma of the bronchus, *J. Am. Med. Assoc.*, 101, 1371, 1933.
3. **Lam S.,** Comprehensive management of lung cancer, *J. Bronch.*, 4, 199-200, 1997.

4. **Mountain C.F.,** Revisions in the international system for staging lung cancer, *Chest,* 111, 1710-1717,1997.
5. **Roberts H.L., Komaki R., Allen P., El Naggar A.K.,** Prognostic significance of DNA content in stage I adenocarcinoma of the lung, *Int. J. Rad. Oncol. Biol. Phys.,* 41, 573-578, 1998.
6. **Naguib R.N., Adams A.E., Horne C.H., Angus B., Sherbet G.V., Lennard T.W.J.,** The detection of nodal metastasis in breast cancer using neural network techniques, *Physiol. Meas.,* 17, 297-303, 1996.
7. **Mango L.J.,** Computer-assisted cervical cancer screening using neural networks, *Cancer Lett.,* 77, 155-162, 1994.
8. **Rosenthal D.L., Acosta D., Peters R.K.,** Computer-assisted rescreening of clinically important false negative cervical smears using the PAPNET testing system, *Acta Cytol.,* 40, 120-126, 1996.
9. **Erler B.S., Hsu L., Truong H.M., Marchevsky A.M.,** Image analysis and diagnostic classification of hepatocellular carcinoma using neural networks and multivariate discriminant function, *Lab. Invest.,* 71, 446-451, 1994.
10. **Cross S.S., Harrison R.F., Kennedy R.L.,** Introduction to neural networks, *The Lancet,* 346, 1075107-9, 1995.
11. **Dybowsky R., Gant V.,** Artificial neural networks in pathology and medical laboratories, *The Lancet,* 346, 1203-1207, 1995.
12. **Eberhart R., Simpson P., Dobbins R.,** *Computational Intelligence PC Tools,* Academic Press, 61-201, 1996.
13. **Truong H., Morimoto R., Walts A.E., Erler B., Marchevsky A.,** Neural networks as an aid in the diagnosis of lymphocyte-rich effusions, *Anal. Quant. Cytol. Histol.,* 17, 48-54, 1995.
14. **Bellotti M., Elsner B., Paez De Lima A., Esteva H., Marchevsky A.M.,** Neural networks as a prognostic tool for patients with non-small cell carcinoma of the lung, *Modern Pathol.,* 10, 1221-1227, 1997.
15. **An C.S., Petrovic L.M., Reyter I., Tolmachoff T., Ferrell L.D., Thung S.N., Geller S.A., Marchevsky A.M.,** The application of image analysis and neural network technology to the study of large-cell liver-cell dysplasia and hepatocellular carcinoma, *Hepatology,* 26, 1224-1231, 1997.
16. **Marchevsky A.M., Patel S., Wiley K.J., Stephenson M.A., Gondo M., Brown R.W., Yi E.S., Benedict W.F., Anton R.C., Cagle P.T.,** Reasoning with uncertainty in pathology: artificial neural networks and logistic regression as tools for prediction of survival in Stage I and II non-small cell lung cancer patients, *Mod. Pathol.,* 11, 618-625, 1998.
17. **Astion M.L., Wilding P.,** The application of backpropagation neural networks to problems in pathology and laboratory medicine, *Arch. Pathol. Lab. Med.,* 116, 995-1001, 1992.
18. **Fletcher J.M., Rice W.J., Ray R.M.,** Linear discriminant function analysis in neuropsychopathy research: some uses and abuses, *Cortex,* 14, 564-577, 1978.
19. **Zimmerman P.V., Hawson G.A., Bint M.H., Parsons P.G.,** Ploidy as a prognostic determinant in surgically treated lung cancer, *The Lancet,* 2, 530-533, 1987.
20. **Fontanini G., Macchiarini P., Pepe S., Ruggiero A., Harding M., Bigini D., et al.,** The expression of proliferating cell nuclear antigen in paraffin sections of peripheral, node-negative, non-small cell lung cancer, *Cancer,* 70, 1520-1527, 1992.
21. **Cibas E.S., Melamed M.R., Zaman M.B., Kimmel M.,** The effect of tumour size and tumour cell DNA content on the survival of patients with stage I adenocarcinoma of the lung, *Cancer,* 63, 1552-1556, 1989.
22. **Kawai T., Suzuki M., Kono S., Shinomiya N., Rokutanda M., Takagi K., et al.,** Proliferating cell nuclear antigen and Ki-67 in lung carcinoma. Correlation with DNA flow cytometric analysis, *Cancer,* 74, 2468-2475, 1994.

23. **Hall P.A., Levison D.A., Woods A.L., Yu C.C.W., Kellow D.B., Watkins J.A., Baenes D.M., Gillet C.E., Complejohn R., Dover R., Wassem N.H., Lane D.P.N.,** Proliferating cell nuclear antigen (PCNA) immunolocalization in paraffin sections: an index of cell proliferation with evidence of deregulated expression in some neoplasms, *J. Pathol.,* 162, 285-294, 1990.
24. **Horio Y., Takahashi T., Kuroishi T., Hibi K., Suyama M., Niimi T., et al.,** Prognostic significance of p53 mutations and 3p deletions in primary resected non-small cell lung cancer, *Cancer Res.,* 53, 1-4, 1993.
25. **Suzuki H., Takahashi T., Kuroishi T., Suyama M., Aariyoshi Y., Ueda R.,** p53 mutations in non-small cell lung cancer in Japan: association between mutations and smoking, *Cancer Res.,* 52, 734-736, 1992.
26. **Ebina M., Steimberg S.M., Mulshine J.L., Linnoila R.I.,** Relationship of p53 overexpression and up-regulation of proliferating cell nuclear antigen with the clinical course of non-small cell lung cancer, *Cancer Res.,* 54, 2496-2503, 1994.
27. **Muers M.F., Shevlin P., Brown J.,** Prognosis in lung cancer: physicians' opinion compared with outcome and a predictive model, *Thorax,* 51, 894-902, 1996.
28. **Pieper J.,** El ocio y la vida intelectual, *Rialp S.A., Madrid*, 21-22, 1974.

Chapter 5

THE USE OF A GENETIC ALGORITHM NEURAL NETWORK (GANN) FOR PROGNOSIS IN SURGICALLY TREATED NONSMALL CELL LUNG CANCER (NSCLC)

M.F. Jefferson, N. Pendleton, S.B. Lucas, and M.A. Horan

I. INTRODUCTION

Nonsmall Cell Lung Cancer (NSCLC) accounts for approximately three quarters of all lung cancer histologies. Surgical resection is the preferred treatment and approximately 50,000 operations are performed in the United States alone each year [1]. The overall prognosis for resected NSCLC is poor with fewer than a third of patients who undergo resection still alive 5 years later [2].

Neural networks are mathematical models that have been shown to be more efficient than standard statistical approaches in predicting the behaviour of pathophysiological systems [3]. For cancer prognosis, Baxt has reviewed how neural networks have been used to predict outcome measures in prostate, breast, and ovarian cancer [4] and we have applied this approach to the study of NSCLC outcome after surgery [5].

A criticism of clinical neural network studies has been that their workings and results are arcane [6]. Using neural networks with clinical data, we have previously demonstrated that when a genetic algorithm [5,7] is used with a neural network (a genetic algorithm neural network: GANN) there are two benefits: firstly, a significant increase in predictive efficiency and lack of overlearning phenomenae [8] and secondly, the capacity to produce an "understandable" list of key predictive variables from categorical and continuous data [5,7].

In examining diagnostic tests with binary indicator outcome measures (such as "life" or "death") Bayes' theorem may be used [9]. It has been successfully applied in a wide range of medical settings to take into account the effect of prevalence (prior odds) on diagnostic test results [10]. Where such a method is used to predict life or death outcome at discrete time points, this may be considered as a diagnostic test. The aim is to give a clinician more information about the outcome of a case than was known previously (i.e., increase posterior odds).

In this chapter, we discuss the efficacy of a novel development of the genetic algorithm neural network method using Bayes' theorem to predict patient outcome after resection of NSCLC.

0-8493-9692-1/01/$0.00+$1.50

II. METHOD

A. THE NSCLC DATA

Between 1980-1992, 886 pulmonary resections from NSCLC patients were received by the Department of Histopathology, Broadgreen Hospital, Liverpool, UK. Patients were accepted solely on the basis of operability; age did not contribute to the assessment.

The specimens were then examined macroscopically by a histopathologist whose examination included measurement of the maximum tumour diameter in three dimensions using a vernier calliper. Tumour volume was estimated by multiplying the three maximum dimensional measurements. Material from the specimens was taken from representative areas for subsequent light microscopic examination, which was performed by two histopathologists within the department.

Each report generated from the department of histopathology included the following data: identification number; date of operation; date of birth; sex; specimens received; description of the macroscopic and microscopic findings including tumour site, dimensions, tumour cell type, and nodal metastasis. Cell type was reported following the World Health Organisation criteria [11] and nodal metastasis by the nodal score according to TNM classification criteria [12]. Staging was performed according to the UICC criteria [13]. Only cases of squamous cell and adenocarcinoma were included in this study (n=531). An independent histopathological review of cell-type diagnosis was performed in a random group of 90 cases (13%).

Outcome was determined by obtaining certified dates of death from the National and Mersey and Cheshire Regional Cancer Registries. The end-point for follow-up was January 1996. From this, duration in the study and status (alive or dead) were recorded. No cases were lost to follow-up.

III. MATHEMATICAL METHOD: THE GENETIC ALGORITHM NEURAL NETWORK

A. SELECTION OF PREDICTORS BY GENETIC ALGORITHM

For n predictors selected r at a time, the probability of selection of the ith variable is

$$p_i = r / n$$

with the probability of not being selected (q_i), therefore:

$$q_i = 1 - p_i$$

For g generations, where the ith variable has been selected n_i times as an optimal predictor for a given generation, the probability ($p(n_i)$) that this variable was not selected by chance is therefore given by:

$$p(n_i) = \sum_{j=0}^{n_i} \left(C_j^g . p_i^j . q_i^{g-j} \right)$$

where C_j^g is the number of combinations of g generations taken j at a time. This weighting was used to select variables for the information genome. The probability (p_{gi}) of selection of the ith variable as one of the optimal classifiers in an information genome after g generations being

$$p_{gi} = \frac{p(n_i)}{\sum_{i=1}^{n} p(n_i)}$$

B. CLASSIFICATION

The efficacy of the variables in a genome was calculated from the classification matrix. The function optimised (at the cutoff point), s_c, was for the case of two categories considered in this study:

$$s_c = \text{Sensitivity} + \text{Specificity}$$

C. CHOOSING THE OPTIMAL GENOME FOR USE WITH A NEURAL NETWORK

The range of the values of outputs of the neural network (0-1) for a given genome was divided into parts and a cutoff point was used to assign the cases to target categories. The optimal position of division between categories was determined by using nested loops to maximise the value of the optimising function (s_c).

D. UPDATING THE OPTIMAL INFORMATION GENOME

The information genome that gave the maximum value of s_c in a given generation was selected as the optimal predictive genome for that generation (s_{oc}) by updating according to the conditions:

$$\text{IF:} \quad s_c > s_{oc} \qquad \text{THEN:} \quad s_{oc} = s_c$$

E. DEFINING THE NEURAL NETWORK ARCHITECTURE

A multilayer feedforward back-propagation of error neural network was used. The architecture of the neural network was determined by the following rules:

1. The number of neurons in the input layer = number of case variables in the genome.
2. The number of neurons in the output layer = one (the predicted outcome result).
3. The number of neurons in the hidden layers = the geometric means rounded to the nearest integer of a geometric progression of four terms with a common ratio 0.5, where the first term is the number of variables in the input layer, and the last term is the number of outputs (one).

F. TRAINING THE NEURAL NETWORK

The neural network was used to predict the next case from the data of preceding cases. A prediction was made for each case of the data set after the first case. The efficacy of the network was assessed after each cycle of predictions by the value of s_c.

G. STOPPING RULE FOR THE TRAINING PROCESS

The stopping rule for the training process was controlled by the changes in s_c. The error δs_c, for the *t*th training loop was

$$\delta s_c = \frac{s_{ct} - s_{ct-1}}{s_{ct-1}}$$

An iteration counter (m) was set to zero at the beginning of each training loop. The training loop was also controlled by a maximum iteration counter m_t. The maximum iteration for loop t $(m_{\max})$ was given by the geometric progression:

$$m_{\max} = 2^{j-1}$$

The training loop was terminated if:

$$m \geq m_t \qquad \text{OR} \qquad m_t \geq m_{\max} \qquad \text{OR} \qquad \delta s_c = \delta s_{ct}$$

When the training loop terminated, the values of s_{t-1} became the optimal value for that genome.

H. CLASSIFICATION SOLUTION

The solution to the classification process consisted of the genome that was the optimal classifier over all generations and the trained neural network for that genome.

I. APPLICATION OF BAYES' THEOREM

The 2 by 2 classification matrix used to predict s_c was used to calculate a likelihood matrix. The probability that a patient who had the test result would experience the outcome was then calculated, by Bayes' theorem, from the prior probabilities obtained from the database. This assumed that both the database and the subset of cases on which the likelihoods were based were sufficiently large to give good estimates of both the priors and the likelihoods.

J. COMPUTATIONAL METHOD

The method described required a large amount of computational power which was achieved with a 120-MHz Pentium IBM-PC-compatible computer. The software to implement the method was written in Visual Basic for DOS (v1.0).

IV. STATISTICAL METHODS

For survival analysis, zero time for each subject was designated as the date of resection. The end point of the follow-up period was January 1996. Certified dates of death were obtained from the National and Mersey and Cheshire Regional Cancer Registry. No cases were lost to follow-up.

Kaplan-Meier (product-limit) estimates computed for the overall survival function unadjusted for any covariate factors.

A. PREDICTIVE STATISTICS

Logistic regression was performed in a forward stepwise manner with entry testing based on significance of score statistic <0.05, and removal testing based on probability of likelihood ratio statistic >0.10. Categorical covariates were contrasted with reference to the last category. Statistical tests were performed using SPSS for Windows (SPSS release 6.1).

B. COMPARISON OF PREDICTIVE STATISTICS

Predictive methods were compared by examining the efficiency of classifying outcomes correctly. Target outcomes comprised actual outcomes (alive or dead) at 6, 9, 12, 15, 18, and 24 months after operation. Control experiments used logistic regression on the same data. Sets of paired outcome predictions were compared by the McNemar test.

V. SURVIVAL

Of the 531 cases, 283 (53.30%) had been recorded as dead by the end of the follow-up period. Median survival time was 43.23 months (95% C.I.: 28.46, 57.96). Survival of cases is illustrated in the Kaplan-Meier survival plot in Figure 5.1 and the distribution of case variables by survival categories is shown in Table 5.1. There were 248 (46.70%) patients alive at the end of the follow-up period. No cases were lost to follow-up by 24 months from time of surgery.

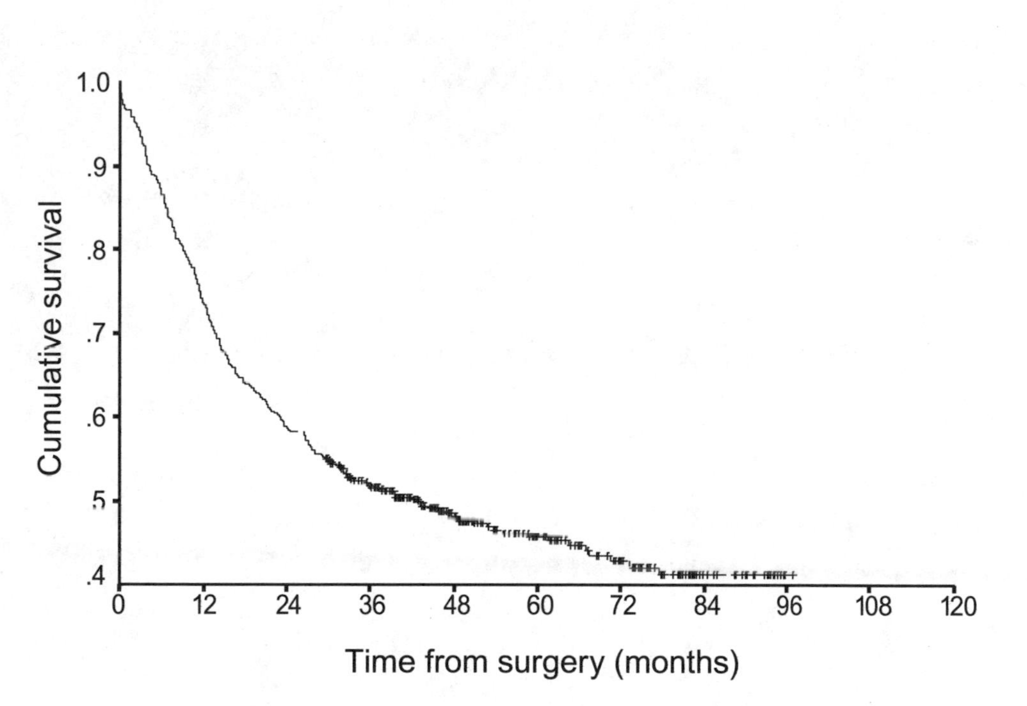

Censored cases are shown by a line across the survival function line.

Figure 5.1 Kaplan-Meier survival function for cases in study.

Table 5.1 The distribution of case variables Age, Gender, Stage, Cell type, N-score, and LN Vol by 6, 9, 12, 15, 18, and 24-months survival categories.

	Mean Age	Gender		Stage			Cell-type		N -score			Mean LN Vol
		female	male	I	II	IIIa	Adeno-	Sqaum	0	1	2	
6 months												
alive	63.8	151	311	283	75	104	198	264	305	79	78	1.61
dead	63.7	15	54	30	12	27	31	38	33	16	20	1.76
9 months												
alive	63.8	143	285	269	67	92	184	244	289	71	68	1.58
dead	64	23	80	44	20	39	45	58	49	24	30	1.81
12 months												
alive	63.6	132	259	252	62	77	167	224	268	63	60	1.55
dead	64.3	34	106	61	25	54	62	78	70	32	38	1.84
15 months												
alive	63.6	123	237	235	56	69	149	211	251	56	53	1.52
dead	64.3	43	128	78	31	62	80	91	87	39	45	1.86
18 months												
alive	63.5	116	224	224	53	63	139	201	238	54	48	1.5
dead	64.5	50	141	89	34	68	90	101	100	41	50	1.85
24 months												
alive	63.6	109	204	213	49	51	127	186	226	49	38	1.5
dead	64.1	57	161	100	38	80	102	116	112	46	60	1.81

A. SURVIVAL CLASSIFICATION BY LOGISTIC REGRESSION

Variables selected by stepwise logistic regression with p and R values for the regression according to time from surgery categories are shown in Table 5.2.

B. SURVIVAL CLASSIFICATION BY GANN

Case variables selected by the genetic algorithm neural network and posterior odds for the classification are shown in Table 5.3.

C. COMPARISON OF LOGISTIC REGRESSION AND GANN FOR CLASSIFICATION OF SURVIVAL

Sensitivity, specificity, positive predictive value, and odds ratio for classification by GANN and logistic regression is shown in Figure 5.2. Sensitivity for classification by GANN was less than logistic regression at all time points. However, specificity for classification by the GANN was greater than for logistic regression at all time points. This difference was greater than that for sensitivity.

Positive predictive value and odds ratios were greater than prevalence and prior odds for all time points for the GANN, and for all time points except 9 months for logistic regression. Positive predictive value and odds ratio for GANN were greater than logistic regression at all time points.

Significant differences in classification between GANN and logistic regression were found at the 9-, 12-, and 15-month time points (McNemar tests, $p < 0.01$). From the plots of positive predictive value and odds ratios, it can be seen that at these time points, this represents a significant *improvement* in classification by the GANN method compared to logistic regression.

Table 5.2 Distribution variables selected by stepwise logistic regression with p and R values for the regression according to time from surgery categories.

Prediction time	Predictor variable	p	R
6 months	Stage	0.0082	0.117
9 months	LN vol	0.0059	0.1033
	Stage	0.0035	0.1185
12 months	LN vol	0.0001	0.1455
	Stage	0.0004	0.1382
15 months	LN vol	<0.0000	0.2078
	N	0.0003	0.1345
18 months	LN vol	<0.0000	0.2127
	N	0.0005	0.1281
24 months	LN vol	<0.0000	0.1904
	N	<0.0000	0.1682

Table 5.3 Case variables selected by the genetic algorithm neural network and posterior odds for the classification.

Time from surgery	Predictor variables	Posterior odds
6 months	LN vol Age Cell type	6.67
9 months	Cell type N score Age	4.66
12 months	LN vol Stage Cell type	5.65
15 months	LN vol Gender Age	2.97
18 months	LN vol Stage Age	2.47
24 months	LN vol N-score Stage	2.18

Figure 5.2 (a)

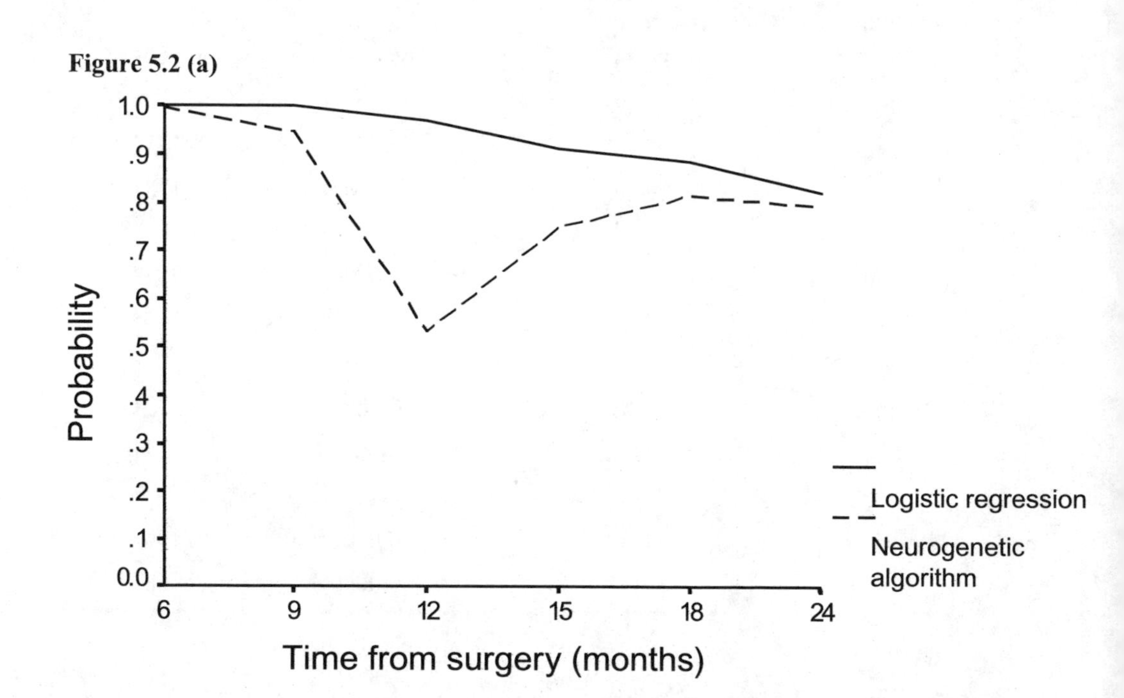

Figure 5.2 (b)

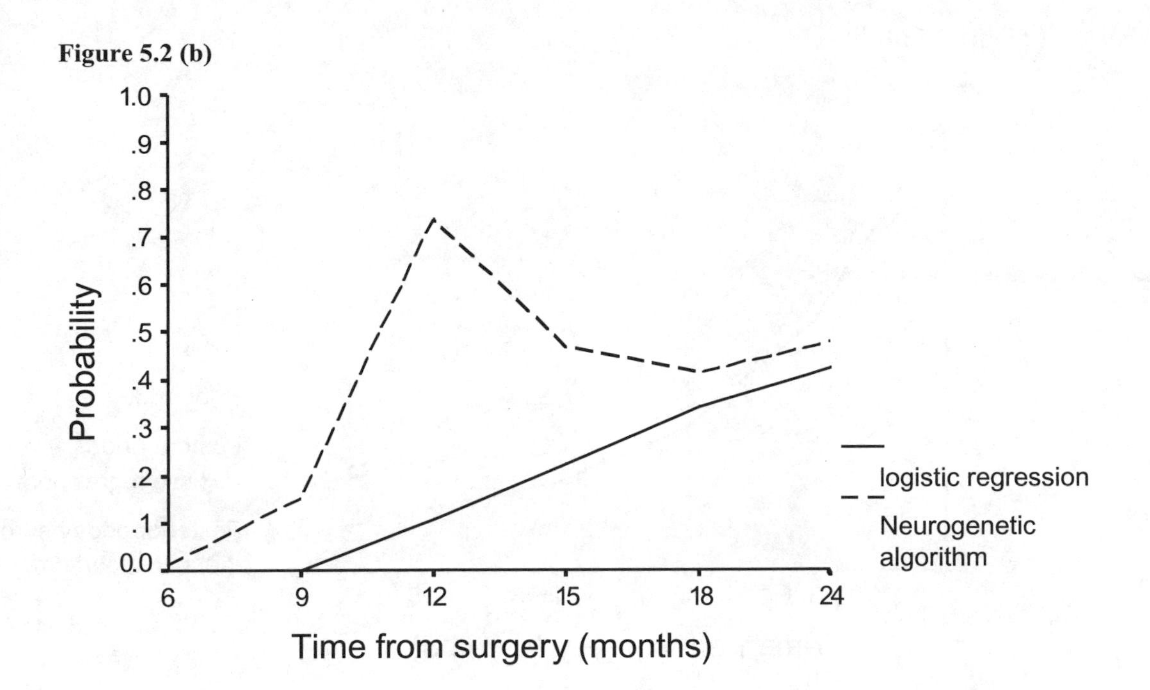

Figure 5.2 (c)

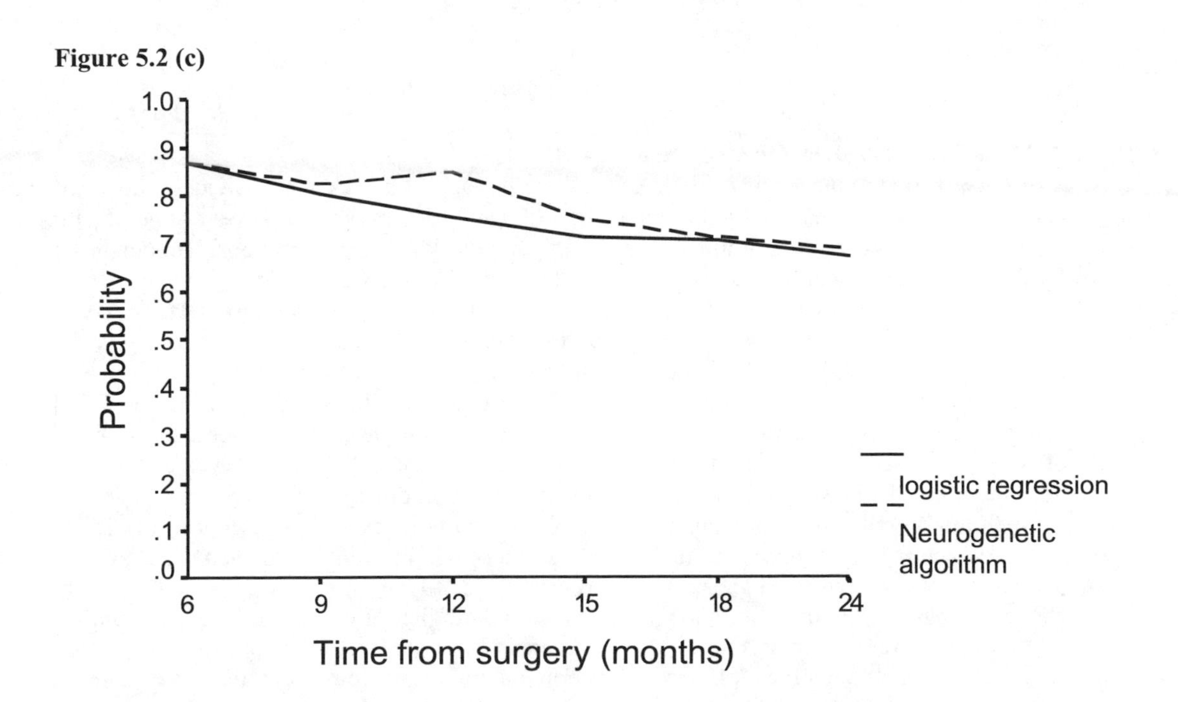

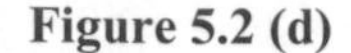

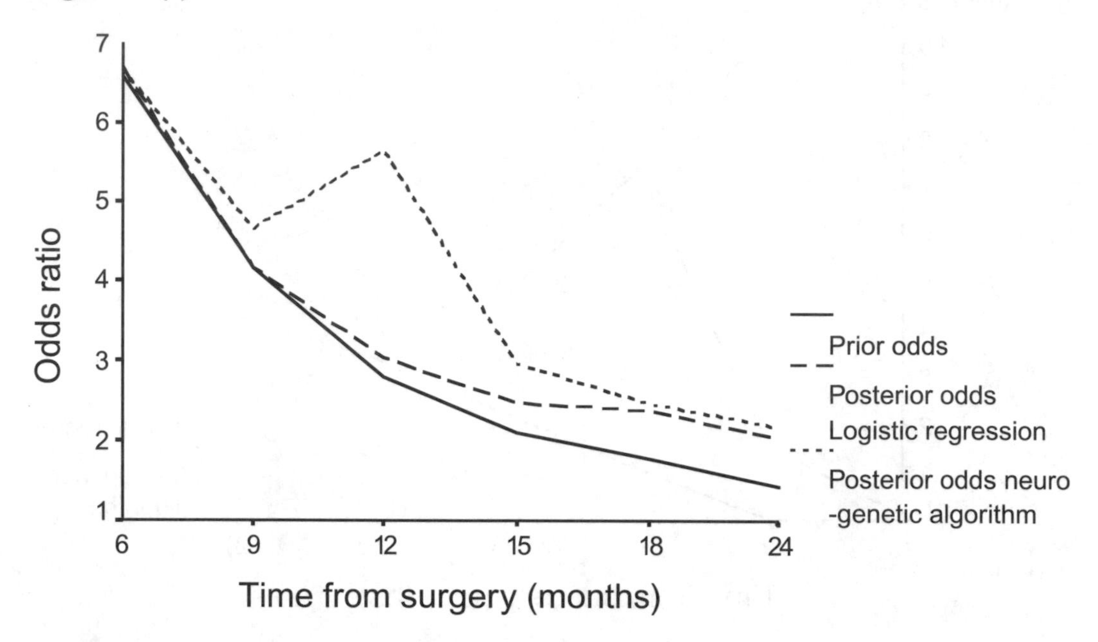

Figure 5.2 Sensitivity (a), specificity (b), positive predictive value (c), and odds ratio of classification (d) of survival by logistic regression and genetic algorithm neural network at 6 categories of time after surgical resection for NSCLC.

VI. DISCUSSION

A. INTERPRETATION OF CLINICAL FINDINGS

Cancer is one of the leading causes of death worldwide. Lung cancer is divided into small cell (SCLC) and nonsmall cell lung cancer (NSCLC) and surgery is the treatment of choice for NSCLC. The factors determining survival of an individual case are poorly understood. Further understanding of lung cancer biology is thus relevant to disease sufferers.

Lung cancer is divided into SCLC and NSCLC by histological morphology. Determination of tumour WHO classification is a key step in determining management, as surgery is the treatment of choice for NSCLC, while chemotherapy is preferred for SCLC.

Cases with stage I, II, or IIIa tumours are considered suitable for surgery [1]. Although the chances of patients presenting with localised disease suitable for curative resection are much higher than in SCLC, surgically treated patients account for only 15% of all cases of NSCLC. For those treated with surgery, two thirds will suffer recurrent disease within 5 years [5,14].

In common with some previous reports [16], this study gives indirect evidence of effects of NSCLC cell type on survival as this factor was chosen on occasion by the genetic algorithm neural network to predict prognosis. Furthermore, the cell-type measure was more frequently chosen at earlier time points, and gross clinicopathological measures (stage and tumour volume measures) at later ones. This is consistent with the clinical impression that "aggressive" histopathology affects short-term outcome and long-term outcome is most affected by gross measures of progression.

Once histological diagnosis has been established, determination of TNM classification and UICC stage of tumours has emerged as the single most important criterion for management [17], such as surgical resection [1]. In common with other studies [13], this study found *stage* to be an extremely significant independent predictor of survival, superseding other factors examined in a multivariate model.

Within the TNM scale, the development of mediastinal metastasis has been shown to be a critical transition affecting survival [18] and respectability [13]. This corresponds to the development of UICC stage IIIa from stage II.

Stage has been shown consistently to be able to group patients with the same cell type into categories with similar prognosis [19,20]. The prognostic significance of this information has proved useful for physicians needing to select treatment [21]; however, there is considerable heterogeneity in survival patterns for different stages, and variance in outcome of similar stages [21]. This has been observed as similar patterns of first observed recurrence independent of stage or cell type. Further, while these factors may correlate well for large cohorts of patients, they do not correlate well with behaviour in individual cases. Indeed, it has not been able to demonstrate that these measures can be used to predict the outcome of individual cases with high efficiency [22].

Survival in NSCLC is regarded as a function of both TNM stage and histopathological cell type, and "the value of the TNM staging lies in its ability to provide guidance and direction for management of the patient" [13], but neither of these measures can predict survival for individuals. Such analyses are difficult because of the biological variability in tumour behaviour. Considerable biological variability in aggressiveness is seen indepen-dent of stage, as is explained by the wide range of tumour doubling times [23]. This produces an extremely unpredictable natural history [1], which has been observed as similar patterns of first observed recurrence independent of stage, or cell type [21]. Thus, while these factors may correlate well for large cohorts of patients, they do not do so very well for the behaviour of individual cases. The consequence of this variability in outcome is difficulty in applying standard statistical methods [22].

To address this, research has focused on the examination of other factors or measures that may have prognostic significance. Tumour biomarkers, in particular, have received a great deal of investigation. The majority of these studies, however, have been on small groups of patients and do not all take into account other prognostic factors, such as staging. Whilst the inclusion of biomarker measurements in multivariate models has been shown to increase prognostic efficiency [24], their measurement has not gained widespread clinical acceptance.

In the case of tumour biomarkers, major contributors to lack of uptake have been expense and lack of availability outside a few special centres. A more fruitful approach might be to investigate whether the information generally recorded could be used more effectively. Our study suggests that the genetic algorithm neural network method may be very suitable for this, and may allow prediction of outcomes for individual cases with a high degree of accuracy, which therefore needs assessment of evidence for accuracy, generality, and effectiveness [25] in a prospective study.

B. METHODOLOGICAL CONSIDERATIONS

1. Classification of survival outcome

It is generally better to avoid summarising survival as outcomes at discrete, arbitrary, time points [26]. There are three main reasons for this:

(a) Censored data and missing values

If survival is classified categorically only noncensored data may be used [9]. The disadvantage of this is that if censored data is removed, many data sets (with large numbers of lost cases) may simply not be left with enough cases for survival to be predicted. As traditional statistical techniques such as Cox's proportional hazard model are unable to use censored data to produce predictions with a high degree of accuracy [22], such data sets are not suitable for prediction by standard methods. Whether a genetic algorithm neural network method could use censored data requires further study.

The advantage for prediction methods where non-censored data is available is that no manipulations are required to account for the loss of cases. As all such procedures necessarily make assumptions about the lost cases, for the purposes of predictive model building, it is best to avoid the need to use these procedures. In theory, since neural network methods can deal with data sets with missing values, the genetic algorithm neural network method should be able to account for case censoring, but this requires further study.

2. Losses and gains in information

If outcome data is divided arbitrarily into categories, some of the information in the data is lost. For survival data, this can be misleading for individual cases, e.g., a case living 6 months and 1 day being treated differently to a case living 6 months. However, the division of continuous variables into categories is common, e.g., division of time into minutes and hours. In lung cancer this is demonstrated if clinicians are asked to predict prognosis; it is found that predictions tended to be at "round numbers" such as 12, 24, or 36 months [22]. The advantages to clinicians' understanding of results as categories rather than dimensions are that they offer greater familiarity, are easier to understand, remember and use, provide a prelude to action, and they "do not strain the resources of a largely innumerate profession" [27]. Such considerations are important if it is appreciated that the endpoint of these methods should be a procedure that is useful for clinicians [25].

The process of reducing survival to a small number of categories also influences the accuracy of predictions that can be made. While reducing input data will produce poorer predictions because of loss of predictive information, reducing target data (e.g., survival outcome) will not necessarily do so. Indeed, as variability in response is the main limit leading to poor efficiency of outcome prediction with the Cox's model [22], reduction in this variability could increase predictive efficiency. Examination of whether this is the case requires further study.

(b) Comparisons and results

Summarising survival as outcome in a small number of categories should not be used to compare samples, e.g., treated and nontreated groups in a randomised trial of lung cancer therapy. In order to do this, proportional hazard models should be used [9]. However, categorising outcome does not affect comparisons of predictive methods using such data, as in this study. Indeed, as paired predictions for the same data are obtained, a product of this design is that the predictive methods can be directly compared by the McNemar test, and p values derived to test the significance of differences.

In this study, a categorical survival outcome design is used to test the significance of differences in predictive performance between the genetic algorithm neural network method and logistic regression. This is particularly important as few neural network studies in cancer make comparison with other predictive methodologies [5,28]. In the experi-mental setting, this is analogous to quoting the results of an experimental group but not the control group. The reasons for not comparing predictive methods are not clear as appro-priate methods, such as logistic regression, are readily available, easily applied, and have already been used to make comparisons with outcome results from neural networks [29].

However, an effect of the design in this study is that quantitative interpretation of the efficiency of survival classification compared with other studies, is difficult. Firstly, it is not surprising that prediction of survival to lie within a 6-month category is easier than prediction of the continuous survival time. Secondly, as error from the latter will appear greater (since cases with actual survival times in the middle of a 6-month category, error in prediction must be $> \pm 3$ months to produce an error in classification).

Summarising survival outcome into discrete arbitrary categories is thus generally best avoided but has advantages for predictive methods and has been the approach used in the majority of neural network studies [30-32]. Alternative solutions that have been investigated appear to require greater compromises such as nonstandardised data transformation [33]. For the purpose of evaluating and comparing predictive methods, these are probably best avoided.

(c) Assumptions of prior odds and Bayes' theorem

To implement Bayes' theorem where data is not available on the population it must be assumed that prior probabilities derived from the database are representative of the population. Because of the selection bias outlined above it is certain that in this study this is not the case. However, given the size and duration of the database in this study, the table of likelihoods derived by the genetic algorithm neural network for this one centre should be representative of that centre. Thus, while not applicable to the population, the table of likelihoods from the optimal predictive genetic algorithm neural network solution should produce predictions of equal efficiency to those in this study for the centre from which the data was obtained. Determination of this requires prospective study.

As other neural network cancer outcome studies do not apply Bayes' theorem and take into account prior frequency of the positive test result case (i.e., prevalence), errors on application to different samples from the same population are likely to be a particular problem. Further, such approaches mean that the general significance of the results presented cannot be interpreted [9]. Given that an "Achilles heel" of neural networks used in isolation is difficulty in generalisability, the likely exacerbation of this is particularly unfortunate. Furthermore, a consequence of such designs is that they do not allow the examination of pre- and post-test odds, which is the preferred method for evaluating the usefulness of competing predictive methods [9].

3. Adaptability and retraining

Problems relating to the determination of likelihood tables discussed above are examples of training set problems. As was alluded to when these problems were introduced, the only solution to this is to maintain adaptability of the predictive method by periodic retraining.

It was the inability to retrain that led to some of the difficulties encountered by De Dombal [34]. The need to retrain arises once significant amounts of new data have been added to the database. This is vital in order to ensure that new relationships that may have subsequently arisen can be incorporated, and that the table of likelihoods remains representative of the centre. Where reduced sets of the sample data are used (e.g., if a selection procedure such as a genetic algorithm is used), then retraining on the sample data becomes increasingly important as the potential for nonrepresentation will increase in proportion to the amount the sample data is reduced by the selection.

Two important differences between the situation De Dombal et al. faced now mean that the need to retrain can be solved easily by methods such as the one implemented in this study. These are, firstly, neural network methods have the ability to learn by experience and evolve to optimal systems for the data with which they are used. Secondly, computing equipment is now generally available and inexpensive. Further, the cheapness and availability of powerful computing equipment means that, unlike the situation faced by De Dombal and his contemporaries, computational activity can take place at the site where the system is to be used. Such systems can then evolve to match particular institutions and doctors. The availability of computing equipment is so universal that there is no longer any need to attempt to provide a single set of system parameters that will match all doctors and all institutions. Indeed, a single set of system parameters (such as a set of likelihoods), which will be the final and complete answer, is unlikely given the wide variability of subjective clinical data. Furthermore, it may not be desirable, as a system dependent upon a single set of system parameters may not have the ability to adapt to changing circumstances [35]. This problem is the mathematical analogue of the problem of biological overspecialisation. An organism may be so well adapted for a given environ-ment and have so little capacity to change that it fails to survive should it face a somewhat different environment.

A solution to the specialisation dilemma is to continually retrain the network as data is added. This is simulated in the genetic algorithm neural network method by the n+1 case handling for predictions. This may be thought of as simulating an ongoing evolutionary process. Such processes are important as the institution to which they must be applied (hospitals) are dynamic entities that change with time, and thus need both the database and the table of likelihoods to change too. Thus, a set of predictor variables together with the matrix of network weights may produce a genetic algorithm neural network that is optimal for an institution at a given time. However this method risks overspecialisation. These variables may not be the optimal variables at some future time in the same institution and may be quite inadequate now for a different doctor in the same institution. The testing of whether the genetic algorithm neural network method can overcome overspecialisation requires further study.

4. Variable selection by the GA

While neural networks may be considered as "black-boxes" [6], their function may be made more accessible by informing users of which variables are influential. Procedures to do this may also be used to eliminate uninfluential input. This is particularly important for maximising a neural network's ability to generalise, especially when faced with a limited amount of data [35,36]. A variety of empirical stepwise procedures have been suggested to achieve this [30,32,36]. The genetic algorithm procedure used in this study can be thought of as formalising a competitive learning rule, which while also empirical, has the advantage of having been proved robust across a variety of optimisation problems [37].

5. Performance of genetic algorithm neural network compared with logistic regression

The prediction results in this NSCLC sample show the magnitude of improvement produced by the genetic algorithm neural network over logistic regression was large; the ability to classify cases is more than doubled. The high degree of concordance between the variables selected by both methods implies that the same data is being used in a different way. This may be because neural networks identify relationships that violate distribution, linearity, or proportionality assumptions [33], and the genetic algorithm scours the search surface so that optimisation is not arrested in local minima [38].

6. Adaptations in the genetic algorithm neural network method: simulating pre-processing in basic neural systems

The adaptations used in the genetic algorithm neural network method over basic feed-forward back-propagation of error neural networks have been shown to produce advantages in reduced training sample and signal-noise problems [5,7,39]. These advantages may be seen as simulating the preprocessing that is known to occur in biological neural systems. For example, in the visual system, "lateral inhibition" in the lateral geniculate body and the retina reduces signal noise and accentuates salient features before cortical processing of images in the striate cortex. The use of a genetic algorithm can thus be thought of as furthering the biological analogy of neural networks by simulating preprocessing to remove training sample noise before processing by the neural network. As was alluded to in the introduction to neural network architectures, feed-forward back-propagation of error neural networks are only one of several neural network designs that simulate various biological neuronal architectures [40]. Whether the adaptations made here could be applied to these, and what benefits this might bring is not known.

7. Components of methodological performance

Some of the reasons that may explain why the genetic algorithm neural network method out-performed logistic regression in this study are outlined above. However, the determination of which particular parts of the procedure that imparted this performance advantage requires further study. This is important as it will direct the further evolution of the method.

VII. CONCLUSIONS

Standard statistical methods cannot accurately predict the survival of individual cancer patients. Neural networks require adaptation to overcome training-sample and signal-noise problems. This may be done with the application of a genetic algorithm and Bayes' theorem. The factors that affect outcome of patients with NSCLC are unclear. From the sample of NSCLC cases treated with surgery in this study one main conclusion may be drawn: the genetic algorithm neural network method is demonstrated to be able to classify outcome with a high degree of efficiency, and is significantly and considerably better than the appropriate standard statistical method (logistic regression) and further development of this approach is warranted.

REFERENCES

1. **Lederle F.A., Dennis E., Niewoehner M.D.,** Lung cancer surgery, *Arch. Intern. Med.,* 154, 2397-2400, 1994.
2. **Humphrey E.W., Smart C.R., Winchester D.P., Steele G.D. Jr, Yarbro J.W., Chu K.C., Triolo H.H.,** National survey of the pattern of care for carcinoma of the lung, *J. Thorac. Cardiovasc. Surg.*, 100, 837-843, 1990.
3. **Cross S.S., Harrison R.F., Kennedy R.L.,** Introduction to neural networks, *The Lancet*, 346, 1075-1079, 1995.
4. **Baxt W.G.,** Application of artificial neural networks to clinical medicine, *The Lancet*, 346, 1135-1138, 1995.
5. **Jefferson M.F., Pendleton N., Lucas S.B., Horan M.A.,** Comparison of a genetic algorithm neural network with logistic regression for predicting outcome after surgery for patients with non-small cell lung cancer, *Cancer*, 79, 7, 1338-1342, 1997.
6. **Hart A., Wyatt J.,** Evaluating black-boxes as medical decision aids: issues arising from a study of neural networks, *Med. Info.*, 15, 229-236, 1990.
7. **Jefferson M.F., Pendleton N., Mohamed S., Kirkman E., Little R.A., Lucas S.B., Horan M.A.,** Prediction of haemorrhagic blood loss with a genetic algorithm neural network, *J. Appl. Physiol.*, 84,1, 357-361, 1998.
8. **Narayanan M.N., Lucas S.B.,** A genetic algorithm to improve a neural network to predict a patient's response to warfarin, *Meth. Inf. Med.*, 32, 55-58, 1993.
9. **Altman D.G.,** *Practical Statistics for Medical Research*, Chapman & Hall, London, 1995.
10. **Macartney F.J.,** Diagnostic logic, *Br. Med. J.*, 295, 1325-1331, 1987.
11. **WHO** (The World Health Organization), The World Health Organization histological typing of lung tumours, *Am. J. Clin. Pathol.*, 77, 123-136, 1982.
12. **Hermanek P., Sobin L.H.** (Eds.), *TNM Classification of Malignant Tumours*, 4th ed., Springer-Verlag, Berlin, 1987.
13. **Mountain C.F.,** Lung cancer staging classification, *Clin. Chest Med.*, 14, 43-51, 1993.
14. **Splinter T.A.W.,** Therapy for small cell and non-small cell lung cancer, *Curr. Opin. Oncol.*, 4, 315-332, 1992.
15. **Martini N.,** Surgical treatment of lung cancer, *Semin. Oncol.*, 17, 9-10, 1990.
16. **Rosenthal S.A., Curran W.J.,** The significance of histology in non-small cell lung cancer, *Cancer Treat. Rev.*, 17, 409-425, 1990.
17. **Greenberg S.D., Fraire A.E., Kinner D.M., Johnson E.H.,** Tumour cell type versus staging in the prognosis of carcinoma of the lung, *Pathol. Ann.*, 22, 387-405, 1987.

18. **Wantanabe Y., Hayashi Y., Shimizu J., Oda M., Iwa T.,** Mediastinal nodal involvement and the prognosis of non-small cell lung cancer, *Chest*, 100, 422-428, 1991.
19. **Gloeckler L.A.,** Influence of extent of disease, histology and demographic factors on lung cancer survival in the SEER population-based data, *Semin. Surg. Oncol.*, 10, 21-30, 1994.
20. **Hilsenbeck S.G., Raub W.A., Sridhar K.S.,** Prognostic factors in lung cancer based on multivariate analysis, *J. Clin. Oncol.*, 16, 301-309, 1993.
21. **Mountain C.F.,** New prognostic factors in lung cancer: biologic prophets of cancer cell aggression, *Chest*, 108, 246-254, 1995.
22. **Henderson R.,** Problems and prediction in survival analysis, *Stats Med.*, 14, 161-184, 1995.
23. **Geddes D.M.,** The natural history of lung cancer: a review based on rates of tumour growth, *Br. J. Dis. Chest*, 73, 1-17, 1979.
24. **Walop W., et al.**, The use of biomarkers in the prediction of survival in patients with pulmonary carcinoma, *Cancer*, 65, 2033-2046, 1990.
25. **Wyatt J.C., Altman D.G.,** Commentary — Prognostic models: Clinically useful or quickly forgotten, *Br. Med. J.*, 311, 1539, 1995.
26. **Peto R., Pike M.C., Armitage P., et al.,** Design and analysis of randomized clinical trials requiring prolonged observation of each patient — II: analysis and examples, *Br. J. Cancer*, 35, 1-39, 1977.
27. **Kendall R.E.,** *The Role of Diagnosis in Psychiatry*, Blackwell, Oxford, 1975.
28. **Jefferson M.F., Pendleton N., Lucas S.B.,** Neural networks, *The Lancet*, 346, 1712, 1995.
29. **Doig G.S., et al.,** Modelling mortality in the intensive care unit: comparing the performance of a back-propagation, associative learning neural network with multivariate logistic regression, *Proc. Symp. Computers Applied to Medical Care*, 361-365, 1993.
30. **Kappen H.J., Neijt J.P.,** Advanced ovarian cancer — neural network analysis to predict treatment outcome, *Ann. Oncol.*, 4, s31-34, 1993.
31. **Burke H.B.,** Artifical neural networks for cancer research: outcome prediction, *Semin. Surg. Oncol.*, 10, 73-79, 1994.
32. **Snow P.B., Smith D.S., Catolona W.J.,** Artificial neural networks in the diagnosis and prognosis of prostate cancer: a pilot study, *J. Urol.*, 152, 1923-1926, 1994.
33. **Ravdin P.M., Clark G.M.,** A practical application of neural network analysis for predicting outcome of individual breast cancer patients, *Breast Cancer Res. Treat.*, 22, 285-293, 1992.
34. **De Dombal F.T., Staniland J.R., Clamp S.E.,** Geographical variation in disease presentation, *Med. Decis. Making*, 1, 59-69, 1981.
35. **German S., Bienstock E., Doursat R.,** Neural networks and the bias/variance dilemma, *Neural Comp.*, 4, 1-58, 1992.
36. **Wilding P., Morgan M.A., Grygotis A.E., Shoffner M.A., Rosato E.F.,** Application of backpropagation neural networks to diagnosis of breast and ovarian cancer, *Cancer Lett.*, 77, 145-153, 1994.
37. **Goldberg D.E.,** *Genetic Algorithms in Search, Optimization and Machine Learning*, Addison Wesley, New York, 1989.
38. **Holland J.H.,** Genetic algorithms, *Sci. Am.*, 267, 1, 44-50, 1992.
39. **Jefferson M.F., Pendleton N., Lucas C.P., Lucas S.B., Horan M.A.,** Evolution of artificial neural network architecture: prediction of depression after mania, *Meth. Inform. Med.*, 37, 220-226, 1998.
40. **Chuchland P.S., Sejnowski T.J.,** *The Computational Brain,* MIT Press, Cambridge, MA, 1994.

Chapter 6

THE USE OF MACHINE LEARNING IN SCREENING FOR ORAL CANCER

P. M. Speight and P. Hammond

I. EPIDEMIOLOGY

Ninety five percent of malignancies in the oropharyngeal region are squamous cell carcinomas arising from the surface epithelium. In England and Wales, oral cancer affects about 3000 individuals per year [1]. This is a similar number to cervical cancer, but mortality from oral cancer is greater and more people die of it each year. Intraoral cancer has a mortality rate of more than 50% and there has been no improvement in survival for decades. A recent report of a large series in Liverpool [2] shows a crude 5-year survival of 34% with an adjusted actuarial figure of 47%. There is good evidence that these persistently poor survival figures are due to poor detection of small lesions and late presentation. Overall, more than 70% of patients present with large lesions (>2 cm), which have a significantly worse prognosis [3,4]. Added to this, it is now known that oral cancer registrations and incidence are increasing throughout Europe and in the UK [5,6]. Registrations in England and Wales have increased from 2305 in 1985 to 2988 in 1992 (about 30% increase) [1,7]. Careful analysis of this data has shown that the greatest increases have been among males aged 35-64 (i.e., a younger age group): for intraoral cancer, mortality increased from 1.67 per 100,000 in 1966-70 to 2.91 in 1986-90 with a corresponding increase in incidence rates from 3.61 to 5.52 [5]. These data confirm that oral cancer is a serious and worsening health care problem. This is surprising because the disease is easy to detect and treatment for small lesions is relatively simple and effective.

II. CLINICAL FEATURES AND DIAGNOSIS

Oral cancer is most often seen as a persistent ulcer with raised edges and a firm indurated base. Typically the lesion is painless, but patients usually state that the lesion has been present for some time, often months. At this stage, the lesion presents little diagnostic challenge to the experienced clinician; however, these ulcerated lesions are probably late in the natural history of the disease and at time of diagnosis the prognosis is already poor with over 60% of patients having loco-regional lymph node metastases [3]. A major goal for the prevention of mortality and morbidity is early detection of oral cancers and of potentially malignant lesions. Early lesions of oral cancer are often subtle and may easily be missed both by patients and clinicians. Most often, small lesions present as red patches (erythroplakia) or as speckled red and white lesions (speckled or nonhomogeneous leukoplakia). Although typical of early cancer, such

0-8493-9692-1/01/$0.00+$1.50

appearances may also be seen as a result of other, nonmalignant, oral diseases. These lesions are often therefore dismissed as trivial and ignored. Precancerous lesions are usually white patches on the oral mucosa (leukoplakia), but other conditions may result in a similar appearance and white patches overall may be quite common. The problem for dentists and other clinicians is to decide which white patches are significant and which are due to simple causes such as frictional trauma. True leukoplakias which are regarded as potentially malignant are rare in the general population and of these, only about 5% overall may progress to malignant disease.

The challenge therefore is to improve early detection of disease while at the same time ensuring that only relevant lesions are detected and referred for specialist management.

III. SCREENING FOR ORAL CANCER

Poor statistics relating to the incidence and mortality of oral cancer have received considerable attention within the dental profession and, over the last decade, there have been repeated calls for screening and prevention of oral cancer. The purpose of screening is to apply a test to the population to sort out people who probably have a disease from those who probably do not [8]. This involves the application of a test to apparently healthy individuals in the hope of detecting preclinical disease at a stage when it is still curable. In the case of cancer the aim is to detect early lesions that can be cured, or precancerous lesions that can be treated before they progress.

In 1991 a UK working group on screening for oral cancer and precancer was established, with the remit of examining the current literature and advising on the feasibility of screening for oral cancer in the UK [9]. They found that oral cancer met many of the criteria for a screenable disease: it is easy to detect, there is a detectable precursor lesion, and early lesions are curable. A screening test is also relatively easy and involves a systematic examination of the mouth to identify relevant lesions. However, littie is known of the natural history of the disease. Although potentially malignant lesions can de detected, only about 5% overall become malignant [3], and there are no tests currently available to specifically identify this minority. The working group's report [9] did not recommend population screening for oral cancer, but made recommendations for further research including evaluation of screening tests and pilot screening programmes. Other groups have made similar recommendations [10] and have suggested that opportunistic screening of high risk groups may be beneficial [11].

Recently we have carried out a number of pilot screening programmes in hospital, medical practice, and industrial environments. In these studies dentists were able to detect relevant lesions with a sensitivity and specificity similar to that obtained in other screening programmes [12,13]. There was some variability between the different programmes which may reflect the experience of the examiners (Table 6.1). In the hospital and medical practice projects, 2027 individuals were examined with an overall sensitivity and specificity of 0.74 and 0.99, respectively [12]. In the medical practice invitational programme however, compliance for the oral examination was only about 25% which, in association with the low prevalence of the disease in the general population, further confirmed that invitational population screening for oral cancer may not be cost-beneficial [14].

This view has been reiterated in a number of recent reviews and reports. Many of these have suggested that we should seek to implement secondary prevention programmes which screen a selected subset of the population who can be identified as being at a high risk of the disease [8,9,11,15].

Table 6.1 The performance of dentists in detecting relevant lesions in three pilot oral cancer screening programmes. The programme in the dental hospital was opportunistic, while those in the medical practice and company headquarters were invitational.

Screening programme	*Reference*	*n*	Sensitivity	Specificity
Medical practice	Jullien et al., 1995 [12]	985	0.64	0.99
Dental hospital	Jullien et al., 1995 [12]	1042	0.81	0.99
Company headquarters	Downer et al., 1995 [13]	309	0.71	0.99

IV. SELECTION OF HIGH-RISK GROUPS USING A NEURAL NETWORK

In the two pilot screening programmes mentioned above, 2027 individuals over the age of 40 years were examined. Each was screened and subsequently examined by a hospital specialist to confirm the diagnosis and to provide a gold standard for the sensitivity and specificity calculations. Each subject also completed an interview questionnaire regarding personal details, dental attendance, and smoking and drinking habits. This information was collected because age, gender, and tobacco and alcohol use are known to influence oral cancer risk. Thus we had a large database of more than 2000 subjects containing details of their high risk habits and whether or not they had a cancer or precancerous lesion. The overall prevalence of lesions in this group was 2.7% (54 subjects).

This data was used to prepare a neural network designed to predict the likelihood of an individual having a precancer or cancer of the mouth [16]. The neural network software was written by a postgraduate student [17] in the Turbo Pascal programming language (Borland International Inc., California) and was able to input data directly from a commonly used database (Paradox, Borland International Inc., California). Two groups of subjects were randomly generated, each with the same prevalence of positive cases. These comprised a training set of 1662 individuals (44 positives) and a test set of 365 individuals (10 positives).

V. TRAINING AND TESTING THE NEURAL NETWORK

For training the network, ten items of personal information relating to age, gender, and habits were selected from the questionnaire data (Table 6.2) and used as input variables for each of the 1662 individuals in the training set along with the result of the specialist oral examination as positive (cancer or precancerous lesion present) or negative. Each variable, except age, was presented to the network in binary form. Gender was represented as two separate Boolean variables, male and female. Age was represented as a normalised continuous variable, between 0 and 1, commencing at age 40 years. For a variety of reasons, a 1-out-of-*N* encoding scheme for age, for example based on age decade, was rejected.

The neural network model used was a standard three layer feed-forward network, trained with the back-propagation algorithm. A sigmoid activation function was employed throughout. Two measurements of error were used: mean square error during training and percent error (for both positive and negative cases) during testing. The former was chosen to give feedback on occurrence of local minima and network paralysis. The latter seemed more appropriate as an indication of the network's overall decision-making ability. The best results were obtained with one output node, three nodes in a single hidden layer, a learning rate of 0.01, a momentum constant of 0.05 and initial weights and biases set randomly between -0.03 and +0.03. During training, fine-tuning improvements in performance were achieved by altering the learning rate and momentum constant and by biasing the selection of negative over positive cases from the training set. For example, the initial optimal performance (based on percent error) occurred after 600,000 patterns were presented to the network. At this point, the mean square training error was 0.12 and the overall percentage correct in the test set was 71%. Training was interrupted at this point and the learning rate and momentum constant were reduced to 0.001 and 0.01, respectively, whereupon training was continued. Further experimentation established a bias rate of 4/5 for negative cases as achieving a new optimal performance with an associated mean square training error of 0.08 and a test set success rate for negative and positive cases of 83% and 73% , respectively.

Table 6.2 Input variables used to train the neural network. Data obtained from the questionnaire database of personal information of the screened population.

Question	Definition
Male	
Female	
Nonsmoker	Never smoked for more than 10 years
Moderate smoker	< 20 cigarettes/day
Heavy smoker	≥ 20 cigarettes/day
Nondrinker	Never drinks or < 5 units a week
Moderate drinker	Female ≤ 14, Male ≤ 21 units a week
Heavy drinker	Female > 14, Male > 21 units a week
Age	Continuous variable from 40 years
Irregular dental attendee	Has not visited a dentist in the last year

The state of optimum performance was evaluated by plotting receiver operating characteristic (ROC) curves [18] which plot the true positive (sensitivity) against the false positive (1-specificity) rates at different decision-making thresholds and determine a test's ability to differentiate between normal and abnormal. Assessment of performance (diagnostic accuracy) is represented by the area under the curve where a perfect test gives an area of 1.0 and a random classification produces a value of 0.50. An optimum performance was achieved with an ROC area of 0.84 [16].

The performance of the network in identifying individuals with lesions is summarised in Table 6.3. The best performing network had a sensitivity and specificity of 0.80 and 0.77 compared to 0.74 and 0.99 for the dental screeners who evaluated the same group of subjects. The likelihood ratio, which represents the odds of a positive decision being correct, was 3.48 for the network compared to 74.00 for the dental screeners. Although there were 23% false positives, this may be acceptable for a system which is intended to act as a prescreen filter. Those identified as at risk by the network would then be referred for a detailed oral mucosal examination.

Table 6.3 The performance of the neural network in predicting the presence of oral cancer or precancer compared to the gold standard specialist diagnosis.

		Specialist Diagnosis		
		Positive	Negative	Total
	Positive	8	82	90
Neural Network	Negative	2	273	275
	Total	10	355	365

Lesion prevalence:	(10/365)	= 2.74%
Sensitivity :	(8/10)	= 0.80
Specificity :	(273/355)	= 0.77
Likelihood ratio:	(0.80/0.23)	= 3.48

A criticism of neural network analysis is its black box nature, reflecting the lack of symbolic and hence human-interpretable output. Some effort was made to examine and interpret the best performing network's internal representation. For example, a technique of Saito and Nakano [19] can be used to compare the effects of individual input nodes. First, it is necessary to derive arithmetic differences in output node activation between the situation with all inputs set to 0, and then with one input node set at 1 and the remainder at 0. This is repeated for each input node and is meant to reflect the influence of one input node on the output independent of the other input nodes (row 1 of Table 6.4). Second, when presenting an example case to the network with its corresponding input values, one can measure the same arithmetic difference in output activation between the two situations when just one of the inputs is given the values 0 and 1. An average of these differences over all input patterns can be computed for each input node. This is meant to reflect the influence of a particular input node on the output node, but this time in the context of all other inputs (row 2 of Table 6.4).

It can be seen from Table 6.4 that gender and age appear to have no significant influence given the low values for the calculations in row 2. These also suggest that having been a smoker in the last 10 years has a negative effect on output node activation, but perhaps the inherent error in the model can explain this. Smoking factors related to high consumption and an extensive period of smoking appear to have a stronger influence on a positive output. The kind of alcohol consumed appears to have a fairly weak effect whereas the amount of alcohol is one of the two strongest factors. The most influential factor appears to be irregular dental attendance, perhaps reflecting a lack of concern for oral health.

Overall the network identified 25% (90 subjects) of the test set as being at high risk. This subset contained 80% of the lesions in the general population with a prevalence of 9% — three times greater than the 2.7% seen in the cohort as a whole. For the first time, this shows that a neural network can identify individuals at high risk of oral cancer and suggests that such a system may be useful in predicting disease in a general population. In medical or dental practice, simple lifestyle data could be entered into the computer and only those identified as high-risk need proceed to a screening examination.

VI. COMPARISON OF NEURAL NETWORKS AND OTHER MACHINE LEARNING TECHNIQUES

In the previous section, we described how a neural network was hand-crafted, with considerable fine-tuning, by a computer science postgraduate as part of an individual MSc project [17]. After the project was complete, the neural network was not readily available for reuse in a clinical environment or even for demonstration. The decision was taken, therefore, to repeat the machine learning analysis but this time using a commercial data mining package that is user friendly, robust, and that can export induced models in the form of executable procedures. The CLEMENTINE system (Integral Solutions Ltd.) supports a range of machine learning techniques, including simple decision tree and rule induction algorithms based respectively on ID3 [20] and C4.5 [21] (C5.0 in the later version of CLEMENTINE). It also supports feed-forward and Kohonen neural networks, and in addition enables models to be exported as C programs. The availability of these other techniques in CLEMENTINE allowed us to include comparison of their performance as part of the repeated analysis. As for the first study, the work was carried out by a postgraduate MSc student [22].

Table 6.4 Relative measures of influence on output node activation for each input node. Row 1 summarises difference when all nodes inputs are 0 and relevant column node has input 1. Row 2 gives mean over all input node patterns for difference in output node activation when particular column node has input 0 and 1.

	Male	Female	Age	Smoke in last 10 yrs	Smoke > 20 cigs. per day	Smoke > 20 yrs	Beer or wine	Fort. wine or spirits	Over weekly drink limit	Not visited dentist for 1 yr
1	0.27	0.38	0.16	-0.20	0.79	0.41	-0.10	-0.02	0.79	0.64
2	-0.02	-0.06	0.04	-0.11	0.28	0.40	0.13	0.19	0.58	0.73

VII. DATA VISUALISATION IN CLEMENTINE

The visual programming interface in CLEMENTINE can be used for preliminary data visualisation and subsequent machine learning. Icons representing data files and operations are selected from a palette and placed on a drawing area in the style of computer-aided design systems (Figure 6.1).

Sequences of operations are connected together by streams, and data is viewed as flowing from source data files through streams to a destination. Destination nodes are executed to generate tables, histograms, graphs, decision trees, neural networks, etc. Thus, an end-user need not be an experienced programmer to develop models and prototypes, and can easily modify or re-engineer existing models. Figure 6.2 illustrates the iconic representation of a source file of patient data and three nodes supporting data visualisation. Visual inspection of datasets promotes a better understanding of the variations to be found and may even encourage useful preprocessing of the data before models are induced. Before selecting training and test sets, it can be helpful to visualise distributions of major fields, such as age or gender, to identify any biases that may need to be taken into account, or to boost confidence in the results of the induced models. Figure 6.3 shows the tabular representation generated by the "execution" of the node labelled "table" in Figure 6.2. Similarly, Figures 6.4 and 6.5 illustrate the "execution" of the nodes labelled "time_smoke" and "age_years" which produce a distribution and histogram for the entire dataset showing respectively the male-female distribution for period of smoking and their age distribution. Being able to present histograms quickly and simply helps identify the likely importance of some fields or the granularity at which they should be analysed. For example, Figure 6.5 may influence the choice of measurement of age in terms of years or five yearly intervals, or even decades.

These visualisation capabilities prove to be particularly useful and contribute to the user friendliness of the CLEMENTINE system. An unexpected benefit of the preliminary visualisation of the dataset was the detection and elimination of some redundant and unacceptably noisy negative cases.

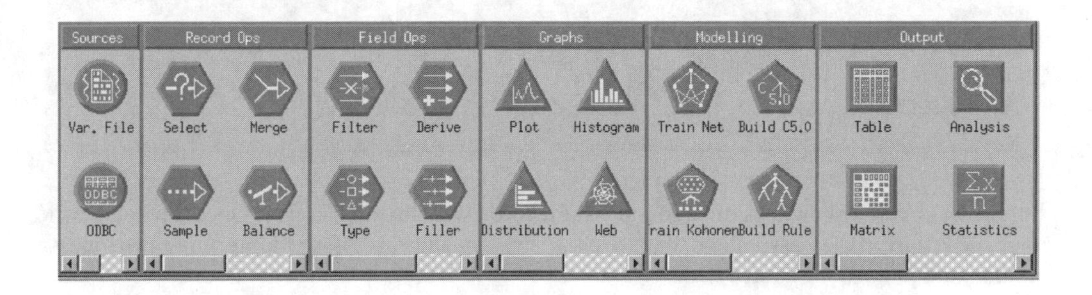

Figure 6.1 CLEMENTINE's palette of nodes for representing data sources, data processing and modelling.

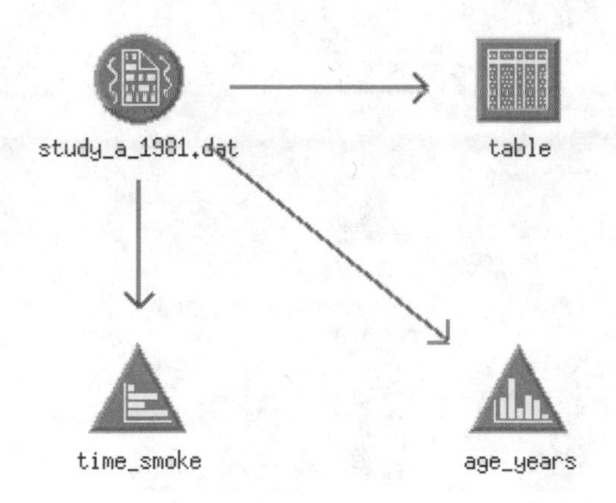

Figure 6.2 A CLEMENTINE "stream" representing a data source and three visualisation operations. Data flows from the source data file object (upper left) to a table object (upper right) and distribution and histogram charting objects (lower left and right, respectively).

table (1981 records)

Table Generate

smoke_cigars	smoke_rollup	smoke_pipe	drinker	beer	wine	fortified	spirits	dental_visit
N	N	N	Y	N	Y	N	N	2
N	N	N	Y	N	N	N	Y	1
N	N	N	Y	N	Y	N	N	1
N	N	N	Y	Y	N	N	Y	1
N	N	N	Y	N	Y	Y	N	1
N	N	N	Y	N	N	Y	N	2
N	N	N	N	N	N	N	N	2
N	N	N	Y	N	N	N	Y	1
N	N	N	Y	N	Y	N	N	2
N	N	N	Y	Y	N	N	N	1

Figure 6.3 Table showing collection of data records with labelled fields. Once the source file node in Figure 6.2 is associated with a data file, "execution" of the table node produces a tabular summary of the source data.

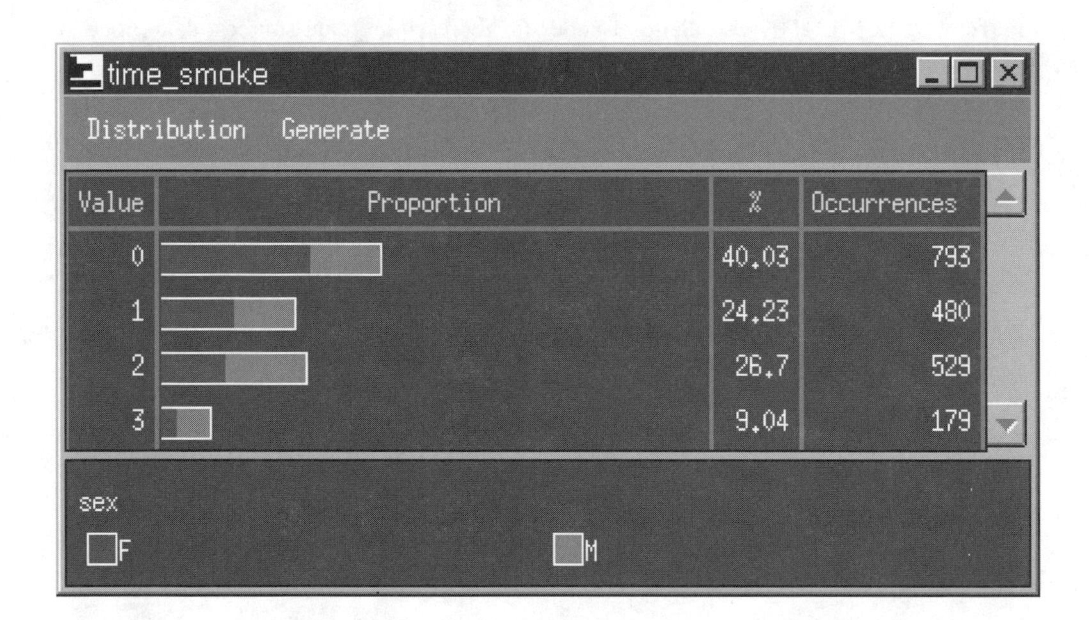

Figure 6.4 Distribution showing time smoked overlaid by sex of patient. The chart identifies the asymmetry between male and female patients in terms of the period of smoking. A larger proportion of female subjects have never smoked (*time_smoke = 0*); whereas, a smaller proportion have smoked for 20 or more years *(time_smoke = 3)*.

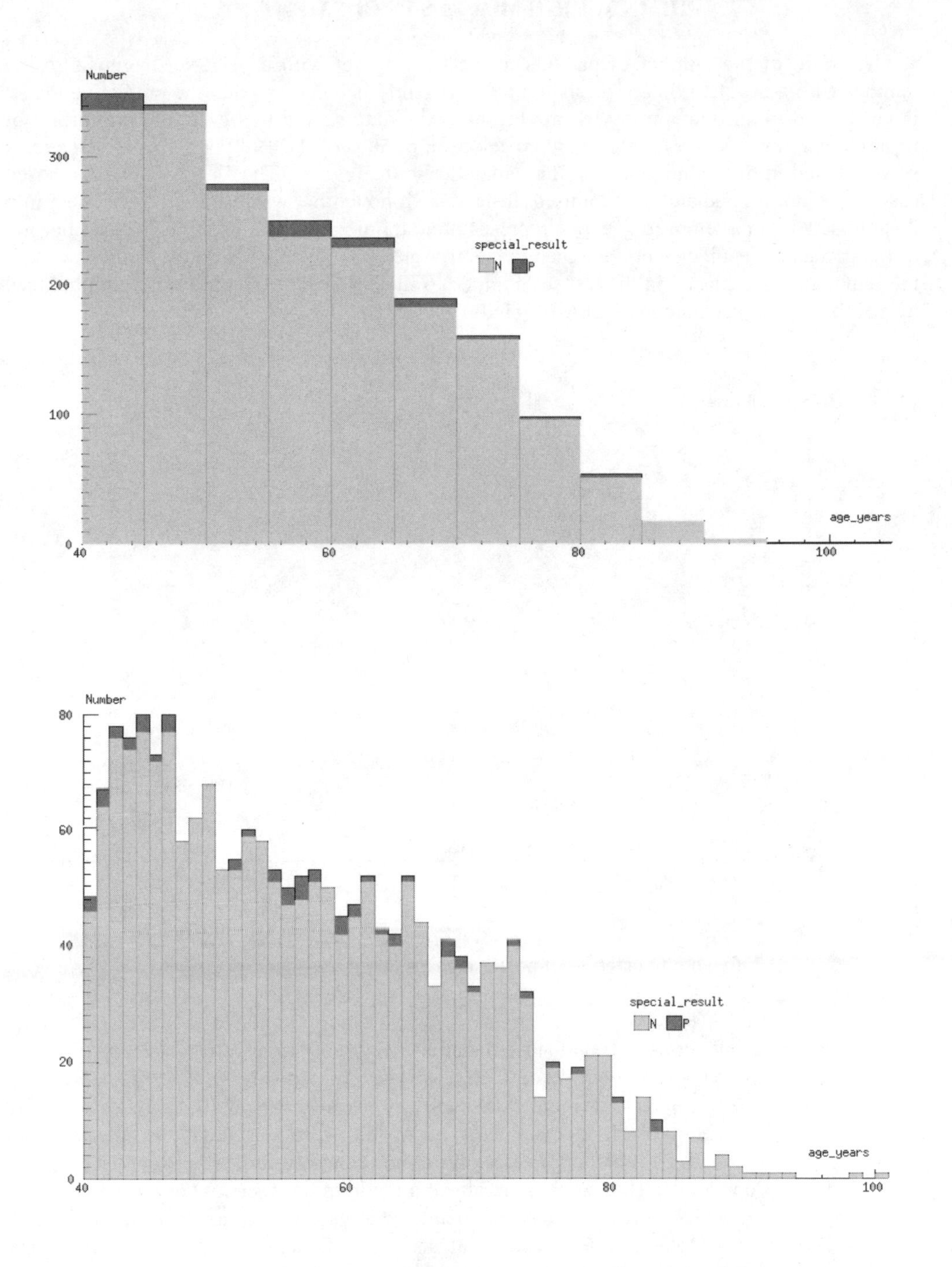

Figure 6.5 Histograms of age distribution overlaid by specialist classification (positive or negative).

VIII. INDUCING MODELS IN CLEMENTINE

The ratio of the number of patients in the training set with a positive diagnosis to the number with a negative diagnosis should be sufficiently balanced so that the predictive model is not biased to an outcome by its proportion in the data set. In this case, the proportion of negative diagnoses was 97.3%. A random selection of 50% of the 1900 or so negative patients was included in the training set and the remainder in the test set. The 54 positively diagnosed cases were not immediately randomised. Instead, a Kohonen net was used to cluster them into disjoint sets in an attempt to generate representative training and test examples. A proportion of the patients in each cluster were then randomly selected for inclusion in the training set and the remainder was placed in the test set. Figure 6.6 illustrates an example clustering produced by a Kohonen net generated in CLEMENTINE.

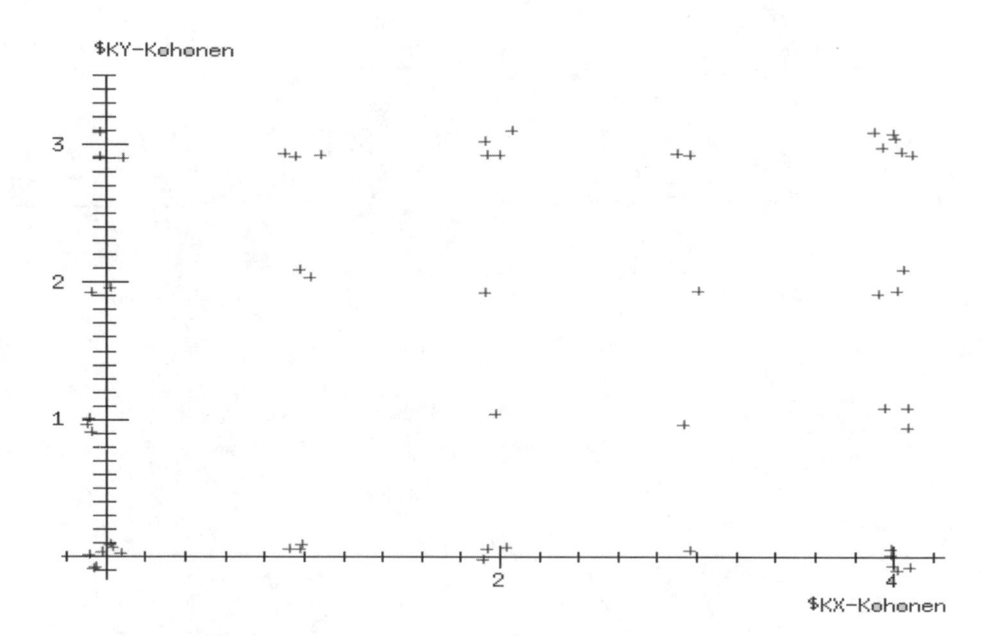

Figure 6.6 Clustering of positive cases using a Kohonen network.

The final training set used contained 991 patient records (948 negative; 43 positive) and the test set contained 132 patient records (121 negative; 11 positive). The most effective balance of positive to negative training examples was found to be 60:40. Experiments were conducted with a number of data sets, all of which were derived from the original questionnaire data obtained in the pilot screening programmes described in previous sections: a larger data set containing 18 unaltered variables; a medium data set containing 10 variables of which 8 were new derived variables (equivalent to that used in the first study); and a small data set of 8 variables selected after further analysis of risk factors described in the literature. On average, the medium data model (see Table 6.2) performed best in both studies.

The results of the second study are given in Table 5. Although still encouraging, they are not as good as the performance of the first neural network. However, direct comparison is not possible since the actual training and test datasets used in the first study were no longer available. In addition, the significant benefits of using a commercial, user-friendly, and robust data mining package are obviously offset against restricted access to its internal workings, thus reducing the kind of fine-tuning during training that was possible in the first study.

Table 6.5 Summary of results for second study.

Second Study	Sensitivity	Specificity	Likelihood Ratio	Pred. +ve	Pred. -ve
Decision tree (medium)	0.64	0.72	2.26	0.17	0.96
Neural network (small)	0.64	0.68	1.97	0.15	0.95
C4.5 rule set (medium)	0.73	0.56	1.66	0.13	0.96

Neural networks lack symbolic output in a form meaningful to domain experts. By comparison, a useful feature of decision tree and rule-based induction algorithms is their meaningful output. Tables 6.6 and 6.7 illustrate a decision tree and a set of rules generated by the CLEMENTINE software.

The decision tree (Table 6.6) is shown in two halves, with the topmost influencing factor being *smoked_in_last_10_yrs*, with a *normalised age of 0.267* (about 56 years of age) and *smoking_over_20_yrs* being other influential parameter values. Although a decision tree format is potentially more meaningful than the numerical output of a neural network, when it is as large as the tree shown, it is not straightforward to interpret. Tree pruning facilities are provided in most inductive environments and can help to reduce complexity, potentially at the cost of accuracy on the test data set. To be fair, the data fields available for this induction exercise are not linked closely enough with possible causative effects to give any deep insight. For example, if data were available on pathological effects on cells, then a more meaningful interpretation might be feasible. The first in the pair of numbers in brackets preceding a classification to Positive or Negative represents the number of test set cases satisfying the accumulated list of conditions from root to the current point. The single number in brackets at the end of other lines records the same value. The second number in the pair labelling the assigned classification reflects the confidence in that rule and is the proportion of the cases satisfying the conditions that receive a correct classification. For example, the first 5 lines of the tree could be transformed into the rule:

```
IF      smoked_in_last_10_yrs T (455)
AND     norm_age  < 0.267 (214)
AND     smoking_over_20_yrs T (101)
AND     norm_age  < 0.05 (43)
AND     drinks_fort_or_spirit T (27)
THEN    POSITIVE (0.963)
```

Table 6.6 A decision tree produced in CLEMENTINE using the ID3 induction algorithm.

```
smoked_in_last_10_yrs T (455)
  norm_age < 0.267 (214)
    smoking_over_20_yrs T (101)
      norm_age < 0.05 (43)
        drinks_fort_or_spirit T (27, 0.963) -> P
        drinks_fort_or_spirit F (16)
          norm_age < 0.009 (13, 1.0) -> P
          norm_age >= 0.009 (3, 1.0) -> N
      norm_age >= 0.05 (58, 1.0) -> N
    smoking_over_20_yrs F (113)
      dentist_in_last_12_mth T (91)
        male T (50)
          drinks_fort_or_spirit T (3, 1.0) -> N
          drinks_fort_or_spirit F (47, 0.872) -> P
        male F (41)
          drinks_fort_or_spirit T (15, 0.933) -> P
          drinks_fort_or_spirit F (26)
            norm_age < 0.088 (19)
              norm_age < 0.06 (4, 1.0) -> N
              norm_age >= 0.06 (15, 0.933) -> P
            norm_age >= 0.088 (7, 1.0) -> N
      dentist_in_last_12_mth F (22, 0.364) -> N
  norm_age >= 0.267 (241)
    norm_age < 0.395 (135)
      smoking_over_20_yrs T (27)
        drinks_beer_or_wine T (9, 1.0) -> N
        drinks_beer_or_wine F (18, 0.778) -> P
      smoking_over_20_yrs F (108, 0.907) -> P
    norm_age >= 0.395 (106)
      smoking_over_20_yrs T (35, 0.8) -> P
      smoking_over_20_yrs F (71)
        drinks_beer_or_wine T (43)
          dentist_in_last_12_mth T (20, 0.3) -> N
          dentist_in_last_12_mth F (23, 0.609) -> P
        drinks_beer_or_wine F (28, 0.5) -> N
smoked_in_last_10_yrs F (556)
  smoking_over_20_yrs T (63, 0.571) -> N
  smoking_over_20_yrs F (493)
    drinks_over_limit T (15, 0.933) -> P
    drinks_over_limit F (478)
      dentist_in_last_12_mth T (371)
        drinks_beer_or_wine T (211)
          drinks_fort_or_spirit T (76)
            norm_age < 0.242 (31)
              norm_age < 0.146 (10, 1.0) -> N
              norm_age >= 0.146 (21, 0.667) -> P
            norm_age >= 0.242 (45)
              norm_age < 0.333 (35, 0.8) -> P
              norm_age >= 0.333 (10, 1.0) -> N
          drinks_fort_or_spirit F (135)
            norm_age < 0.133 (54)
              male T (24)
                norm_age < 0.105 (21)
                  norm_age < 0.092 (6, 1.0) -> N
                  norm_age >= 0.092 (15, 0.867) -> P
                norm_age >= 0.105 (3, 1.0) -> N
              male F (30, 0.467) -> P
            norm_age >= 0.133 (81, 0.667) -> N
        drinks_beer_or_wine F (160)
          male T (28, 0.464) -> P
          male F (132)
            norm_age < 0.256 (52)
              norm_age < 0.026 (29, 0.931) -> P
              norm_age >= 0.026 (23, 1.0) -> N
            norm_age >= 0.256 (80)
              norm_age < 0.511 (43)
                norm_age < 0.434 (25, 0.48) -> N
                norm_age >= 0.434 (18, 0.778) -> P
              norm_age >= 0.511 (37)
                norm_age < 0.55 (16)
                  norm_age < 0.536 (2, 1.0) -> N
                  norm_age >= 0.536 (14, 1.0) -> P
                norm_age >= 0.55 (21, 0.333) -> N
      dentist_in_last_12_mth F (107)
        male T (72)
          norm_age < 0.365 (12, 1.0) -> N
          norm_age >= 0.365 (60, 0.7) -> P
        male F (35, 0.6) -> N
```

Table 6.7 Rules produced in CLEMENTINE using the C4.5 induction algorithm.

```
Rule #1 for N:
    if norm_age > 0.105
    and norm_age <= 0.227
    and smoked_in_last_10_yrs == F
    and drinks_fort_or_spirit == F
    then -> N (30, 0.939)

Rule #2 for N:
    if male == F
    and smoking_over_20_yrs == T
    and drinks_over_limit == F
    then -> N (28, 0.937)

Rule #3 for N:
    if norm_age > 0.235
    and norm_age <= 0.379
    and smoked_in_last_10_yrs == F
    and drinks_fort_or_spirit == F
    then -> N (27, 0.932)

Rule #4 for N:
    if smoking_over_20_yrs == T
    and drinks_fort_or_spirit == F
    and dentist_in_last_12_mth == T
    and norm_age <= 0.477
    then -> N (13, 0.93)

Rule #5 for N:
    if male == T
    and norm_age > 0.191
    and norm_age <= 0.323
    and smoked_in_last_10_yrs == F
    then -> N (9, 0.9)

Rule #6 for N:
    if norm_age <= 0.052
    and norm_age > 0.0
    and smoked_in_last_10_yrs == F
    then -> N (15, 0.888)

Rule #7 for N:
    if norm_age <= 0.191
    and norm_age > 0.0
    and smoked_in_last_10_yrs == F
    and drinks_fort_or_spirit == T
    then -> N (11, 0.881)

Rule #8 for N:
    if norm_age > 0.548
    and norm_age <= 0.704
    and smoked_in_last_10_yrs == F
    and drinks_fort_or_spirit == F
    then -> N (14, 0.881)

Rule #9 for N:
    if smoked_in_last_10_yrs == F
    and smoking_over_20_yrs == T
    and drinks_fort_or_spirit == F
    then -> N (3, 0.873)

Rule #10 for N:
    if norm_age > 0.339
    and norm_age <= 0.439
    and smoked_in_last_10_yrs == F
    and drinks_fort_or_spirit == T
    then -> N (8, 0.81)
```

```
Rule #1 for P:
    if norm_age <= 0.0
    then -> P (36, 0.949)

Rule #2 for P
    if norm_age > 0.323
    and norm_age <= 0.339
    and drinks_fort_or_spirit == T
    then -> P (34, 0.946)

Rule #3 for P
    if norm_age > 0.439
    and smoked_in_last_10_yrs == F
    and drinks_fort_or_spirit == T
    then -> P (71, 0.933)

Rule #4 for P
    if male == F
    and norm_age > 0.191
    and norm_age <= 0.339
    and smoked_in_last_10_yrs == F
    and drinks_fort_or_spirit == T
    then -> P (37, 0.913)

Rule #5 for P
    if norm_age > 0.227
    and norm_age <= 0.235
    and smoked_in_last_10_yrs == F
    then -> P (18, 0.9)

Rule #6 for P
    if drinks_over_limit == T
    then -> P (36, 0.875)

Rule #7 for P
    If norm_age > 0.052
    and norm_age <= 0.105
    and smoked_in_last_10_yrs == F
    and drinks_fort_or_spirit == F
    then -> P (78, 0.874)

Rule #8 for P
    if male == T
    and smoked_In_last_10_yrs == T
    then -> P (324, 0.856)

Rule #9 for P
    if smoked_in_last_10_yrs == T
    and smoking_over_20_yrs == F
    then -> P (87, 0.852)

Rule #10 for P
    if norm_age > 0.379
    and norm_age <= 0.548
    and smoked_in_last_10_yrs == F
    then -> P (85, 0.774)

Rule #11 for P
    if norm_age > 0.704
    then -> P (23, 0.772)

Default : ->P
```

Only 27 test set cases satisfy the conditions of this rule, 26 of which (i.e., 96.3%) receive the correct classification. The attempt described earlier to interpret the neural network produced in the first data analysis highlighted some peculiarities of the most influential factors. Similar oddities can be found in the decision tree. For example, some arms of the decision tree deal with very small numbers of cases.

The rules produced by CLEMENTINE's C5.0 algorithm (Table 6.7) are relatively compact in comparison to the decision tree and they allow a more focused inspection of the derived classification. Age and recency of smoking (in the last 10 years) appear to be influential in the recognition of positive cases. Gender does not appear to play a significant role in the rule set.

IX. EVALUATING THE POTENTIAL PERFORMANCE OF MACHINE LEARNING FOR DETECTION OF HIGH-RISK INDIVIDUALS

As discussed earlier, a number of expert groups have been unable to recommend the introduction of population screening for oral cancer, largely because of the lack of evidence of its effectiveness or cost benefits. It is acknowledged that the highest form of evidence for the effectiveness of a screening programme would be a randomised controlled trial. However, oral cancer is of low prevalence and the costs and logistical problems associated with such a trial are almost insurmountable. An alternative is to conduct a simulation model of a screening programme. Using decision analysis we constructed a simulation model of an opportunistic oral cancer and precancer screening programme in a hypothetical population of 100,000 individuals over the age of 40 years [23]. The assumptions of the model and the data used to inform it were derived from best evidence, or from our previous pilot screening programmes and are shown in Table 6.8. A simple representation of the model is given in Figure 6.7. The outcome of the screening simulation was expressed as quality adjusted life years (QALYs) or as equivalent lives saved.

Table 6.8 Assumptions of the hypothetical screening model and sources of data.

Population	100,000 adults over age 40 years		
Duration	One cycle of 1 year		
Prevalence of lesions	Oral precancer	2.57%	Jullien et al. [12]
	Oral cancer	0.098%	
Validity of the screening test	Positive predictive value	0.67	Jullien et al. [12]
	Negative predictive value	0.99	
Stage of lesions	*Without screening:*		Speight and Morgan [3]
	Stage 1	60%	
	Stage 2+	40%	
	With screening:		
	Stage 1	40%	
	Stage 2+	60%	
Average survival	Health	20 yrs	
	Precancer	19.2 yrs	
	Stage 1 cancer	14.6 yrs	
	Stage 2 cancer	10.8 yrs	
Health state utilities	Health	1.00	Downer et al. [24]
	Precancer	0.92	
	Stage 1 cancer	0.88	
	Stage 2 cancer	0.68	

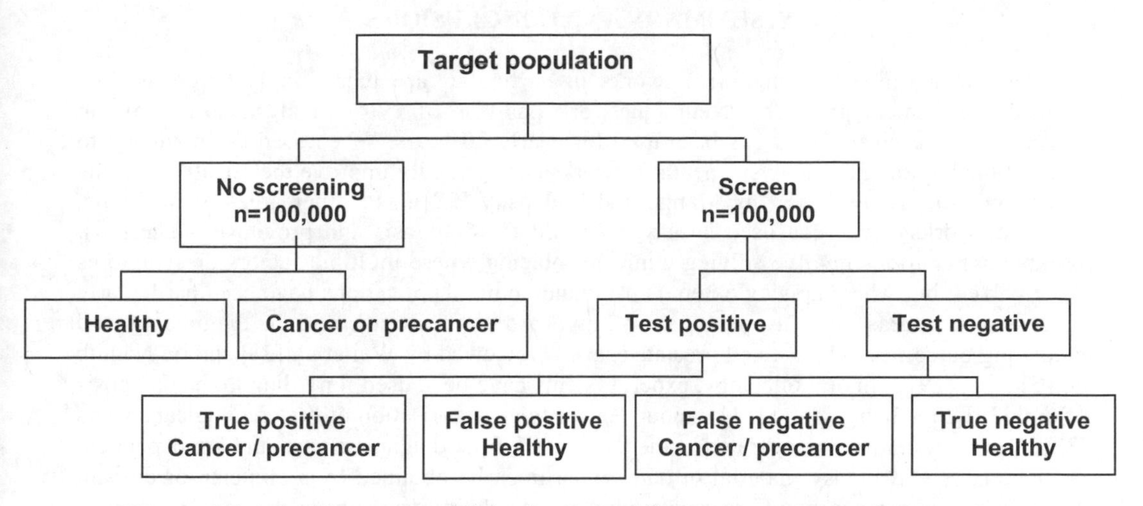

Figure 6.7 A decision tree model for simulation of an oral cancer screening programme.

When the simulation was applied, a single 1-year screening cycle resulted in a total health gain, for the population of 100,000, of 112 QALYs — equivalent to 5.2 lives saved. Since only about 50% of the population is registered with a dentist, this gives a potential gain of only 56 QALYs or 2.8 lives.

In a second experiment, the simulation was repeated on the same hypothetical population but with the intervention of the previously described neural network [16]. In this case the decision model was adapted to a "high-risk" strategy using the data obtained from the neural network study. In this model, 25% of the population was preselected for screening [25]. The prevalence of lesions in this subset was 8.89%, yielding 2222 subjects with lesions. Since the total population contained 2664 lesions (2.7% of 100,000; Table 6.4), this means that 442 lesions were missed in the nonselected group. When the simulation was applied there was a total gain of 312 QALYs — equivalent to 15.6 lives saved. If we again assume a 50% compliance, this represents a potential gain of 8 lives saved.

A model of this sort is only a very simplistic representation of reality; nevertheless, it can provide a general insight into a health care intervention and gives a crude indication of whether a strategy is likely to be of any benefit. In this case, the application of the model to the total population of 100,000 resulted in only a modest gain of 3 lives, whereas the use of the machine learning model to preselect only those individuals likely to be at high risk yielded a gain of about 8 lives. Moreover, to achieve this gain only one quarter of the population would need to be actually examined. This is the first study to demonstrate the potential efficacy of machine learning in oral cancer screening and suggests that it is a promising strategy for a cost-effective screening programme. Although a detailed cost-benefit analysis has not been carried out, it is possible to make some crude estimates based on the cost of a dental examination. In the UK NHS at the present time the extra cost of an "extensive" clinical examination is about £3. In the scenario suggested by the model, assuming 50% attendance, the additional cost of opportunistically screening 50,000 people would be £150,000, compared to only £37,500 to screen the 12,500 individuals identified as high-risk. This is equivalent to about £5,000 per life saved. This compares well to the estimated costs of £80,000 and £300,000 per life saved for breast and cervical cancer, respectively [26].

X. SUMMARY AND CONCLUSIONS

Machine learning, and neural networks in particular, are increasingly being used in mainstream clinical practice. Neural network analysis of cytological smears to aid in screening for cervical cancer has been used for nearly 20 years. When used as an adjunct to conventional cytological analysis, neural networks can markedly improve the sensitivity of the screening process (reviewed by Mango and Radensky [27]). In other areas of medicine, neural networks have been used largely as an aid for diagnosis and prognosis. The most suitable applications involve solving clinical problems where multiple factors or symptoms are involved, but where no single item is pathognomonic. Applications have been particularly successful in areas such as diagnosis of myocardial infarction and in diagnosing and predicting outcomes in breast and prostate cancer (reviewed by Wei et al. [28] and by Naguib and Sherbet [29]). In oral oncology, expert systems have been used for aiding in the diagnosis of oral [30], or salivary gland [31] tumours, or for the categorisation of oral cytological smears [32]. These systems have operated at the distal end of the diagnostic tree, and are dependent on the analysis of biopsy material or data which must be obtained by a clinician or domain expert. Their purpose is to aid in the determination of a definitive diagnosis.

No systems have yet been described which utilise machine learning for the prediction of risk of cancer as an adjunct to population screening. The models described in this chapter are novel in that they are intended to operate at the very start of the diagnostic process and may even be operated by the potential patient, with no intervention from a medical expert. The purpose is to provide a "pre-screen filter" that can be applied to a general, apparently healthy, population to identify those at risk of disease. Selected individuals may then proceed into the expert diagnostic process, commencing with a screening examination. It is envisaged that such a system may be used in the public domain or opportunistically in a health care environment.

Many potentially useful expert and knowledge-based systems have failed to be taken up in clinical practice simply because they were not integrated with available clinical information systems, or they were too difficult to use. Clinicians rightly reject decision-support systems that require re-entry of data that are already recorded. Therefore, no matter how well machine learning models perform, they will only be successfully adopted if they are well integrated or at least demonstrably useful in a clinical environment. In our case, this can be achieved by linking the induced models with dental practice management systems so that risk screening can be carried out on initial data capture, the assumption being that patients will cooperate and supply relevant information on their smoking and drinking habits.

REFERENCES

1. ONS Cancer Statistics, Registrations 1992, Office for National Statistics, Series MB1, No. 25, Her Majesty's Stationery Office, London, 1998.
2. **Jones A.S.,** Prognosis in mouth cancer: tumour factors, *Oral Oncol., Eur. J. Cancer,* 30B, 1, 8, 1994.
3. **Speight P.M., Morgan P.R.,** The natural history and pathology of oral cancer and precancer, *Comm. Dent. Health,* 10, suppl. 1, 31-41, 1993.
4. **Platz H., Fries R., Hudec M.,** Prognosis of oral cavity carcinomas — results of a multi-centre retrospective operational study (the DOSAK study), Munich: Hanser, 1996.
5. **Hindle I., Downer M.C., Speight P.M.,** The epidemiology of oral cancer, *Br. J. Oral Maxillofac. Surg.,* 34, 471-476, 1996.
6. **Macfarlane G.J., Boyle P., Evstifeeva T.V., Robertson, C., Scully C.,** Rising trends of oral cancer mortality among males worldwide: the return of an old public health problem, *Cancer Causes and Control,* 5, 259-265, 1994.

7. OPCS Cancer statistics, Registrations 1985, Office of Population Censuses and Surveys, Series MB1, No. 18, Her Majesty's Stationery Office, London, 1990.
8. **Chamberlain J.,** Evaluation of screening for cancer, *Comm. Dent. Health*, 10, Suppl. 1, 5-11, 1993.
9. **Speight P.M., Downer M.C., Zakrzewska J.,** Screening for oral cancer and precancer: report of the UK working group on screening for oral cancer and precancer, *Comm. Dent. Health,* 10, Suppl. 1, 1993.
10. **Boyle P., Macfarlane G.J., Blot W.J., Chiesa F., Lefebvre J.L., Mano Azul A., de Vries N., Scully C.,** European school of oncology advisory report to the european commission for the Europe against cancer programme: oral carcinogenesis in Europe, *Oral Oncol. Eur. J. Cancer,* 31B, 2, 75-85, 1995.
11. **Warnakulasuriya K.A.A.S., Johnson N.W.,** Strengths and weaknesses of screening programmes for oral malignancies and potentially malignant lesions, *Eur. J. Cancer Prev.*, 5, 93-98, 1996.
12. **Jullien J.A., Downer M.C., Zakrzewska J.M., Speight P.M.,** Evaluation of a screening test for the early detection of oral cancer and precancer, *Comm. Dent. Health,* 12, 3-7, 1995.
13. **Downer M.C., Evans A.W., Hughes-Hallet C.M., Jullien J.A., Speight P.M., Zakrzewska J.M.,** Evaluation of screening for oral cancer and precancer in a company headquarters, *Comm. Dent. Oral Epidemiol.*, 23, 84-88, 1995.
14. **Jullien J., Zakrzewska J.M., Downer M.C., Speight P.M.,** Attendance and compliance at an oral cancer screening programme in a general medical practice, *Oral Oncol., Eur. J. Cancer,* 31B, 202-206, 1995.
15. **Speight P.M., Zakrzewska J., Downer M.C.,** Screening for oral cancer and Precancer, *Oral Oncol., Eur. J. Cancer,* 28B, 45-48, 1992.
16. **Speight P.M., Elliot A.E., Jullien J.A., Downer M.C., Zakrzewska J.M.,** The use of artificial intelligence to identify people at risk of oral cancer and precancer, *Br. Dent. J.*, 179, 382-387, 1995.
17. **Elliot A.E.,** The use of neural networks in medical systems analysis, MSc Dissertation, Southbank University, UK, 1993.
18. **Altman D.G., Bland J.M.,** Diagnostic tests 3: receiver operating characteristic plots, *Br. Med. J.*, 1994, 309, 188, 1993.
19. **Saito, Nakano,** Medical diagnostic expert systems shell based on PDP model, *Proceedings of the IEEE International Conference on Neural Networks,* 1988.
20. **Quinlan J.R.,** Induction of decision trees, *Machine Learning,* 1, 81-106, 1986.
21. **Quinlan J.R.,** *C4.5: Programs for Machine Learning*, Morgan Kaufman, San Mateo, Ca., 1993.
22. **Elliot C.G.,** The use of inductive logic programming and data mining techniques to identify people at risk of oral cancer and precancer, MSc Dissertation, Brunel University, UK, 1996.
23. **Downer M.C., Jullien J.A., Speight P.M.,** An interim determination of health gain from oral cancer and precancer screening: 2. Developing a model of population screening, *Comm. Dent. Health,* 14, 227-232, 1997.
24. **Downer M.C., Jullien J.A., Speight P.M.,** An interim determination of health gain from oral cancer and precancer screening: 1. Obtaining health state utilities, *Comm. Dent. Health*, 14, 139-142, 1997.
25. **Downer M.C., Jullien J.A., Speight P.M.,** An interim determination of health gain from oral cancer and precancer screening: 3. The effect of preselection of high-risk group, *Comm. Dent. Health,* 15, 72-76, 1998.
26. **Roberts C.J., Farrow S.C., Charney M.C.,** How much can the NHS afford to spend to save a life or avoid a severe disability? *The Lancet,* I, 89-91, 1985.
27. **Mango L.J., Radensky P.W.,** Interactive neural network-assisted screening: a clinical assessment, *Acta Cytol.*, 42, 233-245, 1998.

28. **Wei J.T., Zhang Z., Barnhill S.D., Madyastha K.R., Zhang H., Oesterling J.E.,** Understanding artificial neural networks and exploring their potential applications for the practising urologist, *Urology,* 52, 161-172, 1998.
29. **Naguib R.N.G., Sherbet G.V.,** Artificial neural networks in cancer research, *Pathobiology,* 65, 129-139, 1997.
30. **Zhizhina N.A., Prokhonchukov A.A., Yermolov V.F., Pelkovsky V.Yu.,** Automated computer system for differential diagnosis and laser treatment of benign tumours and tumour-like masses in the oral cavity, *Stomatologica (Moscow — in Russian),* 3, 61-65, 1998.
31. **Firriolo F.J., Levy B.A.,** Computer expert systems for the histopathological diagnosis of salivary gland neoplasms, *Oral Surg. Oral Med. Oral Pathol. Oral Radiol. Endoc.,* 82, 179-186, 1996.
32. **Brickley M.R., Cowpe J.G., Shepherd J.P.,** Performance of a computer simulated neural network trained to categorise normal, premalignant and malignant oral smears, *J. Oral Pathol. Med.,* 25, 424-428, 1996.

Chapter 7

OUTCOME PREDICTION OF OESOPHAGO-GASTRIC CANCER USING NEURAL ANALYSIS OF PRE- AND POSTOPERATIVE PARAMETERS

J. Wayman and S.M. Griffin

I. INTRODUCTION

Cancers of the oesophagus, stomach, and oesophago-gastric junction have important implications for health resources now and in the future. The only hope for cure in these patients is radical surgical resection with or without adjuvant chemotherapy or radiotherapy. These treatments carry significant risk of morbidity and mortality. Added to this is a protracted period of rehabilitation following surgery in which the patients' quality of life can remain poor. All too frequently, patients deemed curable by surgery by conventional analysis undergo this radical therapy only to develop and succumb to recurrence of disease, sometimes within months of treatment. If such early recurrence could be predicted, patients may be spared exhaustive and possibly hopeless therapy in favour of a nonsurgical treatment. Indeed they may be offered additional therapy prior to surgery with the intention of preventing such recurrence. Several studies have sought to use artificial neural networks to predict outcome in other malignancies and more recently this has been utilised in oesophago-gastric cancer.

Data from patients undergoing potentially curative resection of adenocarcinoma of the oesophago-gastric junction has been collected prospectively and analysed by an artificial neural network system. Preoperative data have been used as input variables to the network. A separate neural structure has been designed for use with selected additional postoperative parameters. Output variables for both systems were recurrence at 12, 18, and 24 months. Correct prediction of recurrence at 12, 18, and 24 months using preoperative data alone had specificity of 60%, 62%, and 60% and sensitivity of 100%, 80%, and 80%, respectively. Inclusion of postoperative parameters improved the sensitivity of prediction at 18 months to 90% and at two years to 93%, while specificity improved to 72.7% at 12 months, 66% at 18 months, and 62.2% at 24 months.

Artificial neural networks are able to reliably predict, even with limited clinical pre-operative information, patients destined to fail when treated by surgery alone. This approach may have a role in assisting clinicians to achieve more appropriate selection of patients for surgery and neo-adjuvant therapy. Further research in this important area may allow even better selection of patients. Nevertheless, significant improvements in prognosis will only result if patients with oesophago-gastric cancer can be diagnosed earlier in the course of disease. It is impractical to screen all patients for cancer, but it is likely that among the vast

0-8493-9692-1/01/$0.00+$1.50

number of patients suffering from dyspepsia there are some with an underlying cancer. The next challenge of neural networks should be to attempt to identify such patients at an earlier stage in the cancer sequence and thus improve the overall outcome.

II. ARTIFICIAL NEURAL NETWORKS FOR THE PREDICTION OF OUTCOME OF OESOPHAGO-GASTRIC CANCER

Oesophago-gastric oncological practice in the West has altered with an overall reduction in the incidence of gastric cancer [1] and the emergence of adenocarcinoma of the oesophagus. Several reports have suggested that the rising trend in adenocarcinoma of the lower oesophagus is mirrored by adenocarcinoma of the gastric cardia and oesophago-gastric junction. Much evidence for this has been derived from analysis of cancer registry data from various regions and countries including North America [2], Scandinavia [3], UK [4-6], Australia and New Zealand [7], and from retrospective series [8-11]. More recent evidence from the Northern and Yorkshire Cancer Registry and Information Service (NYCRIS) of the United Kingdom has demonstrated that this trend continues with a similar increase in the incidence of adenocarcinoma of the lower oesophagus adenocarcinoma (Figure 7.1) and gastric cardia (Figure 7.2) relative to other oesophago-gastric sites and histological types [12]. These findings are borne out still further by the findings of a prospective audit in the Northern Oesophago-Gastric Cancer Unit, a specialist centre for the treatment of patients with oesophageal and gastric cancer, which confirms the continuing rise in proportion of cancers diagnosed around the gastro-oesophageal junction (Figure 7.3).

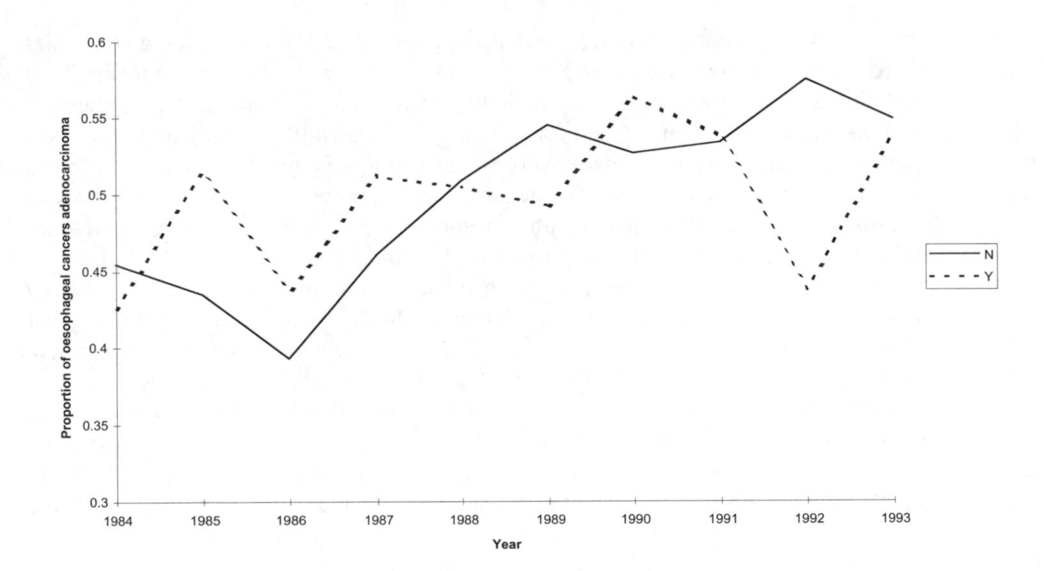

Figure 7.1 Graph showing the proportion of patients with oesophageal cancer diagnosed as adenocarcinomas rather than squamous carcinoma in the Northern (— N) and Yorkshire (- - - - Y) regions (1984-1993). Data from the NYCRIS.

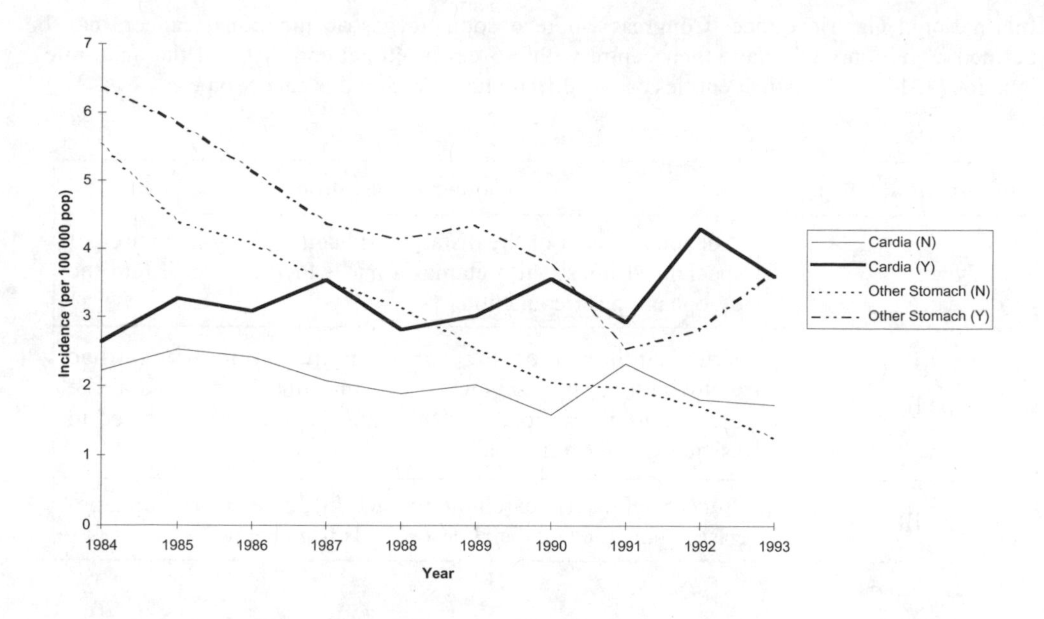

Figure 7.2 Graph showing the age standardised incidence of proximal, cardia cancers (Type 2 junctional cancers) compared with all other recorded gastric cancer subsites in the Northern (N) and Yorkshire (Y) regions (1984–1993). Data from the NYCRIS.

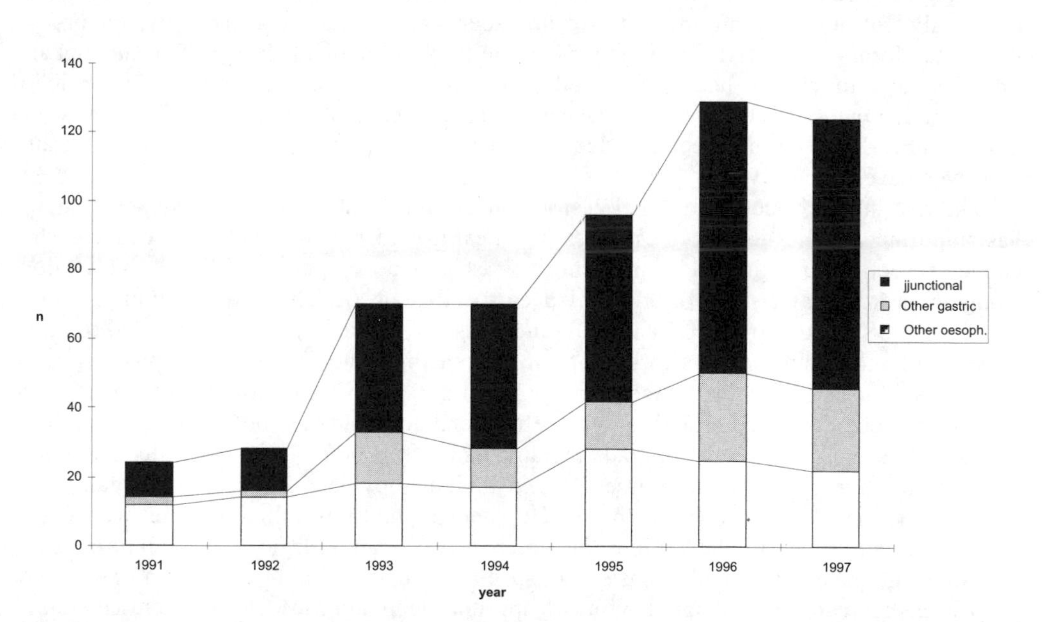

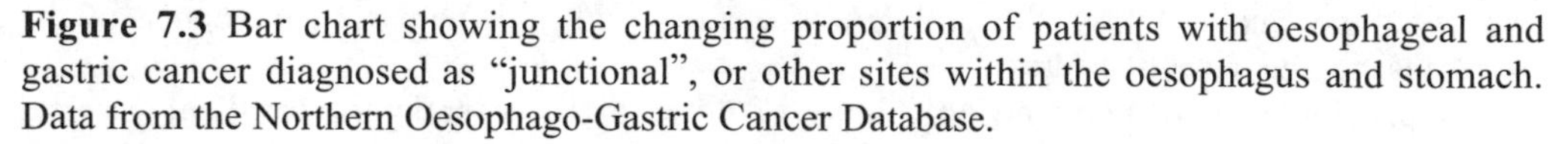

Figure 7.3 Bar chart showing the changing proportion of patients with oesophageal and gastric cancer diagnosed as "junctional", or other sites within the oesophagus and stomach. Data from the Northern Oesophago-Gastric Cancer Database.

Recently, clarification by consensus has been sought for the classification of tumours arising in the area of the oesophago-gastric junction. A system has been suggested by the

International Gastric Cancer Congress where oesophago-gastric junctional cancers can be defined as tumours that have their centre within 5 cm proximal and distal of the anatomical junction [13]. Three distinct entities can be differentiated within this cancer type.

Junctional Type	Cancer Description
Type I	Adenocarcinoma of the distal oesophagus arising in an area of specialised intestinal metaplasia and which may infiltrate the oesophago-gastric junction
Type II	True carcinoma of the cardia arising from the cardiac epithelium or short segments with intestinal metaplasia at the oesophago-gastric junction; this entity is also often referred to as "junctional carcinoma"
Type III	Subcardial gastric carcinoma which infiltrates the oesophago-gastric junction and distal oesophagus from below

There is no clear explanation for the continued rise in the relative incidence of adenocarcinoma of the gastric cardia and adenocarcinoma of the lower oesophagus. A columnar lined oesophagus (Barrett's oesophagus) is known to increase the risk of developing adenocarcinoma of the lower third of the oesophagus. Barrett's oesophagus is in turn often presumed to be a consequence of gastro-oesophageal reflux. Case-control studies show a twofold relative risk of developing adenocarcinoma of the oesophagus with reflux and oesophagitis [14], and a trend for using drugs known to relax the gastro-oesophageal sphincter has paralleled the increasing incidence of this adenocarcinoma. Socioeconomic factors are implicated for proximal gastric cancers [15]; a role for western diet [16] as well as alcohol and tobacco have inevitably been postulated and a weak association shown. The role of *Helicobacter pylori* has been well rehearsed for distal gastric cancer, but its role in proximal gastric cancer may be more complicated with recent reports suggesting that certain strains may even have a protective role [17].

The rise in incidence of proximal gastric cancer and distal oesophageal adenocarcinoma has important implications for resources and health care management. Proximal gastric cancer resections require additional surgical expertise compared with relatively more straightforward distal gastric procedures; indeed specific subspecialist surgical training now is mandatory [18]. Additional ITU and HDU facilities and training has to be provided to allow closer and more intense monitoring of the increasing proportion of oesophago-gastric resections which will involve thoracotomy or hiatal dissection. For those patients unsuitable for surgical resection, strategies need to be defined and adequate facilities provided to palliate. These include endoscopic stenting, radiotherapy, and laser therapy. The cost effectiveness of all these treatments needs to be assessed and their deployment and regional organisation planned. It may lead, in turn, to the development of multidisciplinary teams working in specialist centres within the regions in which medical and surgical gastroenterologists, anaesthetists, oncologists, pathologists, and specialist nurses with an interest in oesophago-gastric cancer can be assembled with all appropriate modalities of treatment available. Whatever the final solution, the problem of dealing with the increasing incidence of the disease is one that must be addressed.

As previously indicated, the only hope of cure for these patients is radical surgical resection. This, however, carries a significant risk to patients in terms of operative morbidity and mortality [19,20]. While such risks can be justified if cure is a reasonable expectation, for patients destined to fail due to recurrence of disease these inherent risks associated with radical treatment should be avoided. Currently the decision whether or not to operate is made on the interpretation of preoperative assessments of tumour stage and patient fitness. This evidence is an extrapolation of the anticipated postoperative pathological staging. The correlation between pre- and postoperative findings is frequently poor. Thus, a pathologist postpones definitive statements about prognosis until examination of the resected specimen. Although differences can be demonstrated in prognosis as determined by pathological tumour stage and grade, the prognosis as it applies to individual patients still remains unpredictable.

Time to recurrence following resection of Type I and Type II junctional cancers is similar (Figure 7.4) and is dependent on the degree of local tumour invasion, lymph node involvement (Figure 7.5), tumour grade, and the presence of histological evidence of vascular, perineural, and lymphatic invasion (Figure 7.6). Nevertheless, such prognostic factors by themselves do not allow accurate selection of patients for surgical intervention with or without neo-adjuvant therapy. Not only do existing methods of analysis fail to take account of more subtle nonlinear relationships between these and other variables, but also the accuracy of prediction is related to the accuracy of postoperative pathological resected specimen analysis which is inherently too late for key treatment decisions. What is needed is a means of predicting outcome using less linearly based preoperative data.

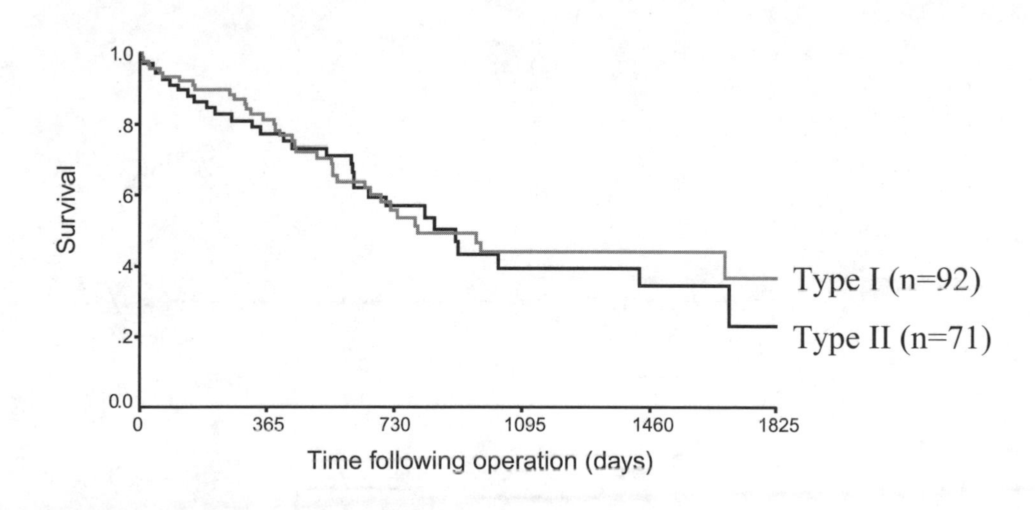

Figure 7.4 Survival following resection of esophago-gastric junctional cancers. Figure demonstrates Kaplan-Meier survival curves for survival of 92 Type I junctional cancer patients and 71 Type II junctional cancer patients following resection. There is no significant difference between the two groups (Log Rank Test).

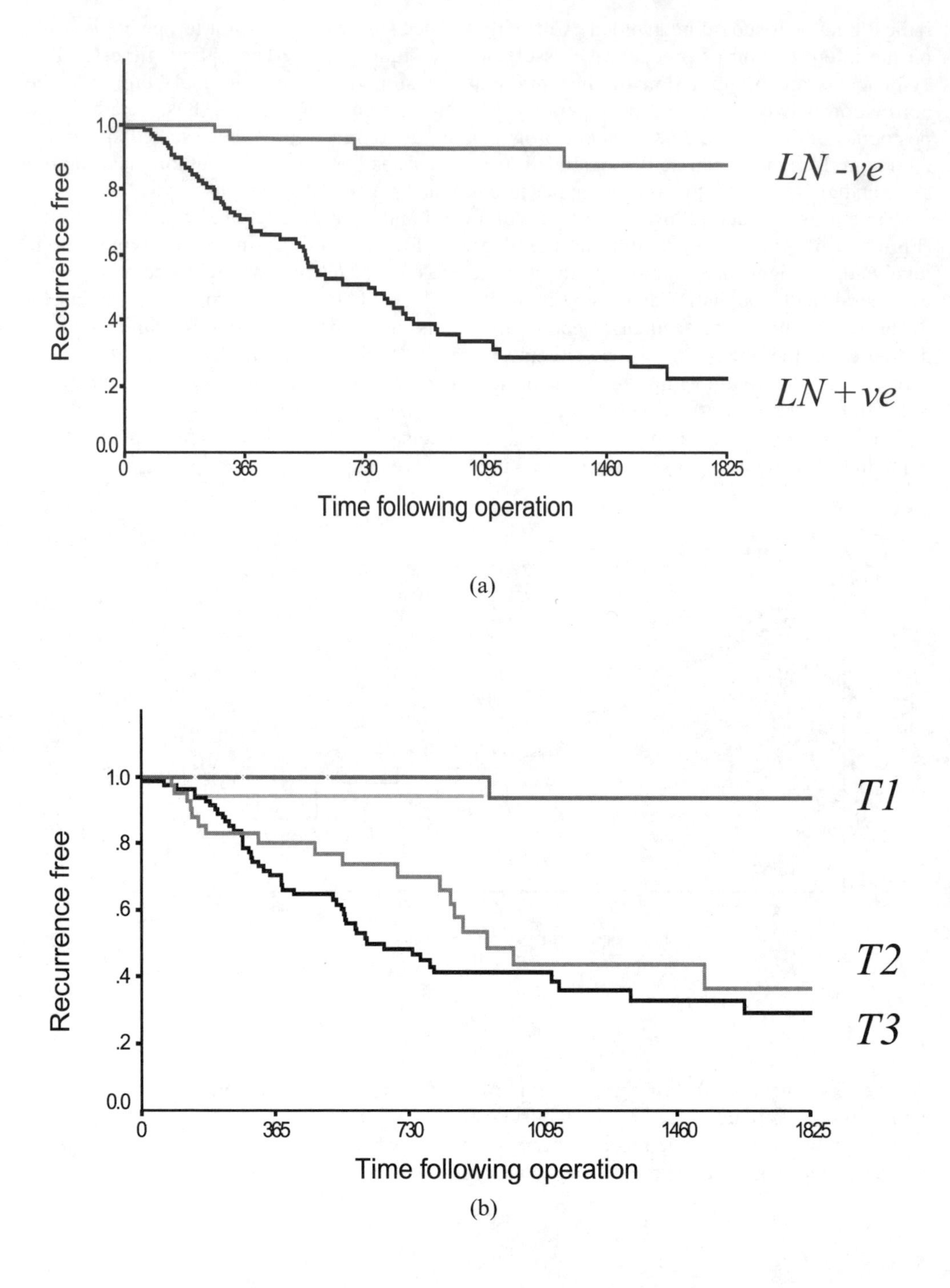

Figure 7.5 Survival following resection of 163 patients with junctional cancers. Figures represent Kaplan-Meier survival curves for patients with lymph node disease compared to those without (a) and for patients with differing depth of local tumour invasion (T-stage), (b) N- and T-stage significantly affect outcome (Log Rank Test).

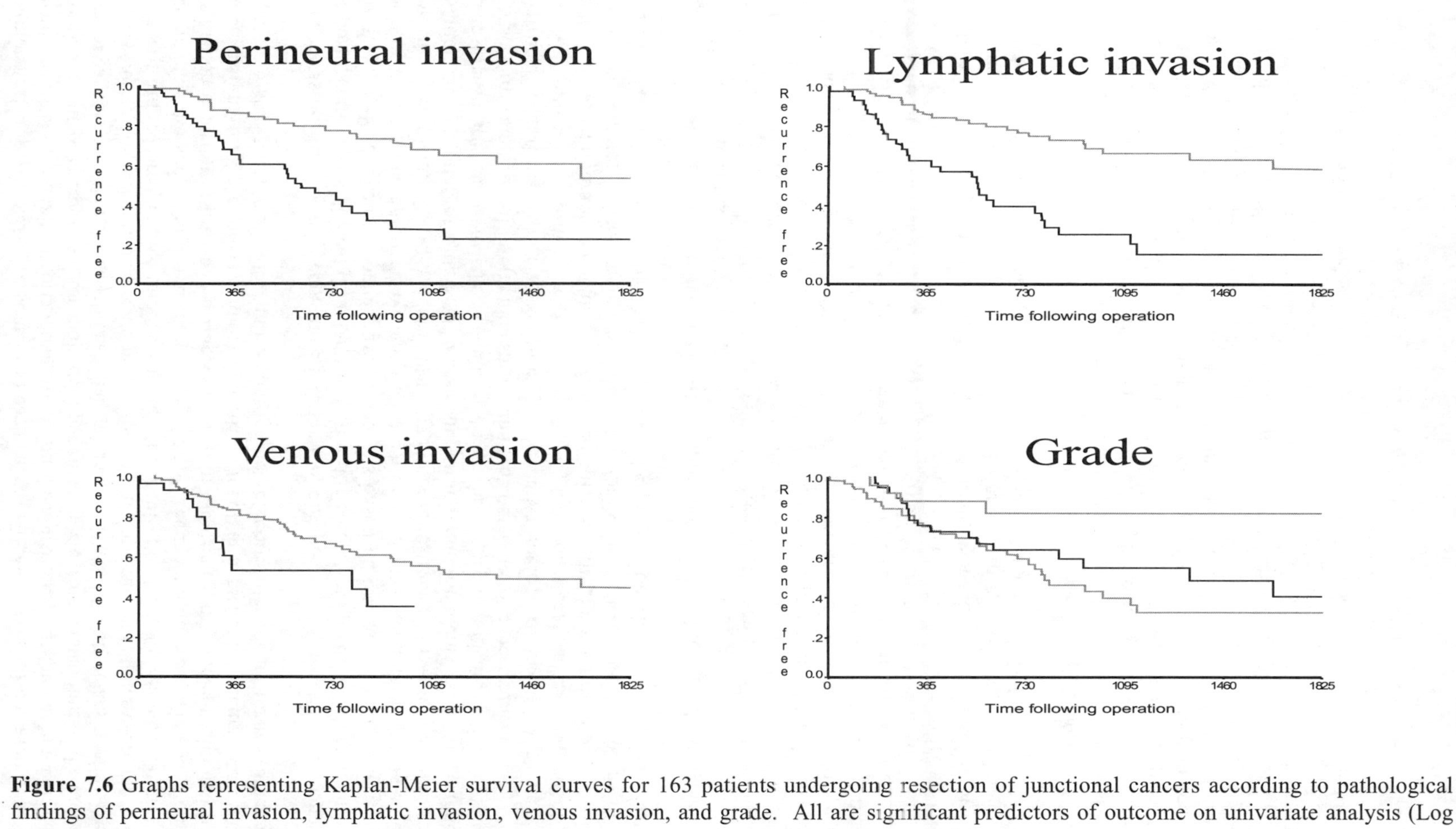

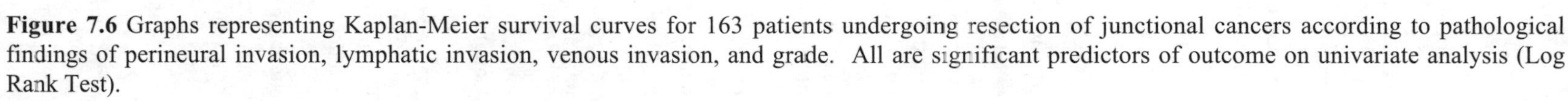

Figure 7.6 Graphs representing Kaplan-Meier survival curves for 163 patients undergoing resection of junctional cancers according to pathological findings of perineural invasion, lymphatic invasion, venous invasion, and grade. All are significant predictors of outcome on univariate analysis (Log Rank Test).

The treatment options available at present (curative intent radical surgery, with or without neo-adjuvant therapy or palliative strategies) each carry different risks and potential benefits for patients. It is of crucial importance in managing these patients that the correct and most appropriate strategy is employed for individual patients. A clear understanding of the natural history of cancers affecting the gastro-oesophageal junction is vital for clinicians treating these patients. Currently, decisions regarding prognosis, and hence treatment strategy, are made on the basis of limited preoperative tumour staging. Inevitably this leads to treatment failures in which patients are subjected to radical surgery and still recur within a year; the operation in this situation contributes little and detracts much from the quality of a patient's limited life. Greater insight into prognosis and likelihood of local and systemic recurrence at the preoperative stage may also allow more appropriate selection of patients for neo-adjuvant therapy.

In contrast to the lack of preoperative information, clinicians are faced with increasingly more postoperative pathological data, but can find it difficult to interpret this information in a useful way. Indeed, even elaborate survival analysis based on univariate, multivariate, and proportional hazard paradigms have not so far culminated in a tangible advancement of prognostic assessment. Such "standard" tests give only an estimate of risk as it applies to a population and are often of little help in assessing an individual patients' risk of recurrence. Such tests also are unable to take account of all of the highly nonlinear relationships that comprise a growing maze of information surrounding the outcome for cancer patients.

Artificial neural networks (ANNs) offer an alternative method of interpreting data that provides a straightforward measure of outcome for an individual case, takes into account all available data, and draws conclusions from complex nonlinear relationships. Unlike conventional statistics, ANNs can interpret more accurately data where relationships are of an unknown function of the variable. This includes the prognostic value of a variable when influenced by another or when it varies with time. In this way, ANNs are a tool that may help clinicians to make sense of the increasingly complex nature of biological systems and malignant disease in particular.

ANNs are parallel information-processing structures that attempt to emulate certain performance characteristics of the biological neural system [21]. ANNs have found an application in several areas of medicine and cancer research in particular [22,23]. Recent work has looked at the role of ANNs in prediction of outcome for patients with colorectal [24], urological [25], and breast cancer [26]. An artificial neural network consists of many processing elements (neurons) which are organised into groups called layers. A typical network consists of a sequence of layers successively connected by full or random connections. There are typically two layers with connection to the outside world: an input layer where data is presented to the network and an output layer which holds the response of the network to a given input. The mathematical model of an artificial neuron and the structure of a generic feed-forward fully interconnected artificial neural network have been described in Chapter 1.

The concept of ANNs has recently been studied in relation to gastric cancer, where a single layer perception had been applied and the prediction of lymph node metastasis assessed [27]. In that study, Bormann classification and depth of invasion were the main factors analysed and, although relatively high sensitivity and specificity values were achieved, the authors rightly stipulated that the integration of a greater number of clinical and pathological factors would be more beneficial in assessing the final outcome. Furthermore, an alternative neural structure, perhaps comprising of at least one hidden layer, would also add to a more effective nonlinear analysis of the interactions between the markers considered.

When compared to traditional statistical approaches, ANNs may provide a more consistent method of predicting outcome for patients with gastric cancer [28]. Using a three-layer neural network design, 60 input variables, a variable number of hidden neurons in the second layer and a single output variable of death or not at 12 months, predictive sensitivity of 62%, specificity of 77%, and overall accuracy of 71% were achievable. In this study, the number of variables analysed was very large relative to the number of cases (133 to train the network and 50 to validate), and the results were not significantly different to those achievable by traditional multivariate analysis.

We have looked at the accuracy with which an ANN can predict outcome following treatment of patients with oesophago-gastric junction cancer. A number of pre- and post-operative factors have been analysed in this regard, and the outcome related to whether tumour recurred within 12, 18, and 24 months of operation.

One hundred and three consecutive patients undergoing radical surgical resection of oesophago-gastric junctional adenocarcinoma were studied. All patients had undergone detailed preoperative assessment prior to selection for surgery. This assessment included appraisal of tumour stage and resectability by chest X-ray, endoscopy, abdominal ultrasound scan and thoraco-abdominal CT scan. Patient fitness for surgery was formally assessed by tests of renal, hepatic, respiratory, cardiac, and psychological function. All patients were deemed fit for radical surgery with a realistic expectation of cure. Pre-operative data was recorded prospectively (Table 7.1). Selected pathological information derived from a detailed standardised assessment of the resected specimen was recorded separately (Table 7.2).

Table 7.1 Preoperative parameters recorded.

Age	
Sex	
Junctional cancer type	*Type I*
	Type II
Endoscopic distance from incisors	
Grade of cancer (from preliminary biopsy specimens)	
Planned operative approach	*Transabdominal*
	Thoracoabdominal
	Ivor-Lewis two stage oesophagectomy
Additional procedures planned	*None*
	Splenectomy
	Splenectomy and pancreatectomy

Table 7.2 Additional postoperative pathological parameters recorded.

Depth of tumour invasion (T-stage)
Nodal status (N-stage)
Total number of lymph node groups involved
Presence of neural invasion
Presence of vascular invasion
Resection margin involvement
Resection margin clearance (cm)

Patients underwent clinical review at 6 weeks after discharge and then three monthly thereafter. Clinical review consisted of history and clinical examination. There was a low threshold for investigation of any potential recurrence. Investigation was dictated by the nature of symptoms and clinical examination but involved endoscopy, plain X-ray, ultrasound, CT scan, radioisotope bone scan, and relook laparotomy as appropriate. Histological confirmation was obtained wherever possible. Autopsy information was available in 10 patients.

Primary outcome was defined as recurrence within 12, 18, and 24 months. The input variables were analysed separately as exclusively preoperative factors (Table 7.1) and then as pre- and postoperative pathological information together (Tables 7.1 and 7.2). A radial basis function artificial neural network structure was simulated in this study and was implemented using the NeuralWorks Professional II Plus neural network package (NEURALWARE, Pittsburgh, PA, USA). Training of the networks involved introducing the input data along with respective outcome information of the presence or absence of recurrent disease by each time point (Table 7.3). Forty-three cases were used to train the network and 60 were used to test it; allocation of cases to training or testing groups was done at random.

We found no significant difference in sex and age distribution for Type 1 and Type 2 junctional adenocarcinomas [male: female 3.4:1 vs. 6.6:1; age 63 (40-77) vs. 70 (42-78)]. Thirty-one patients developed proven recurrent disease. The median time to recurrence was 7(1-28) months and was similar between the types 1 and 2 subgroups.

Of the 103 patients studied, recurrent disease was detectable within the first year in 14 cases, by 18 months in 25 cases, and by 24 months in 31. Using simple univariate analysis there was a highly significant relationship between lymphatic invasion and lymph node involvement and recurrence at each time point assessed. There was no significant relationship between recurrence and any single preoperative parameter recorded (Table 7.4).

Five patients in the test group developed recurrence within one year and were, along with 8 out of 10 recurrences within 18 months and 12 out of 15 recurrences at 2 years, correctly predicted using preoperative data alone (Tables 7.5, 7.6, 7.7). False positive results occurred in 22 cases at one year, 19 at 18 months, and 18 at 2 years using preoperative data alone. Sensitivity and specificity of the ANN was improved by the addition of postoperative parameters into the neural network analysis leading to more accurate prediction of recurrence (Table 7.8). There was a strong correlation between the predictive value of pre- and postoperative findings in individual patients at each time period although this correlation reduced with time (at 12 months, correlation coefficient = 0.6333, $p < 0.0001$; at 18 months correlation coefficient = 0.4873, $p = 0.0083$; at 24 months correlation coefficient = 0.266, $p = 0.0025$) (Figure 7.7).

The results of this albeit small study are encouraging. In our series, all patients had thorough preoperative staging and were selected for surgery with the intention of offering significant improvement in survival. In fact, 14 out of 103 succumbed to recurrent disease (most with distant metastases) within just 12 months of their operation. Had we been able to identify these 14 patients, they might have been spared radical surgery or perhaps selected for neo-adjuvant therapy. Our simple univariate analysis shows that none of the preoperative factors were helpful in predicting first-year failures. The artificial neural structure on the other hand, when tested, selected all patients destined to have recurrence within one year. Potentially, with more cases, the neural network can be retrained to predict not only recurrence but also site of recurrence; such a prediction may allow a yet more refined selection for neo-adjuvant therapy in those patients likely to have early systemic recurrence.

Table 7.3 Table of comparisons between patients with recurrence at 12, 18, and 24 months following operation using chi-square and Mann-Whitney U tests.

	Recurrnece At 1 year	Recurrence-free at 1 year	*p value*	Recurrence at 18/12 months	Recurrence-free at 18/12 months	*p value*	Recurrence at 2 years	Recurrence-free at 2 years	*p value*
N	14	89		25	78		31	72	
Age	66.2 (2.1)	64.0 (1.0)	*0.123*	63.0 (1.89)	64.7 (1.0)	*0.86*	62.2 (1.73)	65.3 (1.05)	*0.9*
Sex									
M	13	74		23	64		29	58	
F	1	15	*0.7*	2	14	*ns*	2	14	*0.8*
Procedure									
IVOR-LEWIS	7	58		16	49		21	44	
TA	1	12	*0.3*	2	11	*0.7*	3	10	*0.8*
TH	6	18		7	17		7	17	
Tumour Level	36.6 (1.2)	34.7 (0.5)	*0.97*	35.7 (0.91)	34.7 (0.5)	*0.83*	35.4 (0.8)	34.8 (0.6)	*ns*
Position									
Oeso.	7	61		16	52		21	47	
Cardia	7	28	*0.18*	9	26	*0.8*	10	25	*0.9*
Grade									
Well	1	17		2	16		4	14	
Mod.	3	30	*0.4*	6	27	*0.5*	8	25	*0.5*
Poor	9	39		15	33		17	31	
Lymphatic Invasion									
Present	10	25		15	20		17	18	
Absent	4	64	***0.002***	10	58	***0.002***	14	54	***0.004***

Table 7.3 *Cont.*

	Recurrnece At 1 year	Recurrence-free at 1 year	*p value*	Recurrence at 18/12 months	Recurrence-free at 18/12 months	*p value*	Recurrence at 2 years	Recurrence-free at 2 years	*p value*
Vascular Invasion									
Present	2	8		4	6		5	5	
Absent	12	79	*0.7*	21	70	*0.3*	26	65	*0.2*
Neural Invasion									
Present	5	57		15	23		18	20	
Absent	9	29	*0.06*	9	53	*0.02*	12	50	*0.01*
Tumour Invasion									
1	1	16		2	15		2	15	
2	5	22	*0.59*	6	21		8	19	*0.7*
3	8	48		17	39	*0.21*	21	35	
LN Groups +ve	2.5 (0.37)	1.2 (0.12)	*0.4*	2.32 (0.26)	1.03 (0.13)	*ns*	2.03 (0.24)	1.04 (0.133)	***0.001***
+ve Donuts	3	6	*0.1*	4	5	*0.2*	4	5	*0.7*
+ve Resection Margin	4	10	*0.09*	5	9	*0.3*	5	9	*0.8*
Additional Procedure									
Splenectomy	1	1		1	1		1	1	
Splenectomy + pancreatectomy	1	0	*ns*	1	0	*ns*	1	0	*0.36*
2 -Team Approach	1	1		1	1		1	1	
Nodal Invasion									
N0	0	37		0	37		3	34	
N1	14	52	***0.003***	25	41	***0.00002***	28	38	***0.0001***

Table 7.4 Numbers of patients with and without recurrence at 12, 18, and 24 months used to train and subsequently test the neural network system.

	Total No.	*Training*	*Testing*
No Recurrence < 1 year	89	34	55
Recurrence < 1 year	14	9	5
No Recurrence < 18 months	25	15	10
Recurrence < 18 months	78	28	50
No Recurrence < 2 years	31	16	15
Recurrence < 2 years	72	27	45

Table 7.5 Number of patients correctly and incorrectly predicted by ANN to develop recurrence by 1 year.

			Actual 1-Year Recurrence	
			Recurrence	**No Recurrence**
ANN Predicted 1-Year Recurrence	*Using Preop Information Only*	**Recurrence**	5	22
		No Recurrence	0	33
	Using Pre- and Postop Information Only	**Recurrence**	5	22
		No Recurrence	0	33

Table 7.6 Number of patients correctly and incorrectly predicted by ANN to develop recurrence by 18 months.

			Actual 18-month Recurrence	
			Recurrence	**No Recurrence**
ANN Predicted 18-Month Recurrence	*Using Preop Information Only*	**Recurrence**	5	22
		No Recurrence	0	33
	Using Pre- and Postop Information Only	**Recurrence**	5	22
		No Recurrence	0	33

Table 7.7 Number of patients correctly and incorrectly predicted by ANN to develop recurrence by 2 years.

			Actual 2-year Recurrence	
			Recurrence	**No Recurrence**
ANN Predicted 2-Year Recurrence	*Using Preop Information Only*	**Recurrence**	5	22
		No Recurrence	0	33
	Using Pre- and Postop Information Only	**Recurrence**	5	22
		No Recurrence	0	33

Table 7.8 Sensitivity, specificity, and accuracy of the ANN at predicting whether or not a case will develop recurrent disease using inputs from pre- and postoperative information.

		Sensitivity (%)	Specificity (%)	Accuracy (%)
At 12 Months	*Preop analysis*	100	60	63.3
	Postop analysis	100	72.7	75
At 18 Months	*Preop analysis*	80	62	65
	Postop analysis	90	66	70
At 24 Months	*Preop analysis*	80	60	65
	Postop analysis	93.3	62.2	70

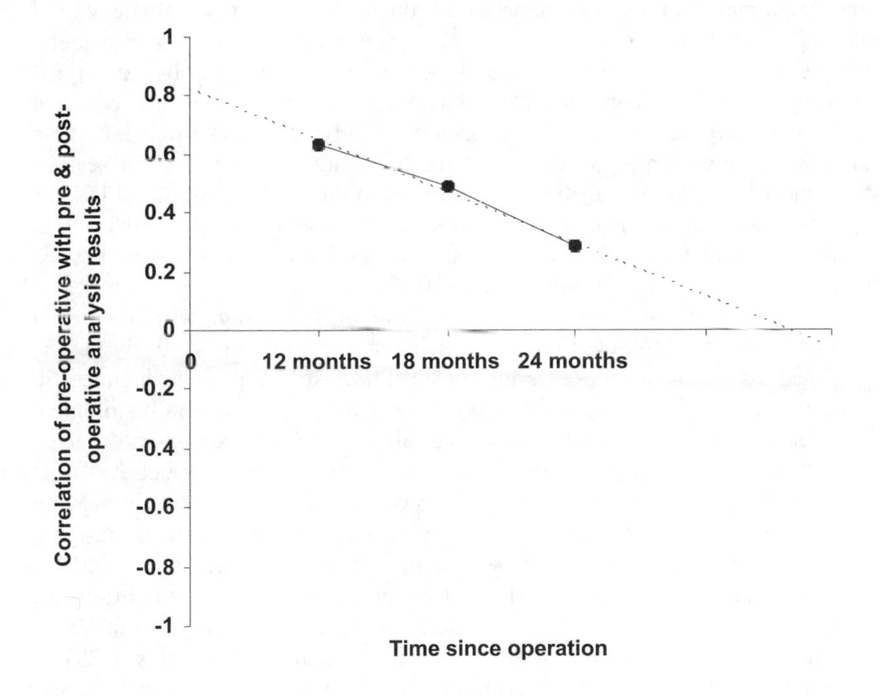

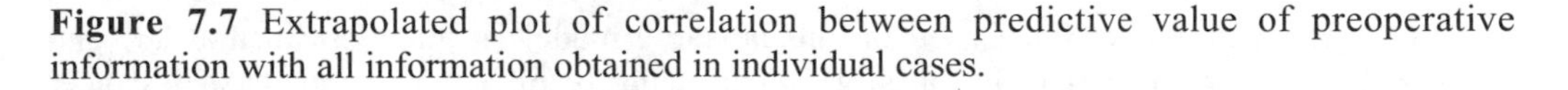

Figure 7.7 Extrapolated plot of correlation between predictive value of preoperative information with all information obtained in individual cases.

From our work, postoperative data seemed more relevant to the prediction of outcome, yet only lymphatic involvement was a significant predictor of outcome in our univariate analysis. Faced with this information, if a clinician considered lymph node positivity as a marker of recurrence, all 14 patients at 1 year, all 25 at 18 months, and 28 of 31 at 2 years would be identified (Table 7.3). Specificity for selecting recurrence on the basis of lymph node positivity equates to only 42% at 12 months and 47% at 18 months and two years. Neural networks, by taking into account complex relationships between available data give a prediction of recurrence which is far more accurate than using postoperative nodal status alone. With respect to the preoperative data included in this study, no prediction using standard statistical methods is possible for comparison.

Our system should not be considered fully developed; it incorrectly predicted failure in a significant minority. Nevertheless, an artificial neural network can continue to be trained on more cases and with additional information, such as various molecular and histopathological parameters that can be obtained from preoperative biopsy specimens. The network, through proper training, determines the usefulness of a particular set of variables and can integrate them either by replacing less important or adding to existing ones. In this way, even if the parameters have unknown or no measurable prognostic significance, their inclusion may still reduce the rate of false positives through their possible nonlinear interactions with more established factors.

Although the use of ANNs as a research tool is growing, their usefulness in clinical practice has yet to be determined. The results do suggest that with further development, neural networks may offer an objective adjunct to surgical decision-making and allow a more appropriate selection of therapeutic modalities for patients.

A greater challenge of current research is the use of ANN to help in the diagnosis of gastro-oesophageal cancer. Although rationalisation of therapy will go some way to improving outcome for patients and avoiding unnecessary operations, the only realistic way of significantly improving outcome is to diagnose the condition at an early stage. Unfortunately, by the time the condition is clinically obvious, the disease is invariably advanced. Oesophago-gastric cancer remains a common disease with a poor survival that has remained unchanged in the West largely because it is diagnosed at an advanced and often incurable stage. In contrast to the improvement in survival reported from individual centres with earlier detection of gastric cancer [29], the overall five-year survival in the United States and UK for patients presenting with gastric cancer is essentially the same today as it was 50 years ago. In Japan, the introduction of population screening with earlier detection of gastric cancer has led to a significant improvement in the overall survival rate [30,31].

The advances in Japan have followed the introduction of screening, with increased detection of early gastric cancer, combined with aggressive surgical practices. Early gastric cancer (EGC) is defined by the Japanese Research Society for Gastric Cancer as a cancer in which the depth of invasion is limited to the submucosal layer of the stomach on histological examination [32]. In Japan, EGC accounts for 35-40% of all newly diagnosed gastric cancers and up to 60% in patients actively participating in screening. It was initially believed that EGC was a disease peculiar to the Japanese, but it has now been described with increasing frequency among Western populations. In the West, the introduction of flexible fibre-optic endoscopy in the early 1970s and subsequent refinement and development of high-resolution video endoscopy has facilitated diagnosis of early gastric cancer allowing identification and biopsy of atypical areas in the stomach [33-35]. The detection rate has increased in the West with awareness of the endoscopic features of EGC. At present in the UK, only 1-2% of gastric cancers are detected early, but these account for 9% of gastric cancers in some specialist units [36].

While population screening based on the Japanese model is unrealistic in the UK and USA, selective screening may be possible. The majority of patients with gastric cancer experience dyspeptic symptoms and investigation of these patients has been shown to result in a higher detection rate of EGC [37]. However dyspepsia is a common condition with a prevalence of over 20% in the community [38-40]. New consultations for dyspeptic episodes account for approximately 2% of general practitioner referrals [41]. The relative simplicity and accessibility of endoscopy, combined with patient expectations, have led to a rapid increase in demand and a concern that it may be overused or used inappropriately. These concerns have led to the establishment of selection criteria for endoscopy. However, while up to 44% of referrals for endoscopy may be deemed inappropriate by these criteria, clinically significant lesions can be found almost as frequently in the inappropriate as in the appropriate group. Neither symptoms nor empirical antisecretory treatments allow adequate selection for patients for endoscopy [39,42]. We know that the likelihood of underlying cancer varies with age and gender (Figure 7.8) but it still remains difficult to predict which patients actually have underlying malignancy. Just as neural networks have been used to help in complex clinical diagnoses such as acute myocardial infarction [43] and pulmonary embolism [44]. The large number of patients and the wealth and complexity of data involved suggest that this should be the next area of research. Such research may allow earlier identification of oesophago-gastric cancer with inevitable significant improvement in prognosis.

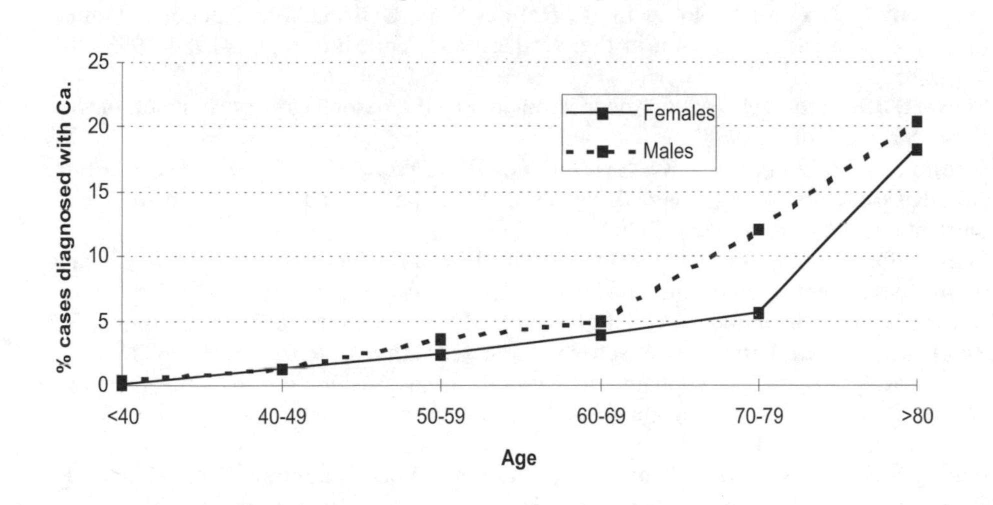

Figure 7.8 Graph representing the change in incidence of cancer findings in patients endoscoped with symptoms of simple indigestion. Data from the Northern Oesophago-Gastric Cancer Unit, Royal Victoria Infirmary, Newcastle upon Tyne, UK.

REFERENCES

1. **Meyers W.C., Damiano R.J., Postlethwait R.W., Rotolo F.S.,** Adenocarcinoma of the stomach; changing patterns over the last 4 decades, *Ann. Surg.,* 205, 1-8, 1987.
2. **Blot W., Devesa S., Kneller R., Fraumeni J.,** Rising incidence of adenocarcinoma of the esophagus and gastric cardia, *J. Am. Med. Assoc.,* 265, 10, 1287-1289, 1991.
3. **Hansen S., Wiig J.N., Giercksky K.E., Tretli S.,** Esophageal and gastric carcinoma in Norway 1958-1992: incidence time trend variability according to morphological subtypes and organ sub-sites, *Int. J. Cancer,* 71, 340-344, 1997.
4. **McKinney P.A., Sharp L., Macfarlane G.J., Muir C.S.,** Oesophageal and gastric cancer in Scotland 1960-1990, *Br. J. Cancer,* 71, 411-415, 1995.

5. **Powell J., McConkey C.C.,** Increasing incidence of adenocarcinoma of the gastric cardia and adjacent sites, *Br. J. Cancer,* 62, 440-443, 1990.
6. **Powell J., McConkey C.C.,** The rising trend in oesophageal adenocarcinoma and gastric cardia, *Eur. J. Cancer Prev.,* 1, 3, 265-269, 1992.
7. **Armstrong R.W., Borman B.,** Trends in incidence of adenocarcinoma of the oesophagus and gastric cardia in New Zealand, 1978-1992, *Int. J. Epid.,* 25, 941-947, 1996.
8. **Pera M., Cameron A., Trastek V., Carpenter H., Zinsmeister A.,** Increasing incidence of adenocarcinoma of the esophagus and esophago-gastric junction, *Gastroenterology,* 104, 2, 510-513, 1993.
9. **Wang H.H., Antonioli D.A., Goldman H.,** Comparative features of esophageal and gastric adenocarcinomas: recent changes in type and frequency, *Human Pathol.*, 17, 5, 482-487, 1986.
10. **Savlon-Harman J.C., Cady B., Nikulasson S., Khettry U., Stone M.D., Lavin P.,** Shifting proportions of gastric adenocarcinomas, *Arch. Surg.,* 129, 381-389, 1994.
11. **Antonioli D.A., Goldman H.,** Changes in the location and type of gastric adenocarcinoma, *Cancer,* 50, 4, 775-781, 1982.
12. **Wayman J., Dresner S., Forman D., Raimes S.A., Griffin S.M.**, Adenocarcinoma of the oesophago-gastric junction in the Northern and Yorkshire region 1984-1993, *Br. J. Surg.,* 85, 31, 1997.
13. **Siewert, J.R. and Stein, H.J.**, Adenocarcinoma of the oesophago-gastric junction, *Br. J. Surg.*, 85, 1457-1459, 1998.
14. **Gao, Y.T., McLaughlin, J.K., Gridley, G., Blot, W.J., Ji, B.T., Dai, Q., Fraumeni, J.J.,** Risk factors for esophageal cancer in Shanghai, China. – II: role of diet and nutrients, *Int. J. Cancer*, 58, 197-202, 1994.
15. **Wu-Williams, A.H., Yu, M.C., Mack, T.M.,** Life-style, workplace, and stomach cancer by subsite in young men of Los Angeles county, *Cancer Res.*, 50, 2569-2576, 1990.
16. **Brown, L.M., Silverman, D.T., Pottern, L.M., Schoenberg, J.B., Greenberg, R.S., Swanson, G.M., Liff, J.M., Schwartz, A.G., Hayes, R.B., Blot, W.J., et al.,** Adenocarcinoma of the esophagus and esophago-gastric junction in white men in the United States: alcohol, tobacco, and socio-economic factors, *Cancer Causes and Control*, 5, 333-340, 1994.
17. **Chow, W.H., Blaser, M.J., Blot, W.J., Gammon, M.D., Vaughan, T.L., Risch, H.A., Perez-Perez, G.I., Schoenberg, J.B., Stanford, J.L., Rotterdam, H., West, A.B., Fraumeni, J.F.J.,** An inverse relation between cagA+ strains of Helicobacter pylori infection and risk of esophageal and gastric cardia adenocarcinoma, *Cancer Res.*, 58, 588-590, 1998.
18. **Sutton D., Wayman J., Griffin S.M.,** The learning curve for oesophageal cancer surgery, *Br. J. Surg.,* 85, 1399-1402, 1998.
19. **Muller J.M., Erasmit T., Stelsner M., Zieren U., Pichlmaier H.,** Surgical therapy of oesophageal cancer, *Br. J. Surg.,* 77, 845-857, 1990.
20. **Fielding J.W.L., Ellis D.J., Jones B.G., et al.,** Natural history of 'early' gastric cancer: results of a ten year regional survey, *Br. Med. J.*, 281, 965-967, 1980.
21. **Naguib R.N.G., Sherbet G.V.,** Artificial neural networks in cancer research, *Pathobiology,* 65, 129-139, 1997.
22. **De Laurentiis M., Ravdin P.,** A technique for using neural network analysis to perform survival analysis of censored data., *Cancer Lett.,* 77, 127-138, 1994.
23. **Cross S.S., Harrison R.F., Kennedy R.L.,** Introduction to neural networks, *The Lancet,* 346, 1075-1079, 1995.
24. **Duthie G.S., Monson J.R.T.,** Artificial neural networks applied to outcome prediction for colorectal cancer patients in separate institutions, *The Lancet,* 350, 469-472, 1997.
25. **Naguib R.N.G., Robinson M.C., Neal D.E., Hamdy F.C.,** Neural networks: a new tool to predict outcome in prostate cancer, *Eur. Urol.,* 30, 73, 1996.

26. **Naguib R.N.G., Adams A.E., Horne C.H.W., Angus B., Sherbet G.V., Lennard T.W.J.,** The detection of nodal metastasis in breast cancer using neural network techniques, *Phys. Meas.*, 17, 297-303, 1996.
27. **Droste K., Bollschweiler E., Waschulzick T., Schütz T., Engelbrecht R., Maruyama K., Siewert J.R.,** Prediction of lymph node metastasis in gastric cancer patients with neural networks, *Cancer Lett.,* 109, 141-148, 1996.
28. **Drew P.J., Bottaci P., Magee P., Macintyre I.M.C., Kerin M.J., Monson J.R.T., Duthie G.S.,** Artificial neural networks for the prediction of outcome following surgery for gastric cancer, *Br. J. Surg.*, 85, 38, 1998.
29. **Sue-Ling H.M., Martin I., Griffith J., Ward D.C., Quirke P., Johnston D. et al.,** Early gastric cancer: 46 patients treated in one surgical department, *Gut*, 33, 1318-1322, 1992.
30. **Murakami T.,** Early cancer of the stomach, *World J. Surg.*, 3, 685-692, 1979.
31. **Maruyama K., Okabayashi K., Kinoshita T.,** Progress in gastric cancer in Japan and its limits of radicality, *World J. Surg.*, 11, 418, 1987.
32. **Sakita et al.,** The development of endoscopic diagnosis of early cancer of the stomach, *Jpn. J. Clin. Oncol.*, 12, 113-128, 1971.
33. **Myren J., Dybdahl J., Serck-Hanssen A., Leitao J.,** Gastroscopy with direct biopsy and routine X-ray examination in the diagnosis of malignancies of the stomach — a retrospective study, *Scand. J. Gastroenterol.*, 10, 193-197, 1975.
34. **Seifert E., Butke H., Gail K., Elster K., Cote S.,** Diagnosis of early gastric cancer, *Am. J. Gastroenterol.*, 71, 563-567, 1979.
35. **Longo W.E., Zucker K.A., Zdon M.J., Ballantyne G.H., Cambria R.P., Modlin I.M.,** Role of endoscopy in the diagnosis of gastric cancer, *Arch. Surg.*, 122, 292-295, 1987.
36. **Sue-Ling H.M., Johnston D., Martin I.G., Dixon M.F., Lansdown M.R.J., McMahon M.J., et al.,** Gastric cancer: a curable disease in Britain, *Br. Med. J.*, 307, 591-596, 1993.
37. **Hallisey M.T., Allum W.H., Jewkes A.J., Ellis D.J., Fielding J.W.L.,** Early detection of gastric cancer, *Br. Med. J.*, 301, 513-515, 1990.
38. **Jones R, Lydeard S.,** Prevalence of symptoms of dyspepsia in the community, *Br. Med. J.*, 298, 30-32, 1989.
39. **Talley N.J., Zinsmeister A.R., Schleck C.D., Melton L.J.,** Dyspepsia and dyspepsia subgroups: a population-based study, *Gastroenterology*, 102, 1259-1268, 1992.
40. **Talley N.J., Zinsmeister A.R., Schleck C.D., Melton L.J.,** Smoking, alcohol, and analgesics in dyspepsia subgroups: lack of an association in a community, *Gut*, 35, 619-624, 1994.
41. **Brown C., Rees W.D.W.,** Dyspepsia in general practice, *Br. Med. J.*, 300, 829-830, 1990.
42. **Bytzer P., Hansen J.M., Schaffalitsky de Muckadell O.B.,** Empirical H2-blocker therapy or prompt endoscopy in management of dyspepsia, *The Lancet*, 343, 811-816, 1994.
43. **Baxt W.G., Skora J.,** Prospective validation of artificial neural networks trained to identify acute myocardial infarction, *The Lancet,* 10, 347, 407-408, 1996.
44. **Patel S., Henry J.W., Ruberfire M., Stein P.D.,** Neural networks in the clinical diagnosis of acute pulmonary embolism, *Chest,* 104, 1685-1689, 1993.

Chapter 8

ARTIFICIAL NEURAL NETWORKS IN UROLOGIC ONCOLOGY

T.H. Douglas and J.W. Moul

I. INTRODUCTION

An artificial neural network (ANN) is a complex computer system that is designed to replicate human decision making by modelling the human neuron [1-3]. The human brain is made of neurons and millions of multiple synapses, and it is believed that with learning, weighting of individual synapses affects the final decisions we make. As input neuronal information is passed through on multiple simultaneous pathways to converge on the final output neuron, it is under the influence of either inhibitory or stimulatory input at each synapse. For a computer to model this process, a neural network is created as a network of many very simple processors, each with its own local memory, linked by unidirectional connections that carry numeric data. The units operate only on their own local data and on the inputs they receive via the connections. Each node receives input from other nodes and, with learning, it changes the weights of the incoming information to produce an output that most closely represents the known outcome. When the sum of the weights exceeds a predetermined threshold, the node fires; otherwise it remains quiet. The combination of the firings of each neuron determines the final decision of the output neuron. Within this system are often hidden layers of neurons that further influence the final outcome. This is unlike conventional computers, where there is a central processor with central memory that processes information sequentially using a defined set of rules. Figure 8.1 represents a model of a neural network [4].

The advantages of neural network information processing arise from its ability to recognise and model nonlinear relationships between data. In biologic systems, clustering of data and nonlinear relationships are more common than strict linear relationships [4]. Conventional statistical methods can be used to try to model nonlinear relationships, but they require complex and extensive mathematical modelling. Neural networks provide a comparatively easier way to do the same type of analysis [5].

In the initial phase of operation the neural network "learns". This is accomplished in the supervised learning method, by showing the network input data and the known outcome. The interwoven weights are adjusted by the training algorithm to reproduce the desired answer.

Initially when a neural network is presented with a pattern, it makes a random guess as to what the answer might be. It then sees how far its answer was from the actual one and makes an appropriate adjustment to its connection weights. This process, known as the backward propagation of error, is repeated until the evolved sets of weights best reproduces the entire training and testing database results in an answer that is most accurate. After the learning phase, the network is given the input data, and it gives its best answer based on prior learning.

0-8493-9692-1/01/$0.00+$1.50

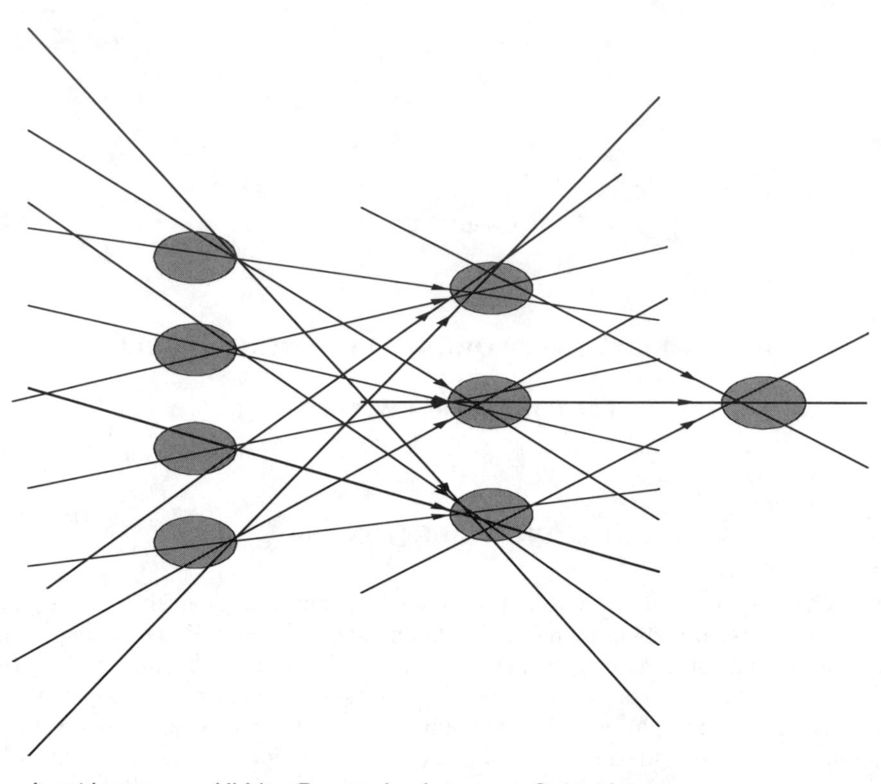

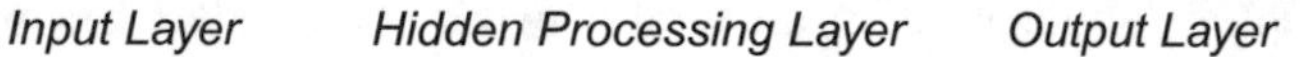

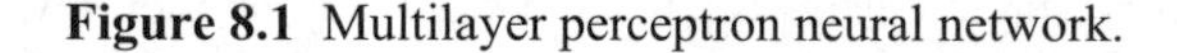

Figure 8.1 Multilayer perceptron neural network.

Neural networks have evolved over the past years, and are used in making financial and weather predictions. Neural networks have been used in a variety of medical applications, mainly in image interpretation [6-12], laboratory studies [13-20], and clinical diagnosis [13,20-26]. One of their most valuable assets is their ability to predict prognosis. Recent studies have shown that, in breast and colon cancer, ANNs are more accurate at predicting prognosis than conventional TNM staging [27]. This chapter summarises the applications of neural networks to urologic oncology.

II. KIDNEY CANCER

Maclin et al. performed some of the earliest applications of neural network in the urologic literature [28]. They trained an ANN to identify renal cell cancer from benign renal cysts in 52 cases by analysing the numeric ultrasound data. On the 47 cases of the test set, the ANN made no mistakes. Since the overall incidence of renal cell carcinoma in cysts is fairly low, the significance of this degree of accuracy is unknown.

III. BLADDER CANCER

Hurst and colleagues used a neural network applied to an image analysis system to identify bladder cells expressing the tumour antigen p300 [29]. In this study, they stained bladder cells with a fluorescent antibody to the p300 tumour antigen. Greyscale images of both positive and false positive cells were digitised and fed into a feed-forward neural network. They trained the network to identify true positive (cancer cells) from false positive (autofluorescence or artefact). When they applied the neural network to high magnification images (50x), they found excellent agreement with the human pathologist's interpretation. For lower power images (12.5x), the ANN was approximately 75% accurate, even though the ANN was only trained on true positives and negatives (no false positives were given to the ANN in the training set). When the ANN was trained on just four input features (as opposed to feeding it raw image data), the ANN was slightly more accurate. This paper demonstrates a powerful feature of neural networks, which is its ability to accurately classify items that humans can accurately classify (e.g., cytology), even when the rules are not clearly definable.

Recently, Pantazopoulos et al. also demonstrated the benefit of using neural networks to improve the speed and accuracy in cytology interpretation [30]. In their study, a back-propagation neural network was applied to a custom image processing system. The nuclei of 45,452 Giemsa stained cells from 470 patients were measured using a custom image processing system. The patients had a variety of genitourinary abnormalities — urolithiasis: 50 patients, inflammation: 61 patients, benign prostatic hyperplasia: 99 patients, carcinoma *in situ*: 5 patients, Grade I bladder carcinoma: 71 patients, and Grades II and III bladder carcinoma: 184 patients. From this data, 13,636 cells were used to train the network to interpret benign and malignant cells. Overall, 141 patients (30%) were used to train the network to predict the benign vs. malignant. This was compared to the cytologic diagnosis rendered by three separate pathologists. The network was able to determine benign from malignant using the morphologic appearance of the nuclei with an accuracy of 90.6%, and suggested the correct patient diagnosis with an accuracy of 96.7% (sensitivity: 94.5%, specificity: 100%) on the remaining training sets.

In a related study, the same authors used a learning vector quantiser (LVQ)-type neural network on the same cellular and patient datasets [31]. An LVQ neural network is optimally designed for classification or pattern recognition tasks. This network is unsupervised and self-organises to cluster similar input patterns together to provide a learned output classification of that data. Using this network, they achieved results similar to their back-propagation network with 90.6% accuracy at predicting cellular classification, and 97.5% accuracy at predicting diagnosis on these patients. These studies demonstrate the neural network's usefulness in complex image interpretation by assisting the pathologist in the cumbersome task of interpreting nuclear cellular architecture.

IV. PROSTATE CANCER

Most of the current work in neural networks in urologic oncology is in the area of diagnosis and treatment outcomes in prostate cancer. The earliest reported work was by Snow et al. [32]. In this study they applied an ANN to a prostate-specific antigen or PSA-1 Washington University of St. Louis prostate screening database of 1787 men with PSA > 4.0 ng/ml to predict positive biopsies based on PSA, digital rectal findings and transrectal ultrasound (TRUS) findings with an accuracy of 87%. They also trained an ANN to predict tumour recurrence in a second database of 983 patients who had undergone radical prostatectomy over a ten-year period [32]. After training, the ANN was able to predict recurrence with 90% accuracy in a test group, using the input variables of age, clinical stage, potency, PSA, and race. These two pilot studies suggested that ANN technology could be applied retrospectively to these databases with better accuracy than conventional statistical modelling.

Our group attempted to improve the neural network's accuracy by including many more variables than Snow et al. used in the previous study [33]. We studied 218 records from our database of 540 radical prostatectomy patients, and trained an ANN to predict organ-confined disease using 38 clinical variables. The variables used included race, age, PSA, prostatic acid phosphatase (PAP), clinical TNM stage, tumour grade, tumour Gleason score, testosterone, creatinine, family history, as well as some unusual variables, such as history of smoking, and medical history questions (history of hypertension, diabetes, etc.). From the 218 records, 129 were used for training, 56 for testing, and finally 33 were used for validation. We had an overall accuracy of 82%, sensitivity of 94%, and specificity of 69%. We also attempted to predict recurrence with the addition of pathologic stage and grade and the 38 clinical variables. The ANN achieved an overall accuracy of 97% with sensitivity of 100% and specificity of 96%.

A further study by Snow and his colleagues using the Prostate Cancer Awareness Week (PCAW) database was reported [34]. This study applied an ANN to a screening database to predict the presence of cancer in 1500 men who had either abnormal digital rectal exam or abnormal PSA. All men underwent prostate biopsy, of which 25% had cancer. The ANN was trained using the 39 clinical and demographic variables and the known outcome. The ANN gave a sensitivity of 72%, a specificity of 78%, and an overall accuracy of 77%. The ANN was able to detect cancer at twice the database average. This suggested the ANN could be used to assist in the decision to proceed with biopsy.

Stamey et al. have reported the results of the ProstAsure™ system, a commercially available neural network to predict prostate cancer risk [35]. In the initial study, the ANN was trained on the input variables of age, PSA (TOSOH), PAP (TOSOH), and creatine kinase isoenzymes (CK-MM, CK-MB, CK-BB) to recognise cancer. The study group was composed of 108 "normal" men (nl DRE, PSA ≤4 ng/ml), 115 with benign prostatic hyperplasia, and 193 untreated cancers (28 Stage T1b, 94 Stage T2a, 34 Stage T3, and 37 Stage M1b). The ProstAsure™ ANN was trained on 65 normal men, 45 men with benign prostatic hyperplasia, and 45 men with cancer. For detection of prostate cancer, the sensitivity was 81% and specificity 92%. For predicting benign prostatic hyperplasia the sensitivity was 63%.

In a recent follow-up report, the ProstAsure™ was applied to men with normal PSA only (PSA ≤4 ng/ml) [36]. Of 298 of these men, 102 had cancer, 108 were normal, and 88 had Benign Prostatic Hyperplasia (BPH). A ProstAsure™ Index (PI) was calculated for each patient based on the same 6 input variables reported in the previous study (age, PSA, PAP, CK-MM, CK-MB, CK-BB). If the PI was ≤ 0.5, no biopsy was recommended. Of the 102 patients with cancer, the PI was > 0.5 in 72 (sensitivity 71%). For the normal patients, 93/108 had PI ≤ 0.5, and for the BPH patients PI ≤ 0.5 in 53/88. This yielded a sensitivity of 86%, assuming no one in these two groups had cancer. These two studies show how a neural net can be used to predict more accurately the presence of cancer independent of the digital rectal exam, even in patients with normal total PSA levels.

Babaian et al. retrospectively compared ProstAsure™ to free PSA in the detection of prostate cancer [37]. In this study, they divided 225 patients into three groups: 94 men with normal digital rectal exam and PSA ≤ 4.0 ng/ml, 77 men with BPH and PSA ≤ 4.0 ng/ml, and 54 men with localised prostate cancer. They calculated PIs and determined free and total PSA on each patient. They found that the ProstAsure™ had a sensitivity of 93% and a specificity of 81%. Using a cutoff of 15%, free PSA had a sensitivity of 80% and a specificity of 74%. In addition, in patients with PSA ≤ 4.0 ng/ml, the ProstAsure™ was less likely to miss prostate cancer than free PSA used with a cutoff of 15% (7% and 20% undetected, respectively). This suggests that the ProstAsure™ is an accurate clinical tool for detecting prostate cancer in the patients with normal PSA. Unfortunately, controlled prospective studies using the PI are not yet available.

Tewari et al. used a probabilistic neural network with a genetic adaptive algorithm to stage prostate cancer patients undergoing radical prostatectomy [38]. A genetic adaptive algorithm is used to find smoothing factors for the variability in input factors. In their study they applied a network to a database of 1200 patients with clinically localised prostate cancer (mean PSA 8.1 ng/ml) from four centres. Their input variables were PSA, biopsy data (unilateral/bilateral/number of positive cores), Gleason score, digital rectal exam stage, presence of perineural invasion on prostate needle biopsy, age, and race. Output variables were margins (positive or negative), seminal vesicles (positive or negative), and lymph nodes (positive or negative). Their network had an accuracy of 76.7% (sensitivity: 81.3%, specificity: 75%) for margins, 73.2% (sensitivity: 100%, specificity: 72.1%) for seminal vesicles, and 72.6% (sensitivity: 83.3%, specificity: 71.8%) for lymph nodes. They proposed the use of this network to determine which patients might benefit from preoperative staging studies, such as bone scan, computerised tomography, or lymphadenectomy. Clinical stage T2a-c accounted for 996 of the 1200 patients, 90 patients had T3 disease, while only 86 patients had stage T1c cancer. In the current era of stage migration and early detection through the use of PSA, this network might not be as accurate a tool for staging the many T1c cancers that are now being treated.

Loch et al. used an ANN to analyse 4mm sequential transrectal ultrasound images, and correlated these findings with the actual whole mount step sections in the corresponding prostatectomy specimens [39]. In 50 patients, there were 381 pathology slides evaluated. The image analysis system correctly identified 99% of the benign images, and there were only 4 false positives. Of 119 pathologically malignant areas, the ANN classified 71% as malignant and 29% as benign. The ANN correctly identified 97% of the isoechoic cancers (34/35). These predictions are much better than TRUS alone.

Krongrad et al. used a neural network to model the emotional component of general quality of life in patients with prostate cancer or BPH [40]. Patients with either prostate cancer or BPH were asked to fill out a quality of life questionnaire (Rand Mental Health Index) at 1- and 6-month intervals. The questions asked were general in nature and were not disease-specific. The data from each patient were then scored and fed into a feed-forward, back-propagation network. The final output neuron predicted if the patient had good or bad quality of life. The neural network's output was compared to conventional statistical analysis. At predicting general quality of life, the ANN had an accuracy rate of 89% at 1 month and 90% at 6 months. Logistic regression was almost as accurate (84% at 1 month, 88% at 6 months), and allowed identification of the most significant predictors. This study demonstrated that an ANN could be used to model general quality of life.

Naguib et al. recently reported the use of a neural network to predict prognosis and outcome in prostate cancer using conventional input variables (age, stage, bone scan findings, grade, PSA, and type of treatment). In addition they performed immunohistochemical staining on tissue specimens for the proto-oncogene, bcl-2 and tumour suppressor gene, p53 [41]. The presence of increased abnormal expression of these genes has been associated with disease progression in prostate cancer [42,43]. Naguib and his colleagues trained a network on 21 patients and tested on 20. The network correctly classified the outcome in 80% of patients. When the immunohistochemical data (p53 and bcl-2 expression) was deleted from the input set, the accuracy fell significantly to 60%. This study showed that these networks can be used to assess the benefit of newer tumour markers. Unfortunately, the sample size was small and prospective validation is needed.

V. TESTICULAR CANCER

Our group used an ANN to predict pathologic Stage I vs. Stage II in patients with clinical Stage I nonseminomatous testicular cancer [44]. The pathologic orchiectomy specimens were retrospectively analysed for the presence of lymphatic, vascular and tunical invasion and the percent of embryonal carcinoma, yolk sac carcinoma, teratoma and seminoma in the tumour. The data was independently given to an ANN expert and a less experienced investigator using a commercially available software package. Using the data from 93 patients, the ANNs were trained to predict pathologic disease on retroperitoneal lymph node dissection. For the ANN expert, using a custom network, the overall accuracy was 92%, sensitivity of 88%, specificity of 96%. For the less experienced researcher, he obtained an overall accuracy of 84.9% if he used only percent embryonal and presence of vascular invasion vs. 79.6% if all seven variables were used as input variables. This study was important for three reasons: first, it confirmed that percent embryonal carcinoma and vascular invasion were risk factors for pathologic disease in nonseminomatous testis cancer; second, it showed that a custom designed neural network was actually better than standard logistic regression analysis (accuracy 85.9%) in predicting pathologic Stage II disease [45]; third, it showed that off-the-shelf ANN packages may not be able to reproduce the excellent results obtained by a custom neural network.

VI. DISCUSSION

As one can see, the applications of ANNs are diverse. The advantages of these ANNs are their relative simplicity compared to conventional statistical analysis, their ability to recognise data relationships between data variables that may either be counter-intuitive or are not obvious to the casual user. As previously stated these neural networks are relatively easy to set up and train, compared with trying to develop statistical models. Excitement abounds for potential uses for these networks. As large databases are organised and collected, these tools can be further refined to assist the urologist in predicting stage, response to therapy, and ultimate survival.

Disadvantages of neural networks arise from the fact that they are an inherent “black box” type of technology. The relationships between the data are often not clear to the user, and most important variables are difficult to identify. Also, if the neural network is overtrained on a small data set, it may lose its ability to be generally applied to new data. It is often not known how to best optimise the network to the data. The number of nodes and number of hidden layers for a given number of input and output nodes are not known. Often this is determined by trial and error [3].

While the study by Moul and colleagues [44] showed that an ANN expert investigator can often achieve better results than a less experienced investigator using off-the-shelf technology, the technology is easily obtainable for general use. There are many commercially available neural network packages, as well as freeware or shareware that can be obtained from the internet. There are even networks that can be accessed directly from the World Wide Web, so that anyone can use this technology [46].

There is a growing base of literature on the use of these systems. However, most of the current reports on neural networks in use in urologic oncology have been done as either retrospective applications on databases or small pilot studies. Since the largest databases exist in prostate cancer, most of the studies have been concentrated in this area. Unfortunately, these databases often include patients treated in the era prior to early detection using PSA. Large prospective applications of neural networks on modern datasets are lacking. Such studies are needed to assess fully the true value of this technology to the urologic oncologist.

REFERENCES

1. **Wasserman P.D.,** *Neural Computing: Theory and Practice*, Van Nostrand Reinhold, New York, 1989.
2. **Simpson P.K.,** *Artificial Neural Systems,* Pergamon Press, Oxford, 1989.
3. **Dayhoff J.,** *Neural Network Architectures: An Introduction*, Van Nostrand Reinhold, New York, 1990.
4. **Cross S.S., Harrison R.F., Kennedy R.L.,** Introduction to neural networks, *The Lancet*, 346, 1075, 1995.
5. **Baxt W.G.,** Application of artificial neural networks to clinical medicine, *The Lancet*, 346, 1135, 1995.

6. **Sochor H., Dorffner G., Porenta G.,** Classification of thallium-201 scintigrams using a neural network trained by back propagation, *J. Nucl. Med.*, 29, 1314, 1988.
7. **Boone J.M., Sigillito V.G., Shaber G.S.,** Neural networks in radiology: an introduction and evaluation in a signal detection task, *Med. Phys.*, 17, 234, 1990.
8. **Asada N., Kunio D., MacMahon H., Montner S.M., Giger M.L., Abe C., Wu Y.,** Potential usefulness of an artificial neural network for differential diagnosis of interstitial lung diseases: pilot study, *Radiology*, 177, 857, 1990.
9. **Gross G.W., Boone J.M., Greco-Hung V., Greenberg B.,** Neural networks in radiologic diagnosis — II: interpretation of neonatal chest radiographs, *Invest. Radiol.*, 25, 1017, 1990.
10. **Goldberg V., Manduca A., Ewert D.L., Gisvold J.J., Greenleaf J.F.,** Improvement in specificity of ultrasonography for diagnosis of breast tumors by means of artificial intelligence, *Med. Phys.*, 19, 1475, 1992.
11. **Wu Y., Giger M.L., Doi K., Vyborny C.J., Schmidt R.A., Metz C.E.,** Improvement in specificity of ultrasonography for diagnosis of breast tumor by means of artificial intelligence, *Med. Phys.*, 19, 1475, 1992.
12. **Wolberg W.H., Mangasarian O.L.,** Computer-aided diagnosis of breast aspirates via expert systems, *Anal. Quant. Cytol. Histol.*, 12, 314, 1990.
13. **Wolberg W.H., Mangasarian O.L.,** Multisurface method of pattern separation for medical diagnosis applied to breast cytology, *Proc. Natl. Acad. Sci.*, 87, 9193, 1990.
14. **Dawson A.E., Austin R.E., Weinberg D.B.,** Nuclear grading of breast carcinoma by image analysis, *Am. J. Clin. Pathol.*, 95, S29, 1991.
15. **Furlong J.W., Dupuy M.E., Heinsimer J.A.,** Neural network analysis of serial cardiac enzyme data: a clinical application of artificial machine intelligence, *Am. J. Clin. Pathol.,* 96, 134, 1991.
16. **Astion M.L., Wilding P.,** The application of back propagation neural networks to problems in pathology and laboratory medicine, *Arch. Path. Lab. Med.*, 116, 995, 1992.
17. **Cohen, M.E., Hudson D.L., Banda P.W., Blois M.S.,** Neural network approach to detection of metastatic lymphoma from chromatographic analysis of urine, *Proc. Symp. Comput. Appl. Med. Care*, 295-299, 1992.
18. **Bartoo G.T., Lee J.S.J., Bartels P.H., Kiviat N.B., Nelson A.C.,** Automated prescreening of conventionally prepared cervical smears: a feasibility study, *Lab. Invest.*, 66, 166, 1992.
19. **Cicchetti D.V.,** Neural networks and diagnosis in the clinical laboratory: state of the art, *Clin. Chem.*, 38, 9, 1992.
20. **Kratzer M.A.A., Ivandic B., Fateh-Moghadam A.,** Neuronal network anaylsis of serum electrophoresis, *J. Clin. Pathol.,* 45, 612, 1992.
21. **Baxt, W.G.,** Use of an artificial neural network for data analysis in clinical decision making: the diagnosis of acute coronary occlusion, *Neural Comput.*, 2, 480, 1992.
22. **Bounds D.G., Lloyd P.J., Mathew B.G.,** A comparison of neural network and other pattern recognition approaches to the diagnosis of low-back disorders, *Neural Networks*, 3, 583, 1990.
23. **Mulsant B.H.,** A neural network as an approach to the clinical diagnosis, *MD Computing*, 7, 25, 1990.
24. **Baxt, W.G.,** Use of an artificial neural network for the diagnosis of myocardial infarction, *Ann. Intern. Med.*, 115, 843, 1991.
25. **Baxt, W.G.,** Analysis of the clinical variables driving decision in an artificial neural network trained to identify the presence of myocardial infarction, *Ann. Emerg. Med.*, 21, 439, 1992.
26. **Astion M.L., Wilding P.,** Application of neural networks to the interpretation of laboratory data in cancer diagnosis, *Clin. Chem.,* 3, 34, 1992.

27. **Burke H.B., Goodman P.H., Rosen D.B., Henson D.E., Weinstein J.N., Harrell F.E., Marks J.R., Winchester D.P., Bostwick D.G.,** Artificial neural networks improve the accuracy of cancer survival prediction, *Cancer,* 79, 857, 1997.
28. **Maclin P.S., Dempsey J., Brooks J., Rand J.,** Using neural networks to diagnose cancer, *J. Med. Syst.*, 15, 11, 1991.
29. **Hurst R.E., Bonner R.B., Ashenayi K., Veltri R.W., Hemstreet G.P.,** Neural net-based identification of cells expressing the p300 tumor-related antigen using fluorescence image analysis, *Cytometry,* 27, 36, 1997.
30. **Pantazopoulos D., Karakitsos P., Iokom-Liossi A., Pouliakis A., Botsoli-Stergiou E., Dimopoulos C.,** Back propagation neural network in the discrimination of benign from malignant lower urinary tract lesions, *J. Urol.,* 159, 1619, 1998.
31. **Pantazopoulos D., Karakitsos P., Pouliakis A., Iokim-Liossi A., Dimopoulos M.A.,** Static cytometry and neural networks in the discrimination of lower urinary system lesions, *Urology,* 51, 946, 1998.
32. **Snow P.B., Smith D.S., Catalona W.J.,** Artificial neural networks in the diagnosis and prognosis of prostate cancer: a pilot study, *J. Urol.,* 152, 5, Pt. 2, 1923, 1994.
33. **Douglas T.H., Connelly R.R., McLeod D.G., Moul J.W., Snow P.B.,** Neural network analysis of pre-operative and post-operative variables to predict pathologic stage and recurrence following radical prostatectomy, *J. Urol.,* 155, 5, 487A, 1996.
34. **Snow P., Crawford E.D., DeAntoni E.P., Gordon S.,** Prostate cancer diagnosis from artificial neural networks using the Prostate Cancer Awareness Week (PCAW) database, *J. Urol.,* 157, 4, 365, 1997.
35. **Stamey T.A., Barnhill S.D., Zhang Z., Madysatha K.R., Prestigiacomo A.F., Jones K., Chan D.,** Effectiveness of ProstAsure in detecting prostate cancer and benign prostatic hyperplasia in men age 50 and older, *J. Urol.,* 155, 5, 436A, 1996.
36. **Stamey T.A., Barnhill S.D., Zhang A., Madastha K.R., Zhang H.,** A neural network (ProstAsure) with high sensitivity and specificity for diagnosing prostate cancer (PCa) in men with a PSA < 4.0 ng.ml, *J. Urol.,* 157, 4, 364, 1997.
37. **Babaian R.J., Fritsche H.A., Zhang Z., Zhang K.H., Madyastha K.R., Barnhill S.D.,** Evaluation of ProstAsure index in the detection of prostate cancer: a preliminary report, *Urology,* 51, 1, 132, 1998.
38. **Tewari A., Narayan P.,** Novel staging tool for localized prostate cancer: a pilot study using genetic adaptive neural networks, *J. Urol.,* 160, 2, 430, 1998.
39. **Loch T., Leuschner I., Brüske T., Küppers F., Stöckle M., Genberg C.,** Neural network analysis of subvisual transrectal ultrasound data: improved prostate cancer detection, *J. Urol.*, 157, 4, 364, 1997.
40. **Krongrad A., Granville L.J., Burke M.A., Golden R.M., Lai S., Cho L., Niederberger C.S.,** Predictors of general quality of life in patients with benign prostate hyperplasia or prostate cancer, *J. Urol.*, 157, 2, 534, 1997.
41. **Naguib R.N., Robinson M.C., Neal D.E., Hamdy F.C.,** Neural network analysis of combined conventional and experimental prognostic markers in prostate cancer: a pilot study, *Br. J. Cancer,* 78, 246, 1998.
42. **Moul J.W., Bettencourt M.C., Sesterhenn I.A., Mostofi F.K., McLeod D.G., Srivastava S., Bauer J.J.,** Protein expression of p53, bcl-2, and KI-67 (MIB-1) as prognostic biomarkers in patients with surgically treated, clinically localized prostate cancer, *Surgery,* 120, 159, 1996.
43. **Bauer J.J., Sesterhenn I.A., Mostofi F.K., McLeod D.G., Srivastava S., Moul J.W.,** Elevated levels of apoptosis regulator proteins p53 and bcl-2 are independent prognostic biomarkers in surgically treated clinically localized prostate cancer, *J. Urol.,* 156, 1511, 1996.
44. **Moul J.W., Snow P.B., Fernandez E.B., Maher P.D., Sesterhenn I.A.,** Neural network analysis of quantitative histological factors to predict pathological stage in clinical stage I nonseminomatous testicular cancer, *J. Urol.*, 153, 1574, 1995.

45. **Moul J.W., McCarthy W.F., Fernandez E.B., Sesterhenn I.A.,** Percentage of embryonal carcinoma and vascular invasion predict pathologic stage in clinical stage I nonseminomatous testicular cancer, *Cancer Res.,* 54, 362, 1994.
46. **Niederberger C.S.,** Commentary on the use of neural networks in clinical urology, *J. Urol.,* 153, 1362, 1995.

Chapter 9

NEURAL NETWORKS IN UROLOGIC ONCOLOGY

C. Niederberger and D. Ridout

I. INTRODUCTION

Urologic malignancies, which include renal, testis, bladder, and prostate cancers, are a challenging heterogeneous group of malignancies. Controversy exists in almost every aspect of the diagnosis and treatment of these malignancies. Data drawn from studies and experience help to guide physicians' decision-making in the classification, staging, and optimal treatments of patients. As most medical data is inherently "noisy" and nonlinear in character, traditional statistical analysis of this data in many cases falls short of expectations [1-3]. It is not surprising that many pioneers in medical research have increasingly applied artificial neural networks (ANNs) to new and existing medical data to allow a more accurate evaluation.

II. RENAL CELL CARCINOMA

Renal cell carcinoma (RCC) is the third most common urologic cancer and makes up 3% of all adult cancers [4]. Diagnosis is frequently made by serendipitous identification of a renal mass on ultrasound and in fact 35-40% of diagnoses may be made in this manner [4,5]. The 5-year survival has been reported between 35-50% and one-third of patients newly diagnosed present with metastatic disease [6].

Traditional staging of an isolated solid renal mass suspicious for RCC has consisted of a CT scan of the abdomen and pelvis, chest X-ray film, serum alkaline phosphatase, serum calcium, and evaluation of renal function. Other staging tests would be directed toward diagnosis of symptomatic metastasis, i.e., brain or bone metastasis.

The radiological diagnosis of RCC can be difficult due to the large differential diagnosis of the renal mass. In many cases, the preoperative diagnosis is unsure and the final diagnosis is made by the pathologist. This diagnostic ambiguity can lead to unneeded surgery and anxiety for the patient.

The natural history of RCC may be unpredictable. In most cases of RCC, metastases are related to primary tumour size; in a small portion, however, metastases are identified regardless of primary tumour size leading many surgeons to be more aggressive, resecting tumours as small as 1.5 cm routinely [4]. Further complicating the natural history of this disease, spontaneous regression of pleural and intrapulmonary metastases has been reported in

0-8493-9692-1/01/$0.00+$1.50

more than 60 cases [7]. Unfortunately, physicians are unable to prospectively identify these patients and the role of nephrectomy in these patients is to date unclear.

ANNs have been applied to the difficult task of preoperative diagnosis of RCC. In 1991, Maclin et al. used a back-propagation ANN to evaluate pathologic cases based on ultrasound input obtained by radiologists [5]. This model used a learning rate of 1.0, a training tolerance of 0.005, a test tolerance of 0.4, and a smoothing factor of 0.9. With 51 input characteristics, this model had an accuracy of 99.5-99.9% in classifying either renal cyst or renal cancer. In 1994, a similar paper by Chang et al. evaluated the renal mass diagnostic system, which uses a Bayesian probabilistic approach, to evaluate patient information, intravenous pylograms, and retrograde pylograms in diagnosing renal parenchymal tumours and tumours of the renal pelvis [8]. The overall accuracy of the system was 83.3%, which was comparable to an attending physician's judgement in this study.

Our laboratory investigated a neural computational approach to predicting new metastases in patients with renal cancer [9,10]. Because the natural history of renal cancer is so eccentric, with disease often progressing in unpredictable fashion and "jumping" stages, we believed that neural computation's nonlinear modelling approach would benefit this enigmatic problem. We collected data from patients seeking treatment for renal cancer at a large public hospital in Chicago. Records included 232 patients in whom it was known whether metastases did or did not develop on follow-up. Features tracked in the database included patient ethnicity, gender, date of birth, date of diagnosis, if a nephrectomy was undertaken, date of surgery, whether lung or bone metastases were present at diagnosis, tumour histology, tumour size, selected therapy, and date of follow-up. We also entered T-, N-, and M-Stage in the database. In this way, both raw and derived (TNM) data was available for the neural network's training set. The outcome was encoded as a binary variable, 0 if no metastases were present at follow-up, and 1 if a metastasis occurred.

In general, we encoded input variables in three ways. Continuous variables, such as patient age, were normalised to a range of -0.9 to +0.9. Binary variables such as gender were assigned -0.9 or +0.9. Categorical variables were encoded with Q = number of categories. For example, ethnicity was encoded in the input layer as African-American = [-0.9 -0.9 -0.9 +0.9], Caucasian = [-0.9 -0.9 +0.9 -0.9], Hispanic = [-0.9 +0.9 -0.9 -0.9], and other = [+0.9 -0.9 -0.9 -0.9]. Table 9.1 shows the encoded variables. For input variables that were not fully populated in the database, an additional input node was encoded, with -0.9 indicating absence and +0.9 presence of the variable in the training set.

The topology of the neural network was fully interlayer connected with 1 input, 1 hidden, and 1 output layers. Bias nodes were included on both input and hidden layers. The learning rule was canonical back-propagation with a sigmoidal activation function, except that at the output node the error function was chosen to be the cross-entropy error function since the targets were binary-valued [3]:

$$\eta(\mathbf{W}) = -(1/M)\sum_{i=1}^{M} \log\left[t^i o^i + (1-t^i)\, o^i\right]$$

where M is the number of training stimuli, t^i is the known outcome for dataset exemplar i, and o^i is the neural network's output. The learning rate was initially set to 0.05, and network training was terminated when the change in error between iterations was less than 10^{-9}, or if the network error increased over a window chosen to be 6000 iterations. The number of hidden nodes was initially set to 10, and overlearning was identified if the training and test set classification errors diverged when plotted vs. training iterations. We then reduced the number of hidden nodes until the training set and test set classification errors no longer diverged, which occurred with a network with six hidden nodes in the hidden layer.

Table 9.1 Input node type and encoding for renal carcinoma dataset.

Number of Input Nodes	Variable	Value(s)
4	Ethnicity	Categorical
1	Gender	Binary
2	Age at diagnosis	Continuous
2	T-Stage	Continuous
2	N-Stage	Continuous
2	M-Stage	Continuous
1	Nephrectomy	Binary
2	Age at nephrectomy	Continuous
2	Lung metastases	Binary
2	Bone metastases	Binary
10	Cell histology	Categorical
1	Tumour size (cm)	Continuous
7	Treatment choice	Categorical

In order to compare neural computational modelling to linear statistical tools, we used linear (LDFA) and quadratic discriminant function analysis (QDFA) to model the renal cancer dataset. Classification accuracy for all modelling tools was defined by:

$$CA = \left[\frac{C}{C+1}\right] . 100$$

where C is the number of correct network classifications in the data set, and I, the number of incorrect classifications. Results are shown in Table 9.2.

Table 9.2 Neural computational modelling compared to DFA.

Data set	LDFA	QDFA	Neural Network
Training	68.4%	69.0%	92.5%
Test	67.2%	69.0%	84.5%

In all cases, the original dataset was divided into two separate sets, a training set and a test set, so that the test set was not used in training.

Physicians are generally not satisfied with simply a model that predicts outcomes. Rather, physicians generally demand to know the significance of individual features to the predictive model, and for a good reason. To this end, we have been investigating feature extraction using Wilk's generalised likelihood ratio test (GLRT), as described by Golden [11]. This method applies that one may reject the null hypothesis that two networks model the training set the same if:

$$2M\left[\ \eta_2\left(\mathbf{W}^2\right)-\eta_1\left(\mathbf{W}^1\right)\ \right] > \kappa_\alpha$$

where κ_α is the chi-squared constant, $\eta_1\left(\mathbf{W}^1\right)$ is the error at a local minimum for network 1, $\eta_2\left(\mathbf{W}^2\right)$ is the error at a similar local minimum for network 2, and M is the number of members in the training set. The number of degrees of freedom for κ_α is defined to be the difference of the number of connections between networks 1 and 2. In order to use Wilk's GLRT for feature extraction in neural computation, the following procedure is implemented:

1. The full network is trained to a local error minimum.
2. The cross-entropy error $\eta_2\left(\mathbf{W}^2\right)$ for the full network is recorded.
3. The feature to be extracted is "removed" by setting its corresponding input nodes to 0.
4. The resulting subnetwork is retrained, with its initial weights set to the final weights of the full network, to a local error minimum.
5. The cross-entropy error $\eta_1\left(\mathbf{W}^1\right)$ for the subnetwork is recorded.
6. $2M\left[\ \eta_2\left(\mathbf{W}^2\right)-\eta_1\left(\mathbf{W}^1\right)\ \right]$ is calculated, and if it exceeds κ_α for degrees of freedom (number of connections in network 1 minus number of connections in network 2), the feature is found to be significant to the model.

We employed Wilk's GLRT as described to our renal cancer dataset in modelling development of new metastases. The results are shown in Table 9.3.

Thus, patient age, gender, T-Stage, N-Stage and cell histology were significant features to the computational model. That tumour state, nodal status, and cellular histology were significant features is not surprising. However, that neither previous lung or bone metastases predicted future metastases was quite interesting. Surgeons have treated renal cell carcinoma for decades as an exception to the rule that a metastasis precludes definitive surgical cure, resecting solitary lung metastases for example from patients with this tumour. This feature extraction experiment offers some evidence that the treatment option of resecting a solitary metastasis from a patient with renal cell carcinoma is a rational choice.

Table 9.3 Application of Wilk's GLRT for feature extraction. (* $p < 0.05$).

Variable Extracted	***p*-Value**
Ethnicity	1.000
Gender	0.009*
Age	< 0.001*
T-Stage	0.004*
N-Stage	0.007*
M-Stage	0.428
Nephrectomy	1.000
Age at surgery	1.000
Lung metastases	0.807
Bone metastases	1.000
Cell histology	< 0.001*
Tumour size	0.739
Treatment choice	1.000

III. PROSTATE CANCER

Prostate cancer (CaP) is the second leading cause of cancer death in men in the United States and a major cause of morbidity and health care expenditure [12]. Approximately 1.5 billion dollars were spent in 1997 for direct treatment of prostate cancer, while an additional 2.5 billion dollars went indirectly to its treatment [13]. Through the use of ANNs, attempts have been made at improving early diagnosis and staging, thus yielding cuts in the massive economic costs associated with the diagnosis and treatment of CaP. In addition, ANNs have been utilised to examine outcomes data and quality of life issues which are becoming increasingly important in the choice of treatment.

The characteristics of CaP in many cases not only make this disease difficult to treat but also difficult to study. The identification of "clinically significant" tumours has increased the complexity of screening for this disease, as no single investigative method is accurate in classifying a tumour that will progress from one, which will not [14]. Current clinical staging techniques understage CaP 40-60% of the time, demanding need for improvement in this area [15]. Additionally, due to CaP's inclination for slow growth and progression, studies that wish to describe the natural history and outcomes of treatment are required to study subjects over an extended period of time during which methods of diagnosis and treatment continue to change. Finally, definitions of end points in treatment such as cure or recurrence of disease continually change, making comparisons of studies an arduous task. These features make the careful study of CaP a challenge.

In 1994, Snow et al. published a pilot study which attempted to assess the accuracy of ANNs in screening for CaP, and to examine the networks ability to predict recurrence after radical prostatectomy [16]. This study used a back-propagation ANN from the Neuroshell 2 software package (Ward Systems Group, Inc., Fredrick, Maryland). The input data was extracted from a prostate specific antigen (PSA) screening data bank of 1787 men. The inputs for the first ANN were average age of patient, maximum PSA, average PSA over all visits, maximum digital rectal examination (DRE) over all visits, maximum transrectal ultrasound (TRUS) findings, and the square root of the absolute value of the change in PSA. Outputs simply consisted of biopsy result. The accuracy of this system at predicting biopsy result was 87% with a positive predictive value of 73-77%. This is significantly better than the reported accuracy of clinical judgement of 33% [17]. Inputs for the second ANN were age at operation, tumour stage (TNM), grade, preoperative potency, pre-operative PSA, and race. Output consisted of recurrence or no recurrence. The accuracy of this system at predicting tumour recurrence after radical prostatectomy was 90%.

Subsequent review of this published data by Barnhill et al. pointed out that after the initial test set no additional blind test sets were used on the systems, which may have biased their results [18]. In addition, length of follow-up in studies of outcomes in prostate cancer treatment is always a difficult question, just as it is in traditional statistics [2]. Due to the growth and progression characteristics of CaP, it is favourable to have follow-up times in excess of 10 years although this is not easily accomplished. This study collected data over a 5-year period.

In 1998, Tewari et al. published an economically minded paper proposing the use of ANNs to increase the accuracy of clinical staging of CaP in patients with clinically organ confined disease [15]. This study used a probabilistic neural network with a genetic adaptive algorithm to find individual and overall smoothing factors and a dataset of 1200 patients. The inputs for this model were race, DRE finding, size of tumour on ultrasound, PSA, biopsy Gleason score, and biopsy staging information (number of positive biopsies, bilateral cancer, and perineural invasion). Outputs were margin status, seminal vesicle involvement, and lymph node metastasis. The accuracy and area under the receiver operating characteristics (ROC) curve were 76.7% and 0.7940, 73.2% and 0.804, 72.6% and 0.768 for margins, seminal vesicle and lymph nodes, respectively. Of note, the negative predictive values were 92%, 100%, and 98% for margins, seminal vesicle, and lymph nodes, respectively. As the authors point out, such high negative predictive values may make such a model an important screening tool avoiding further costly staging procedures.

In 1997, Naguib et al. attempted to assess in a prospective manner the ability of a feed-forward ANN model to predict the outcome of patients undergoing nonsurgical treatment for CaP [14]. Forty-one men with histologically proven CaP served as the dataset. These patients underwent hormonal treatment, watchful waiting, or radiation. Follow-up ranged between 34-68 months. The inputs used were age, tumour stage (T1-T4), skeletal metastasis (M0-M1), Gleason score, PSA, and treatment (hormonal, external beam radiation, or watchful waiting), p53 protein accumulation, and bcl-2 protein overexpression. Outputs of the system were no response to treatment, relapse after treatment, or sustained response to treatment. Overall accuracy of the system was 80%. The system was compared to multiple discriminate analysis (MDA) which had an accuracy of 75% with the same input variables. The authors then serially omitted p53, bcl-2, and both p53 and bcl-2, retested the neural network system, and compared it to MDA to analyse the significance of the experimental markers p53 and bcl-2. The accuracy of the ANN was 70%, 65%, and 60%, respectively. In comparison, the accuracy of MDA was 65%, 60%, and 65%, respectively.

The ANN's prediction of outcomes in this study artfully exceeded the accuracy of MDA however, due to small numbers, short follow-up, and lack of definition of cure and relapse (i.e., biochemical, clinical, etc.), further study in this area is warranted. In addition, the increase in accuracy of the model when p53 and bcl-2 were used as input vectors revealed its ability to evaluate novel prognostic markers [14].

Krongrad et al., in 1997, published a study that attempted to predict the general quality of life (QoL) in patients with benign prostatic hypertrophy (BPH) and CaP [18]. The investigators used a feedforward, back-propagation ANN that evaluated 55 inputs made up of 17 items from the Rand Mental Health Index and additional items chosen by a focus group consisting of medical and allied professionals with backgrounds in urology, geriatrics, sociology, nursing, radiation oncology, statistics and psychology. Using these inputs, classification of QoL was performed by the neural network using a population of VA patients with documented BPH or CaP at 1 and 6 months. These results were then compared to the logistical regression. The overall accuracy, sensitivity and specificity of the ANN at 1 and 6 months were 89%, 89%, 89%, 90%, 94%, and 85%, respectively. In comparison, the overall accuracy of logistical regression at 1 and 6 months were 84% and 88%, respectively. Post-hoc statistical analysis of the ANN revealed four significant disease nonspecific variables at 1 month. These were judgement of health, satisfaction with medical care, retirement status, and the ability to make meals or perform minor housework. No single input was found significant at 6 months.

This study demonstrated the ability of ANNs to classify patients and to identify significant (heavily weighted) input vectors, which in this case influence patient's QoL. Knowledge of these factors can allow clinicians to focus on the most significant QoL issues in caring for their patients. As the authors point out however, study population is not a random sample and thus limits the model's ability to generalise [19, 20].

In 1996, Stamey et al. published data on the ProstAsure™ Index (PI) (Horus Global HealthNet, Hilton Head Island, South Carolina). The initial data on this subject was soon followed by a number of follow-up articles also looking at its utility in CaP. The PI is an ANN originally designed to predict the presence of BPH and CaP in men older than 50 years of age [21]. This network had six input vectors: age, PSA, PAP, CK-MM, CK-MB, and CK-BB. The training and test sets consisted of men with normal DRE and PSA less than or equal to four, patients with BPH and any PSA, and patients with untreated CaP at varying stages. The system output was simply presence or absence of CaP or BPH. The model's sensitivity and specificity for detection of CaP retrospectively was 81% and 92%, respectively, while the sensitivity for the detection of BPH was 63%.

The favourable result of this model led to a number of publications examining the use of PI as a clinical investigative tool. Stamey et al. followed their initial findings up with a publication in 1997 looking at the ability of the PI to diagnose CaP retrospectively in a population of men age 40-80 with a normal DRE and a PSA less than four [22]. The training and test population consisted of three groups. The first group was made up of men with pathologically confirmed CaP, the second was a group of normal men, and the third group contained men with BPH only. The sensitivity and specificity of this model in the detection of CaP in this population was 71% and 86%, respectively. This study, although retrospective, demonstrates well the potential usefulness of PI in screening this population of men with CaP who are not selected for biopsy with traditional screening.

Barnhill et al. published a study in 1997 attempting to examine the efficacy of PI in the diagnosis of low volume CaP [23]. This study looked at 403 patient status post-radical prostatectomy stratified according to volume of disease. The PI had an overall sensitivity of 95% in identifying the patients as having CaP regardless of tumour volume. In the same publication, the ability of PI to predict stage in a population of men with CaP and a PSA less than or equal to four was studied. The PI values in each group, stratified by stage, were not significantly different [24].

In 1998, the same group compared the ability of PI and percent free PSA ability to reliably predict a CaP diagnosis in a population consisting of three groups of men [25]. The first two groups both had a PSA less than or equal to four. Group 1 consisted of normal men, Group 2 was made up of men with BPH, and Group 3 consisted of men with clinically localised CaP. The PI model analysis of these groups resulted in a sensitivity, specificity and area under the ROC curve of 93%, 81%, and 0.9454 with a deviation of 0.0181, respectively. The percent free PSA sensitivity, specificity and area under the ROC curve at a cutoff of 15% were 80%, 74%, and 0.864, with a deviation of 0.0254, respectively. When the free PSA cutoff was raised to 19% to increase the sensitivity to 93%, the specificity decreased to 59%. Further increases in free PSA to 25% increased the sensitivity to 100%, but sacrificed specificity to a value of 39%. This retrospective study suggests that PI may perform better as a diagnostic tool when compared to free PSA in this population.

As prostate cancer methods of diagnosis, treatment, and screening continue to change, ANNs will prove to be a useful adjunct to our current clinical tools. Although few prospective randomised studies have been published in this area, current studies show great promise for the utility of this instrument in the treatment, diagnosis, and screening of the patient with prostate cancer.

IV. BLADDER CANCER

The American Cancer Society estimated that 54,400 people had been diagnosed with bladder cancer and 12,500 people died of the disease in 1998 alone [26]. About 50-75% of patients diagnosed with transitional cell carcinoma (TCC) have superficial disease; of these, only 15-25% will progress [27]. The remaining 25% of newly diagnosed bladder cancers are invasive and roughly half of these patients have metastasis at diagnosis [28,29].

Treatment of this disease is based on T-Stage and grade. The main stay of treatment of superficial disease consists of transurethral resection with or without intravesical chemotherapy depending on grade [30]. The treatment for locally invasive carcinoma is cystectomy [30]. The importance of early detection and surveillance is paramount, as although cystectomy is rare in patients with low T-Stage and grade cancer, it can be life-saving in higher stage and grade tumours.

The need for more accurate and less invasive surveillance and screening tests is warranted. Recently, a number of assays targeted toward bladder tumour antigen (BTA) have arisen out of the desire to avoid cystoscopy in surveillance and in the attempt to detect TCC with improved sensitivity and specificity when compared to the "gold standard" cytology [30]. However, these tests (BTA, BTAstat, and BTAtrak) have limited sensitivity to low-grade TCC and are inferior to cytology in the detection of high-grade TCC [31]. Another non-invasive diagnostic test that may hold more promise is the nuclear matrix protein 22; however, this test is still experimental at this time [32].

Relatively little use of ANNs has to date been applied to the diagnosis, treatment and screening of bladder cancer. One front on which the use of neural networks is being investigated is their use in automated cytology.

Hurst et al. tested a feed-forward neural network in the recognition of patterns of fluorescence using the M344 monoclonal antibody to the p300 tumour-related antigen in bladder cancer [33]. In this study, the ANN's ability to differentiate true-positive cells from negative cells, false-positive cells, and cell sized artefacts was almost identical to that of human experts at high-power magnification (50X). The ANN was also tested at low-power magnification (12.5X) resulting in a 75% correlation when compared to human experts. Data was analysed using confusion matrices.

Pantazopoulos et al. examined two unique ANNs' ability to make a diagnosis from urine cytology [34]. The study compared a back-propagation ANN to a learning vector quantiser model. Each model had 24 inputs: 5 size descriptors, 6 shape descriptors, 1 density descriptor, and 12 texture descriptors. Six outputs were used: lithiasis, inflammation, BPH, carcinoma *in situ*, grade I, grade II, or grade III TCC. The models were initially tested on randomly selected cells and then on patient cases. The accuracy of the systems using randomly selected cells was 90.5%, while their accuracy when examining cases was 97%, and they were not significantly different from one another.

The favourable results of these studies clearly show a role for ANNs in the cytological diagnosis of bladder cancer in the urologic patient. Investigation of ANNs in this area of urologic oncology, however, is still in its infancy.

V. TESTICULAR CARCINOMA

In the United States, 7,200 new cases of germ-cell carcinoma were diagnosed in 1997 in male patients between the ages of 15 and 34 [35]. Treatment of this disease is guided by histological type of cancer and clinical staging. Great progress has been made in the area of treatment of testicular carcinoma in the last 20 years making the prognosis of these patients very good [36]. This, in great part, is due to the use of cisplatin containing chemotherapy used to cure advanced testicular germ-cell carcinoma. Staging of testis cancer includes serum markers (alpha-fetoprotein, human chorionic gonodotrophin and lactate dehydrogenase), computed tomographic (CT) imaging of the abdomen and pelvis, and a chest X-ray film [37]. Retroperitoneal lymph node dissection (RPLND) is used in select patients depending on histology and clinical stage.

Controversy currently exists concerning the use of RPLND in stage I testis cancer seminomatous and nonseminomatous. 17% and 30% of patients with seminoma and nonseminoma who are placed on observation after radical orchiectomy are expected to have occult retroperitoneal metastasis, respectively [36]. By virtue of this low rate of metastasis at stage I and the risk of surgical complications, some clinicians have opted for observation as an alternative to aggressive surgical staging/treatment.

Moul et al. in 1995 used an ANN to analyse four histological factors to compare the accuracy of this model in the staging of patients with clinical stage I nonseminomatous testicular germ cell tumour (NSGCT) to traditional staging [36]. This group also compared the relative accuracy of a commercially available software package in the hands of an inexperienced user and a custom back-propagation ANN devised by an experienced researcher in neural computation. The population consisted of 93 clinical stage I NSGCT patients, all of whom had undergone RPLND and follow-up to determine true stage. The histological input vectors were vascular invasion, lymphatic invasion, tunical invasion, and quantitative determination of percentage of the primary tumour (i.e., percent embryonal carcinoma, yolk sac carcinoma, teratoma, and seminoma). The accuracy of the expert system was 92% with a sensitivity and specificity of 88% and 96%, respectively, while the accuracy, sensitivity, and specificity of the commercial software package was 79%, 71%, and 81.8%, respectively.

This interesting comparison of two neural network models, while demonstrating their high accuracy and potential use in staging, also demonstrated a wide variation of results. The variation of results between networks in this study underscores the importance of careful construction of the network by an experienced researcher.

VI. CONCLUSION

Research assessing the usefulness of neural networks in urologic oncology, although in its infancy, has demonstrated high accuracy in assessing characteristics of nonlinear datasets, identifying patterns, and generalising what it has "learned" to new datasets. As most medical data is nonlinear in character, it is not surprising that this model, in many cases, outperforms traditional linear analysis. In fact, many of the ANNs examined in current studies compare very favourably and many times exceed the accuracy of traditional multivariate analysis. Not all ANNs are equal, however, and as Moul et al. have shown, may vary widely in accuracy depending on the construction of the network and the software used. Randomised prospective studies are still needed to really identify the efficacy of these models in the clinical setting, but preliminary data is very promising.

REFERENCES

1. **Niederberger C.,** This month in investigative urology — commentary on the use of neural networks in clinical urology, *J. Urol.*, 153, 1362, 1995.
2. **Kattan M., Cowen M., Miles B.,** Computer modelling in urology, *Urology*, 47, 1, 14-21, 1996.
3. **Tewari A.,** Artificial intelligence and neural networks: concept, applications, and future in urology, *Br. J. Urol.*, 80, suppl. 3, 53-58, 1997.
4. **Bono A., Lovisolo J.,** Renal cell carcinoma-diagnosis and treatment: state of the art, *Eur. Urol.*, 31, suppl. 1, 47-55, 1997.
5. **Maclin P., Dempsey J., Brooks J., Rand J.,** Using neural networks to diagnose cancer, *J. Med. Sys.*, 15, 1, 11-17, 1991.
6. **Kavolius J., Mastorakos D., Pavlovish C., Russo P., Burt M., Brady M.,** Resection of metastatic renal cell carcinoma, *J. Clin. Oncol.*, 16, 6, 2261-2266, 1998.
7. **Lokich J.,** Spontaneous regression of metastatic renal cancer — case report and literature review, *Am. J. Clin. Oncol.*, 20, 4, 416-418, 1997.
8. **Chang P., Li Y., Wu C., Huang M., Haug P.,** Clinical evaluation of a renal mass diagnostic expert system, *Comput. Biol. Med.*, 24, 4, 315-322, 1994.
9. **Qin Y., Lamb D.J., Golden R.M., Niederberger C.,** A neural network predicts mortality and new metastases in patients with renal cell cancer, Proc. World Congress on Computational Medicine, Public Health and Biotechnology — Building a Man in the Machine, Pt. III, Series in Mathematical Biology and Medicine, 5, 1325-1334, 1994.
10. **Niederberger C.S., Pursell S., Golden R.M.,** A neural network to predict lifespan and new metastases in patients with renal cell cancer, in *Handbook of Neural Computation*, (Eds. Fiesler E., Beale R.), IOP Publishing and Oxford University Press, Oxford, G5.4, 1-6, 1997.
11. **Golden R.M.,** *Mathematical Methods for Neural Network Analysis and Design*, MIT Press, Cambridge, Massachusetts, 1996.
12. **Boring C., Squires T., Tong T.,** Cancer statistics, *Cancer*, 43, 7, 1993.
13. **Parker S., Tong T., Bolden S., Wingo P.,** Cancer statistics, *Cancer*, 47, 5, 1997.
14. **Naguib R., Robinson M., Neal D., Hamdy F.,** Neural network analysis of combined conventional and experimental prognostic markers in prostate cancer: a pilot study, *Br. J. Cancer*, 78, 2, 246-250, 1998.
15. **Tewari A., Narayani P.,** Novel staging tool for localized prostate cancer: a pilot study using genetic adaptive neural networks, *J. Urol.*, 160, 430-436, 1998.
16. **Snow P., Smith D., Catalona W.,** Artificial neural networks in the diagnosis and prognosis of prostate cancer: a pilot study, *J. Urol.*, 152, 1923-1926, 1994.
17. **Catalona W., Smith D., Ratliff T., Basler J.,** Detection of organ-confined prostate cancer is increased through prostate-specific antigen-based screening, *J. Am. Med. Assoc.*, 270, 948, 1993.
18. **Krongrad A., Granville L., Burke M., Golden R., Lai S., Cho L., Niederberger C.,** Predictors of general quality of life in patients with benign prostatic hyperplasia of prostate cancer, *J. Urol.*, 157, 534-538, 1997.
19. **Cross S., Harrison R., Kennedy R.,** Introduction to neural networks, *The Lancet*, 346, 1075-1079, 1995.
20. **Wei J., Zhang Z., Barnhill S., Madyastha K., Zhang H., Oesterling J.,** Understanding artificial neural networks and exploring their potential applications for the practising urologist, *Urology*, 52, 2, 161-172, 1998.
21. **Stamey T., Barnhill S., Zhang Z., Madyastha K., Pretiyiacomo A., Jones K., Chan D.,** Effectiveness of ProstAsure™ in detecting prostate cancer (PCa) and benign prostatic hyperplasia (BPH) in men age 50 and older, *J. Urol.*, 155, suppl., 436A, 1996.

22. **Stamey T., Barnhill S., Zhang Z., Madyastha K., Zhang H.,** A neural network (ProstAsure™) with high sensitivity and specificity for diagnosing prostate cancer (PCa) in men with PSA < 4.0ng/ml, *J. Urol.*, 157, 4, 364, 1997.
23. **Barnhill S., Stamey T., Zhang Z., Zhang H., Madyastha K.,** The ability of the ProstAsure™ index to identify prostate cancer patients with low cancer volume and high potential for cure, *J. Urol.,* 157, 4, 63, 1997.
24. **Barnhill S., Zhang Z., Madyastha K., Zhang H.,** The ProstAsure™ index is useful in the diagnosis of early prostate cancer but does not predict pathologic state in men with serum PSA level less than 4.0 ng/ml, *J. Urol.*, 157, 4, 462, 1997.
25. **Babaian R., Fritsche H., Zhang Z., Zhang H., Madyastha K., Barnhill S.,** Evaluation of ProstAsure index in the detection of prostate cancer: a preliminary report, *Urology*, 51, 1, 132-136, 1998.
26. **Landis S., Murray T., Bolden S., et al.,** Cancer statistics, 1998, *CA Cancer J. Clin.*, 48, 6-29, 1998.
27. **Heney N., Ahmed S., Flannagan M., et al.,** Superficial bladder cancer: progression and recurrence, *J. Urol.*, 130, 1083-1086, 1983.
28. **Kaye K., Lange P.,** Mode of presentation of invasive bladder cancer: reassessment of the problem, *J. Urol.*, 128, 31-33, 1982.
29. **Prout Jr G., Griffin P., Shipley W.,** Bladder carcinoma as a systemic disease, *Cancer*, 43, 2532-2539, 1979.
30. **Droller M.,** Bladder cancer: state-of-the-art care, *CA Cancer J. Clin.*, 48, 5, 269-284, 1998.
31. **Droller M., et al.,** Commentary on improved detection of recurrent bladder cancer using the Bard BTA test, *J. Urol.*, 159, 601, 1998.
32. **Stampfer D., Carpinito G., Rodriguez-Villanueva J., et al.,** Evaluation of NMP22 in the detection of transitional cell carcinoma of the bladder, *J. Urol.*, 159, 394, 1998.
33. **Hurst R., Bonner R., Ashenagi K., Veltri R., Hemstreet III G.,** Neural net-based identification of cells expressing the p300 tumour-related antigen using fluorescence image analysis, *Cytometry*, 27, 36-42, 1997.
34. **Pantazopoulos D., Karakitsos P., Iokim-Liossi A., Pouliakis A., Dimopoulos K.,** Comparing neural networks in the discrimination of benign from malignant lower urinary tract lesions, *Br. J. Urol.*, 81, 574-579, 1998.
35. **Devasa S., Blot W., Stone B., Miller B., Tarone R., Fraumeni Jr. J.,** Recent cancer trends in the United States, *J. Natl. Cancer Inst.*, 87, 175-182, 1995.
36. **Moul J., Snow P., Fernandez E., Maher P., Sesterhenn I.,** Neural network analysis of quantitative histological factors to predict pathological stage in clinical stage I nonseminomatous testicular cancer, *J. Urol.*, 153, 1674-1677, 1995.
37. **Bosl G., Motzer R.,** Testicular germ-cell cancer, *N. Eng. J. Med.,* 337, 4, 242-253, 1997.

Chapter 10

COMPARISON OF A NEURAL NETWORK WITH HIGH SENSITIVITY AND SPECIFICITY TO FREE/TOTAL SERUM PSA FOR DIAGNOSING PROSTATE CANCER IN MEN WITH A PSA < 4.0 ng/mL

T.A. Stamey, S.D. Barnhill, Z. Zhang, C.M. Yemoto, H. Zhang, and K.R. Madyastha

I. INTRODUCTION

We reported in 1996 on the first successful artificial neural network (ANN) for distinguishing men with palpable cancers from healthy volunteers with prostates that felt normal [1]. We also were able to distinguish volunteer men with normal-feeling benign prostatic hyperplasia (BPH) regardless of the level of their serum prostate specific antigen PSA. This ANN (ProstAsure™) utilises six input variables: age, serum PSA, prostatic acid phosphatase (PAP), and three creatine kinase (CK) isoenzymes (CK-BB, CK-MB, and CK-MM) to produce an age-normalised, continuous single-values ProstAsure™ Index (PI). Details of the training and testing set of serums have been reported [1]; importantly, all of the men with palpably normal prostates on digital rectal examination (DRE) had a PSA < 4.0 ng/mL, and only 24% of the men with BPH had a PSA ≥ 4.0 ng/mL. Using a PI cutoff of 1.0, we achieved an overall sensitivity and specificity of 81% and 92%, respectively, for recognising palpable cancers. The sensitivity for detecting BPH in volunteer, healthy men with an enlarged prostate on DRE was 63%, with lower and upper PI cutoff values chosen at 0.0 and 1.0, respectively [1].

According to the 1993 national screening survey of 33,000 volunteer men 40 to 80 years old, 91% had a PSA ≤ 4.0 ng/mL [2]. In a single institutional experience based on 17,258 men with a PSA ≤ 4.0 ng/mL, 8.3% had a suspicious finding on DRE. Of these, only 10.6% had positive results on systematic biopsies, for an overall detection rate of 152/17,258 or < 1% [3]. A multiple institutional study of 6,630 men showed a similar cancer detection rate of 0.8% for men with a PSA ≤ 4.0 ng/mL [4]. However, in this study, the cancer detection rate for men with a PSA > 4.0 ng/mL was six times higher (4.6%) [4].

These cancer detection rates strongly suggest the need for better techniques than DRE alone to screen men with a PSA ≤ 4.0 ng/mL for prostate cancer, especially since we know that radical prostatectomies in these men have highly favourable characteristics [5]. With this background, we have determined the PI in 457 untreated men who had a serum PSA < 4.0 mg/mL, including 97 who had prostate cancer, and compared the true positive rates and false positive rates in receiver-operating characteristic (ROC) curves at various test cutoff values for PI and the ratio of serum PSA. The focus of this chapter is to treat PI as a composite index of serum tests and to compare it with free/total PSA using an independent test data set.

0-8493-9692-1/01/$0.00+$1.50

II. MATERIAL AND METHODS

A. PATIENT SELECTION

Three groups of men with serum PSA < 4.0 ng/mL were selected. The first group was selected from the first 425 men treated only by radical prostatectomy at Stanford University for clinical stage T1c-T2 cancers, of whom 97 (23%) had a *pre-operative* PSA < 4.0 ng/mL. The second group comprised 224 consecutive healthy volunteers attending the 1991 Stanford screening survey whose prostates were considered to be of normal size and consistency when they were examined in the knee-chest position by senior urologic faculty. The third group comprised 136 men from the same screening survey who had an enlarged, symmetrical, soft prostate on DRE. None of these 425 men were involved in the original development of the PI algorithm.

B. LABORATORY ANALYSIS

All sera were collected before DRE, treatment, and biopsy. The sera were stored at -70°C and thawed only once before being analysed for PSA, PAP, and isoenzymes CK-BB, CK-MB, and CK-MM. Laboratory analyses of the serum specimens related to the PI were performed at the clinical chemistry laboratory of the Johns Hopkins Hospital, Baltimore, Maryland. Results of PSA and PAP were determined by using the AIA-PACK (PSA) and AIA-PACK (PAP) test kits manufactured by Tosoh Medics, Inc., Foster City, California, using an AIA-1200 fully automated immunoassay analyser. The ratio of free/total serum PSA was determined at the Department of Urology at Stanford using the Tosoh assay for total serum PSA and the Diagnostic Products Corporation (Los Angeles, California) assay for free PSA.

The CK isoenzymes were separated by electrophoresis using a Cardio Rep CKI Isoenzyme procedure (Helena Laboratories, Inc., Beaumont, Texas). Although all the PI data in this chapter are based on the three isoenzymes of CK, further experience with the PI has shown that total CK is a perfect substitute for assaying the isoenzymes. Total CK seems to play an important role in detecting prostate cancer with a low serum PSA and, interestingly, the lower the total CK the greater the probability of prostate cancer in the ANN.

To eliminate unintentional bias, patient identifications and known diagnoses were blinded during all laboratory analyses, including the computation of the ProstAsure™ Indices.

C. NEURAL NETWORK INPUTS AND DERIVATION OF THE PI

We use the results of the five serum tests: PSA, PAP, and CK isoenzymes and the patient's age as input values to produce an age-normalised, continuous, single-valued PI. Patients are then classified into four diagnostic groups: normal (PI ≤ 0.0), BPH (PI 0.01–0.5), BPH suspicious for cancer (PI 0.51–1.00), and cancer (PI > 1.00). Patients in the suspicious and cancer categories, in general, are recommended to have transrectal ultrasound-guided systematic biopsies of their prostate including the transition-BPH zone.

III. RESULTS

As shown in Figure 10.1*, the peak incidence for the 97 men with prostate cancer was in the 61–70 year age range, while that for men with normal-feeling prostates was two decades earlier. The distribution of cancers in the four clinical stages among the three categories of serum PSA < 4 ng/mL is shown in Table 10.1. Note that 75% of the cancers were associated with PSA values between 2.0 and 3.9 ng/mL.

---

*Chapter 10, Colour Figure 1 follows page 136.

Since the two primary determinants of failure of radical prostatectomy are cancer volume and the percentage of Gleason grade 4 of the largest index cancer (submitted for publication), the distribution of these two determinants in the three PSA ranges are shown in Tables 10.2 and 10.3. There appears to be no difference in cancer volumes in the PSA ranges of 2.0–2.9 ng/mL (n = 39) and 3.0–3.9 ng/mL (n = 34). As expected, Gleason grade 4/5 cancer — the primary determinant of serum PSA [6,7] — increases with each increase in serum PSA (Table 10.3). The index cancer volumes in Table 10.2 show that most of these cancers were clinically significant, i.e., 0.5 cc or greater [8].

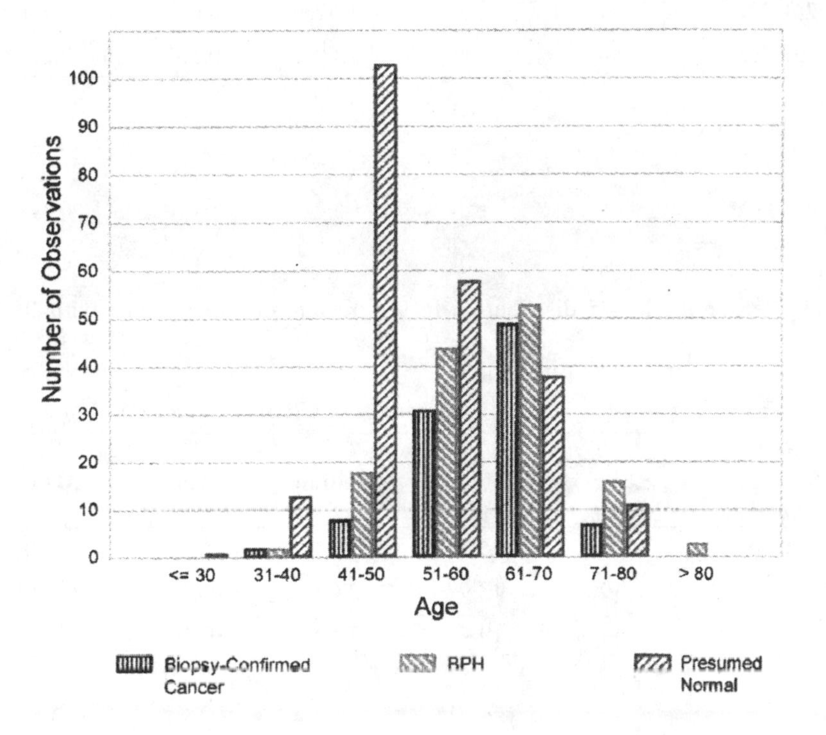

Figure 10.1 Age distribution of 457 test cases with a PSA < 4.0 ng/mL.

Table 10.1 Distribution of 97 cancers with PSA < 4.0 ng/mL according to clinical stage and level of PSA.

PSA (ng/mL)	T1c *n* (%)	T2a *n* (%)	T2b *n* (%)	T2c *n* (%)	Total *n* (%)
0.0–1.9	2 (7)	12 (34)	6 (32)	1 (14)	24 (25)
2.0–2.9	13 (48)	17 (39)	6 (32)	3 (43)	39 (40)
3.0–3.9	12 (44)	12 (27)	7 (37)	3 (43)	34 (35)
Total	**27 (28)**	**44 (45)**	**19 (20)**	**7 (7)**	**97 (100)**

Table 10.2 Cancer volume in 97 prostate patients with PSA < 4.0 ng/mL.

PSA (ng/mL) Range	*n*	*Index Tumour Volume*[†]			
		Mean	**Median**	**Min**	**Max**
0.0–1.9	24	0.97	0.89	0.07	4.33
2.0–2.9	39	2.14	1.57	0.01	11.60
3.0–3.9	34	1.99	1.50	0.35	9.80

[†]Volume of the largest cancer.

Table 10.3 Gleason grade 4/5 distribution in 97 prostate cancer patients with PSA < 4.0 ng/mL.

PSA (ng/mL) Range	*n*	*Percentage of Gleason Grade 4/5 Cancer*			
		Mean	**Median**	**Min**	**Max**
0.0–1.9	24	5.79	0.00	0.00	60.00
2.0–2.9	39	12.97	2.00	0.00	70.00
3.0–3.9	34	19.44	7.50	0.00	90.00

The distribution of the 457 men among the four diagnostic PI zones is shown in Figure 10.2*. The increase in cancer from 3.7% in Zone 1 to 77.1% in Zone 4 contrasts with that in the 224 men with normal-feeling prostates, which decreases from 79% in Zone 1 to 4.2% in Zone 4. The ever-confounding presence of men with BPH, especially in Zones 2 and 3, indicates the diagnostic importance of this group, especially in Zones 3 and 4, which require biopsy of the prostate. Further information on the distribution of the PI zones for the 97 men with cancers is shown in Table 10.4 for the three PSA ranges and in Table 10.5 for the four clinical stages. Table 6 shows the percentage distribution of each of the three diagnostic categories within the four PI zones. Twenty-five of 97 cancers (25.8%) would have been missed, while only 29/224 (13%) normal-feeling prostates would have required biopsy. Fifty-six of 136 (41.2%) men with BPH would have required biopsy (Zones 3 and 4). The overall sensitivity and specificity in these 457 men was 74.2% and 76.4%.

*Chapter 10, Colour Figure 2 follows page 136.

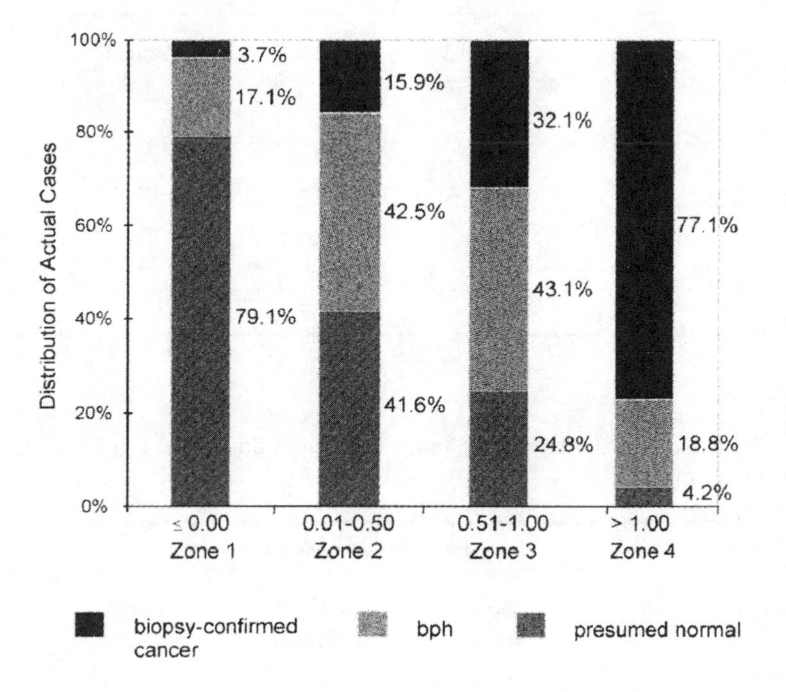

Figure 10.2 Distribution of ProstAsure™ index zones and diagnostic groups of 457 test cases with a PSA < 4.0 ng/mL.

Table 10.4 ProstAsure™ index zones in 97 prostate cancer patients with PSA < 4.0 ng/mL.

		ProstAsure™ Index Zones			
PSA (ng/mL) Range	***n***	**Zone 1 ≤ 0.00**	**Zone 2 0.01-0.50**	**Zone 3 0.51-1.00**	**Zone 4 > 1.00**
0.0–1.9	24	6 (25.0%)	6 (25.0%)	8 (33.3%)	4 (16.7%)
2.0–2.9	39	1 (2.6%)	6 (15.4%)	17 (43.6%)	15 (38.4%)
3.0–3.9	34	0 (0.0%)	6 (17.7%)	10 (29.4%)	18 (52.9%)

Table 10.5 Distribution of cancer stages and ProstAsure™ index zones in 97 prostate cancer patients with PSA < 4.0 ng/mL.

Prostate Cancer Stage	*ProstAsure™ Index Zones*				
	Zone 1 ≤ 0.00	**Zone 2 0.01-0.50**	**Zone 3 0.51-1.00**	**Zone 4 > 1.00**	**Totals**
T1c	1	5	8	13	27
T2a	5	9	12	18	44
T2b	1	3	11	4	19
T2c	0	1	4	2	7
All Groups	**7**	**18**	**35**	**37**	**97**

Table 10.6 Distribution of ProstAsure™ index zones and diagnostic groups in 457 test cases with PSA < 4.0 ng/mL.

Diagnostic Groups	*ProstAsure™ Index Zones*				
	Zone 1 ≤ 0.00	**Zone 2 0.01-0.50**	**Zone 3 0.51-1.00**	**Zone 4 > 1.00**	**Totals**
Biopsy-Confirmed Cancer	**7 (7.2%)**	**18 (18.6%)**	35 (36.1%)	37 (38.1%)	97 (100.0%)
BPH	32 (23.5%)	48 (35.3%)	47 (34.6%)	9 (6.6%)	136 (100.0%)
Presumed Normal	148 (66.1%)	47 (21.0%)	**27 (12.1%)**	**2 (0.9%)**	224 (100.0%)
All Groups	**187**	**113**	**109**	**48**	**457**

Sensitivity = 74.2%   Specificity = 76.4%

As seen in Figure 10.3*, a free/total PSA ratio of ≤ 0.27 includes all but 5 of the 97 cancers (sensitivity of 95%); however, it also includes 270 of the 360 BPH and normal cases for a specificity of 25%. A PI ≥ 0.5 is clearly superior to a free/total PSA ratio of 0.27 in diagnosing prostate cancer, but free/total PSA and PI together are better than either one alone (observe the concentration of cancers in the rectangle bounded by a PI ≥ 0.5 and a free/total PSA of 0.27).

*Chapter 10, Colour Figure 3 follows page 136.

The plot of the estimated ROC curves (CLABROL, Macintosh Version, C.E. Metz, Department of Radiology, The University of Chicago) for the true positive rate (sensitivity) vs. the false positive rate (1 – specificity) is shown in Figure 10.4*. At a 90% sensitivity, the specificity (1 — false positive rate) for free/total PSA is 38%, precisely in the range of many other reported studies on free/total PSA. However, the specificity for the PI index at 90% sensitivity is 57% ($p = 0.0007$ for differences in the area under the two curves in Figure 10.4).

There is a concern about whether cancers detected with a PSA < 4 ng/mL are too small to treat. Of the 97 cancers, 13 (13.4%) were apparently clinically insignificant based on our definition of cancers less than 0.5 cc in volume [8]. Of the 24 cancers in the PSA range of 0–1.9 ng/mL (Table 10.1), 7 (29%) were less than 0.5 cc in cancer volume; five of these seven had no Gleason grade 4/5 cancer. Thus at least five (21%) of the 24 cancers detected in the lowest PSA range were of no clinical significance (small volume, no grade 4). Of the remaining six cancers less than 0.5 cc in volume, four were in the PSA range of 2.0–2.9 ng/mL and two were in the 3.0–4.0 ng/mL range; three of the six contained some Gleason grade 4 cancer (2%, 10%, and 75%).

Of these 13 small cancers, five were in PI Zones 3 and 4. The free/total PSA ranged from 5% to 31% (median 17%, mean 16.5%) in these 13 cancers. The median and mean ages of these 13 men were 62 and 58 years old, respectively.

Interestingly, all seven cancers in the 0–1.9 ng/mL range of PSA were T2a clinically, while all but one of the six cancers in the two higher PSA ranges were T1c tumours.

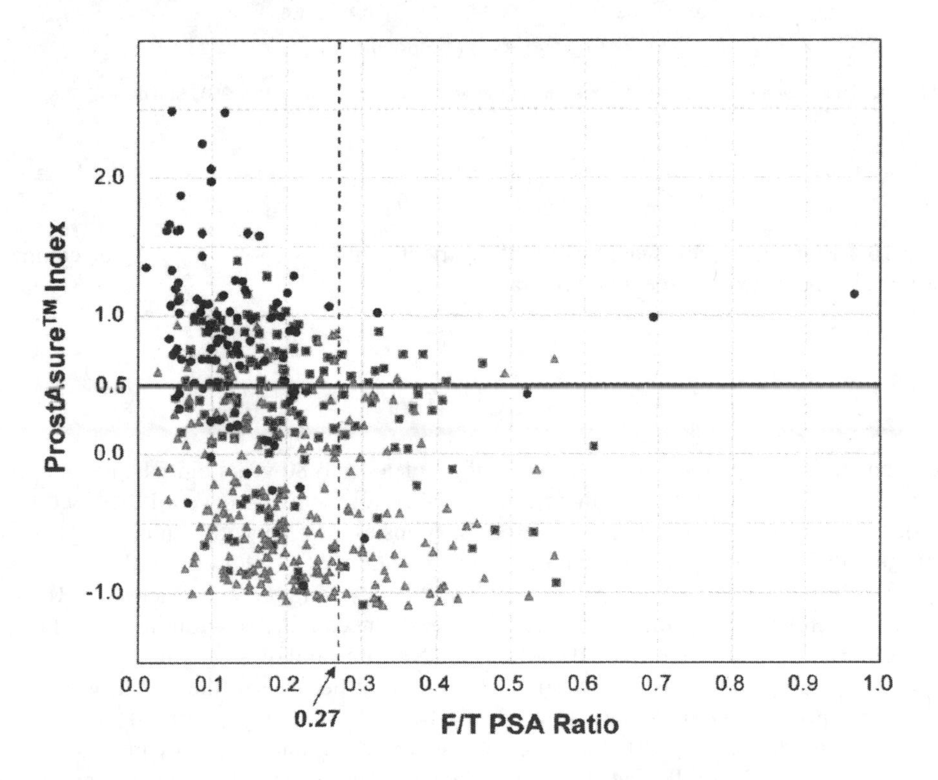

Figure 10.3 Scatterplot of 457 patients with a PSA < 4.0 ng/mL, comparing ProstAsure™ index against free/total PSA ratio.

* Chapter 10, Colour Figure 4 follows page 136.

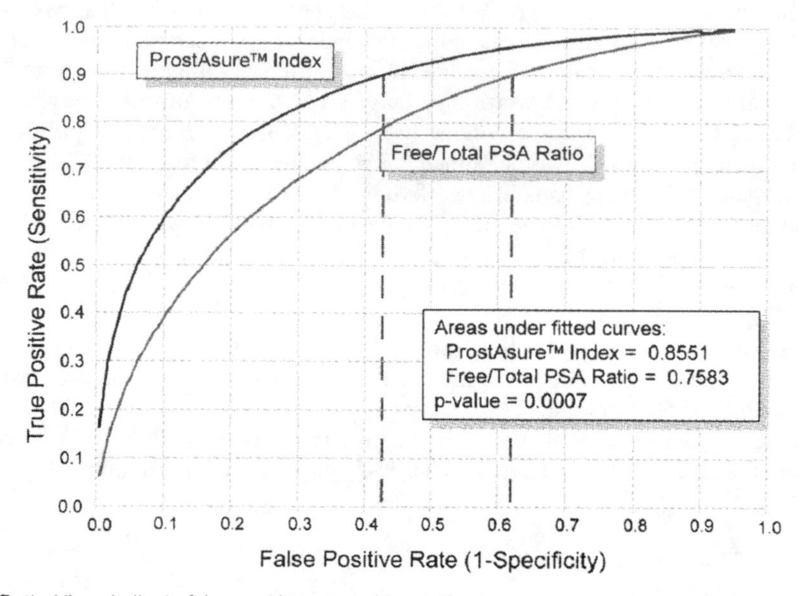

Figure 10.4 ROC curves estimated using 457 patients with PSA < 4.0 ng/mL for comparing ProstAsure™ index against free/total PSA ratio.

IV. COMMENT

Current cancer detection rates in the 90% of all men 40 to 80 years old who have a PSA < 4.0 ng/mL are a fraction (0.8%) of those in the 10% of all men who have a PSA > 4.0 ng/mL (4.6%). The detection rate of 0.8% is based on biopsies in men with a positive DRE who constitute only 8 to 10% of all men with a PSA < 4.0 ng/mL [3,4]. Fowler et al. have recently shown that the cancer detection rate in men with a PSA < 4.0 ng/mL and a normal DRE is one fifth that of men with an abnormal DRE [9]. We clearly need a better serum test to detect men with prostate cancer before it crosses the abnormal PSA threshold of 4.0 ng/mL.

The ProstAsure™ ANN is ideally suited for this task because of the way it was trained. The training process included sera from men who had a soft, symmetrical, normal-sized prostate on DRE during the 1991 PSA screening survey of volunteer healthy men; all of these sera had a PSA < 2.8 ng/mL. The BPH group included men with soft, symmetrical, enlarged prostates on DRE, only 24% of whom had a PSA > 4.0 ng/mL. These controls, therefore, are ideally suited for screening the 90% of all men aged 40 to 80 years with a PSA < 4.0 ng/mL. Moreover, among the cancers used to train the ANN, 76% were T1b and T2 cancers, and most of the T2 cancers were T2a on DRE. We have shown that T2a cancers are similar to T1c cancers in tumour volume and percentage Gleason grade 4/5 cancer [10].

In our original clinical study of 416 men, 193 of whom had prostate cancer, the PI results showed excellent agreement with confirmed cancer and our BPH and normal prostate diagnoses (Kappa statistic = 0.602 ± 0.002) [1]. The PI also demonstrated superiority over diagnoses by PSA alone in ROC curve analysis (PI area under curve of 0.8476 vs. PSA area of 0.7602; $p = 0.0018$). In this chapter, we demonstrate the effectiveness of PI in 457 men with a PSA < 4.0 ng/mL and compare this effectiveness to that of free/total serum PSA. The ROC curves in Figure 10.4 clearly show the superiority of PI over free/total serum PSA; at a 90% sensitivity, the specificity for PI is 57% compared with 38% for free/total serum PSA ($p = 0.0007$). The 38% specificity is well within the range reported for free/total PSA in men with serum PSA > 4.0 ng/mL using other free PSA assays in our laboratories [11,12].

Table 1 shows no advantage to lowering the PSA cutoff from 4.0 to 3.0 ng/mL, as used in the new European cooperative studies [13], because there are just as many cancers in the 2.0-3.0 ng/mL range. Moreover, 25% of the cancers in Table 10.1 were associated with PSA < 2.0 ng/mL. Nevertheless, since this ANN was trained with men with normal prostates and serum PSA < 2.8 ng/mL and men with BPH in whom 76% had a PSA < 4.0 ng/mL, it is likely that the PI will be most useful in men with a serum PSA between 2.0 and 6.0 ng/mL. This has the epidemiologic cost advantage of avoiding the 70% of all men who have a serum PSA < 2.0 ng/mL [2], as well as the 29% (7/24) of men with PSA < 2.0 ng/mL who had cancers < 0.5 cc in volume.

Catalona et al. have recently recommended screening men with a serum PSA of 2.6–4.0 ng/mL with free/total PSA [14]. They biopsied 332 men with a PSA in this range who had benign prostates on DRE; 73 (22%) biopsies were positive for cancer. Using a free/total PSA cutoff of 27%, they detected 90% of the cancers but would have avoided only 18% (specificity) of the 259 benign biopsies. This limited specificity does not compare with the 76.4% specificity of the PI, which includes all men with a PSA < 4.0 ng/mL, not just those with a serum PSA of 2.5–4.0 ng/mL.

The role of CK as a tumour marker is limited to the CK-BB isoenzyme. It is overexpressed in 95% of the cytosols of breast cancer and elevated in the serum of 50% of men with active prostate cancer who have serum PSA > 20 ng/mL [15]. With the advent of highly sensitive assays for the isoenzymes, the decision was made to include the CK in this ANN. As already noted, however, it is the *decrease* in total CK in prostate cancer that adds predictability to the PI.

Finally, the PI was developed to have a high sensitivity for detecting prostate cancer and to specifically distinguish BPH from both normal and cancerous prostates at low levels of PSA (<6.0 ng/mL). This is why this ANN appears so helpful in distinguishing these three categories in men with a PSA < 4.0 ng/mL. With the positive biopsy rate approaching 32% in patients with a PSA > 4.0 ng/mL, systematic biopsies of the prostate are justified in this group without further consideration. The ROC curve plots of PI in Figure 10.4 are directly dependent on the actual composition of the test population. In the ProstAsure™ ANN, the control populations used in ANN development were carefully defined, with a majority having a PSA < 4.0 ng/mL. Thus this ANN was not designed for the 12.5% of all men with palpable BPH seen in our Stanford screens who have PSA levels > 4.0 ng/mL [16]. These men do, however, constitute a substantial fraction of all men referred to urologists to exclude prostate cancer because of an elevated serum PSA. The real diagnostic advantage of the PI, therefore, is its ability to detect early and potentially more curable prostate cancer while the PSA is still < 4.0 ng/mL.

REFERENCES

1. **Stamey T.A., Barnhill S.D., Zhang Z., Madyastha K.R., Prestigiacomo A.F., Jones K., Chan D.,** Effectiveness of ProstAsure™ in detecting prostate cancer (PCa) and benign prostatic hyperplasia (BPH) in men age 50 and older, *J. Urol, (Suppl.)*, 155, Abstract #504, 1996.
2. **DeAntoni E.P., Crawford E.D.,** Prostate cancer awareness week: education, service, and research in a community setting, *Cancer (Suppl.)*, 75, 1874-1879, 1995.
3. **Keetch D.W., Andriole G.L.,** Prostate cancer screening: what are physicians to do? What have we learned?, *Monographs in Urology*, 17, 31-46, 1996.
4. **Catalona W.J., Richie J.P., Ahmann F.R., Hudson M.A., Scardino P.T., Flanigan R.C., deKernion J.B., Ratliff T.L., Kavoussi L.R., Dalkin B.L., Waters W.B., MacFarlane M.T., Southwick P.C.,** Comparison of digital rectal examination and serum prostate specific antigen in the early detection of prostate cancer: results of a multicenter clinical trial of 6,630 men, *J. Urol.*, 151, 1283-1290, 1994.
5. **Noldus J., Stamey T.A.,** Histological characteristics of radical prostatectomy specimens in men with a serum prostate specific antigen of 4 ng/mL or less, *J. Urol.*, 155, 441-443, 1996.
6. **Kabalin J.N., McNeal J.E., Johnstone I.M., Stamey T.A.,** Serum PSA and the biologic progression of prostate cancer, *Urology*, 46, 65-70, 1995.
7. **Noldus J., Stamey T.A.,** Limitations of serum PSA in predicting peripheral and transition zone cancer volume as measured by correlation coefficients, *J. Urol.*, 155, 232-237, 1996.
8. **Stamey T.A., Freiha F.S., McNeal J.E., Redwine E.A., Whittemore A.S., Schmid H.-P.,** Localized prostate cancer: relationship of tumor volume to clinical significance for treatment of prostate cancer, *Cancer (Suppl.),* 71, 933-938, 1993.
9. **Fowler J.E. Jr., Shingleton W.B., Kolski, J.M., Yee D.T.,** Race and prostate cancer detection with PSA < 4.0 ng/mL, *J. Urol. (Suppl.)*, 157, Abstract #248, 1997.
10. **Stamey T.A., Sözen T.S., Yemoto C.M., McNeal J.E.,** Classification of "localized" untreated prostate cancer based on 791 men treated only by radical prostatectomy: common ground for therapeutic trials and TNM subgroups, *J. Urol.*, 1998.
11. **Prestigiacomo A.F., Stamey T.A.,** Can free and total prostate specific antigen and prostatic volume distinguish between men with negative and positive systematic ultrasound guided prostate biopsies?, *J. Urol.*, 157, 189-194, 1997.
12. **Prestigiacomo A.F., Lilja H., Pettersson K., Wolfert R.L., Stamey T.A.,** A comparison of the free fraction of serum prostate specific antigen in men with benign and cancerous prostates: the best case scenario, *J. Urol.*, 156, 350-354, 1996.
13. **Hugosson J., Aus G., Gergdahl S., Frösing R., Lodding P., Fernlund P., Lilja H.,** Results of a population based randomized study of PSA screening for prostate cancer, *J. Urol. (Suppl.)*, 157, Abstract #459, 1997.
14. **Catalona W.J., Smith D.S., Ornstein D.K.,** Prostate cancer detection in men with serum PSA concentrations of 2.6 to 4.0 ng/mL and benign prostate examination, *JAMA*, 277, 1452-1455, 1997.
15. **Zarghami N., Yu H., Diamandis E.P., Sutherland D.J.A.,** Quantification of creatine kinase BB isoenzyme in tumor cytosols and serum with an ultrasensitive time-resolved immunofluorometric technique, *Clin. Biochem.*, 28, 243-253, 1995.
16. **Lui P.D., Terris M.K., Haney D.J., Constantinou C.E., Stamey T.A.,** Prostate specific antigen as a predictor of an abnormal digital rectal examination, *Br. J. Urol.*, 74, 337-340, 1994.

Chapter 11

ARTIFICIAL NEURAL NETWORKS AND PROGNOSIS IN PROSTATE CANCER

F.C. Hamdy

I. INTRODUCTION

When a patient is found to have cancer, there are three main concerns which are translated into crucial questions for the clinician. He/she wants to know how (1) serious the disease is, i.e., how life threatening it is; (2) what the best treatment is with its potential deleterious effects; and (3) the prognosis with or without treatment. Whilst with many cancers there is a first choice treatment and the ideal course of action is clear, for other malignancies, particularly in urology e.g., certain grades and stages of prostate and bladder cancer — treatment decisions are more difficult. Decisions are made usually on the basis of conventional information such as tumour grade, stage, age and co-morbidity, statistical probabilities of disease progression, and an informed discussion between the treating clinician and the patient. For instance, if a man is diagnosed with low-grade and low-stage prostate cancer and he is told that he has a 10-15% risk of progression over a period of 10 years, the clinician is unable to predict exactly which side of the risk fence the patient will fall into. The consequence of such uncertainties could therefore be either overtreatment or undertreatment with their sequelae. Patients with such cancers would benefit greatly from any new methods of predicting outcome that will help them in selecting their treatment, which would be offered with a greater degree of confidence by the physician.

Determining prognosis remains a challenge for clinicians and scientists alike. In addition to conventional parameters as described above, researchers are seeking continuously novel markers, in the laboratory, based on our ever-improving knowledge of disease processes *in vivo* and *in vitro*. These markers are usually tested at three different levels. In patient material (tissue, serum, urine, etc.) to test an association between positivity for this marker and the severity of the disease; in the laboratory *in vitro*, using specific cell lines, ideally of human origin; and *in vivo* in suitable animal models to mimic the human disease situation. Once the value of a specific marker is established, it is then tested again in large cohorts of patients to confirm its role as a prognostic marker, which is likely to have a significant impact on management decisions. These investigations can last many years, and eventually, very few candidate markers reach a significant level of importance in the clinical context of day-to-day practice.

Artificial neural networks (ANNs), as described in Chapter 1, offer a distinct potential of testing these novel markers in conjunction with conventional parameters. The author has been

0-8493-9692-1/01/$0.00+$1.50

involved in the evaluation of ANNs for that particular purpose in both prostate and bladder cancer with promising results. The study described below relates to prostate cancer.

II. PROSTATE CANCER

Prostate cancer is the second most common malignancy in men in the United Kingdom with approximately 14,000 new cases diagnosed and 9,000 men dying from the disease every year. While tumour stage and volume, serum prostate specific antigen levels, histopathological grading and DNA tumour ploidy status have all been shown to correlate with prognosis and survival, none of these methods can predict reliably tumours that are likely to progress and metastasise. Whilst many tumours will remain quiescent and clinically unimportant, some will progress to advanced and metastatic disease resulting in considerable morbidity and mortality. The biggest dilemma in the management of this malignancy is to discriminate cancers that will progress from those that will remain at a latent stage. It is disconcerting that to date, no reliable method to achieve this discrimination exists. The problem is compounded by controversies surrounding the efficacy of aggressive treatment, particularly in the early stages of the disease.

In addition to established clinical prognostic markers, several new factors are emerging which may have a varying degree of significance in predicting outcome. Amongst these novel experimental markers are the genes regulating programmed cell death, otherwise known as apoptosis. These include the tumour suppressor gene p53 and the proto-oncogene bcl-2. It is now evident that the effects of androgen suppression in prostate cancer are mediated via apoptosis. Deregulation of the genetic pathway leading to programmed cell death may confer hormone-resistant prostate cancer which is incurable. Our group has demonstrated previously that the combination of bcl-2 overexpression and p53 nuclear accumulation by immunohistochemistry correlates strongly with hormone refractory prostate cancer [1,2]. In the study described herein, we incorporated experimental with conventional markers to assess the sensitivity of neural networks in predicting outcome following appropriate training. The results were compared with those obtained from conventional statistical methods.

III. PATIENTS AND METHODS

A. PATIENTS

Forty-one men with histologically proven prostate cancer were studied. Their age ranged from 47 to 86 years (median 73 years). Twenty men (49%) had evidence of skeletal metastasis as demonstrated by technetium 99m isotope bone scanning, and received hormone manipulation. Eleven patients (27%) had clinically localised disease and received either “watchful waiting” or external beam irradiation. The remaining 10 men (24%) had locally advanced cancers and received either radiotherapy or hormone manipulation. Follow-up ranged from 34 to 68 months (median 56 months). To date, 25 patients have died from the disease. Of those, 5 had not responded to initial treatment and the remaining 20 developed resistant prostate cancer. The remaining 16 patients were alive and well at the last follow-up.

B. METHODS

1. Immunohistochemistry

Immunohistochemical staining of representative tissue sections was performed using specific antibodies against bcl-2 (Dako, UK), and p53 (DO-7, Dako, UK) as described previously [1]. One thousand cells were counted to detect p53 nuclear protein accumulation and bcl-2 protein overexpression. The intensity of nuclear p53 protein accumulation was classified according to the percentage of cells with strong nuclear staining: "+" = 5-25%, "++" = 26-75%, "+++" = > 75%. Intensity of cytoplasmic staining for bcl-2 in tumour cells was categorised as "+" = focal areas of staining (< 5%), "++" = diffuse staining (5-50%), "+++" = diffuse staining (>50%). Positive controls matching the fixation protocol of the test material were used. These were colorectal carcinoma for p53 and tonsil for bcl-2. In addition, basal cells in benign prostatic glands and lymphocytes which are known to stain positively for bcl-2 were used as internal positive control. Negative controls were performed by omitting the primary antibody in each case.

2. Artificial neural networks

The patients were randomly subdivided into training and test sets consisting of 21 and 20 patients, respectively. The analysis was simulated on the NeuralWorks Professional II/Plus software package (NeuralWare, Pittsburgh, PA, USA). The structure used is of the feed-forward type and based on Kohonen's self-organising maps and the back-propagation of errors.

A total of 8 input neurons were considered. They consist of six conventional factors: patient's age, tumour stage (T1-T4) [3], skeletal metastasis (M0-M1), Gleason score, serum PSA, and treatment (hormonal, external beam irradiation, or watchful waiting), and two experimental markers: p53 and bcl-2 immunostaining. Three output neurons consisting of different outcomes were used: (1) no response to treatment, (2) relapse following initial successful treatment and/or disease progression in untreated patients, and (3) sustained complete response to treatment or no progression in untreated patients.

3. Statistical analysis

In order to evaluate ANNs, the data was analysed in parallel with conventional statistics. The method used was a multiple discriminant analysis (MDA). This was performed using the software programme Unistat 4.5 (Unistat Ltd, UK). Probabilities were tested using Fisher's exact and McNemar's tests; p values less than 0.05 were considered statistically significant.

IV. RESULTS

A. IMMUNOHISTOCHEMISTRY

Twenty-three patients (56%) had positive staining for p53 and 35 (85%) had positive staining for bcl-2. Whilst bcl-2 staining was not significantly related to histological grade or other clinical parameters, p53 staining was related to both histological grade and clinical stage at diagnosis. There were no significant differences between scores of p53 and bcl-2 staining and these parameters (data not shown). Sixteen of 25 patients (64%) who had hormone refractory disease, either at the onset of treatment (n=5) or within 18 months from initiation of hormone manipulation (n=20) were p53 positive, compared with 7 of 16 (44%) who had a sustained response to treatment and were alive and well at follow-up (Fisher's exact test: p = 0.0069). Twenty-two of 25 patients (88%) with hormone resistance and 13 of 16 (81%) who are alive and well were bcl-2 positive with no statistically significant difference between these groups. Thirteen of the 25 patients (52%) who escaped hormonal control were positive for both bcl-2 and p53, compared with 4 of the 16 patients (25%) who are alive and well (Fisher's exact test: $p < 0.0001$). Patient outcome was correlated with immunohistochemical findings. Prediction of outcome was tested using conventional criteria alone and in combination with immunoreactivity for p53 and/or bcl-2.

B. NEURAL NETWORK ANALYSIS

Four separate analyses were performed. In the first, all 8 input markers were considered and the outcomes predicted for the test set of 20 patients. To analyse the respective significance of the experimental markers (p53 and bcl-2) on the results, they were each omitted in turn and the network repeatedly simulated and tested. Finally, in order to assess the combined impact of those two experimental markers on outcome prediction, they were both omitted from the set of input neurons and the network was simulated and validated on the test set of 20 patients. Results of all the above analyses are given in the confusion matrices of Table 11.1 (a-d), along with their Kappa (κ) statistics and 95% confidence intervals (CI).

Table 11.1 (a-d) Confusion matrices showing the relationship between actual and ANN predicted outcomes for the cases when (a) all markers are considered, (b) p53 is omitted, (c) bcl-2 is omitted, and (d) both p53 and bcl-2 are omitted from the analysis. Kappa (κ) statistics with 95% confidence intervals (CI) are also given for each case.

		Actual Outcome			
		No response to treatment	**Sustained response to treatment**	**Relapsed**	**TOTAL**
ANN Predicted Outcome	**No response to treatment**	1	0	0	**1**
	Sustained response to treatment	0	8	3	**11**
	Relapsed	1	0	7	**8**
	TOTAL	**2**	**8**	**10**	**20**

ANN Prediction Accuracy = 80%, κ = 0.6522, CI = 0.3585 <> 0.9459 ($p < 0.00001$)

(a)

		Actual Outcome			
		No response to treatment	**Sustained response to treatment**	**Relapsed**	**TOTAL**
ANN Predicted Outcome	**No response to treatment**	0	0	0	**0**
	Sustained response to treatment	0	6	2	**8**
	Relapsed	2	2	8	**12**
	TOTAL	**2**	**8**	**10**	**20**

ANN Prediction Accuracy = 70%, κ = 0.4444, CI = 0.0992 <> 0.7897 ($p = 0.0058$)

(b)

	Actual Outcome			
ANN Predicted Outcome	**No response to treatment**	**Sustained response to treatment**	**Relapsed**	**TOTAL**
No response to treatment	0	0	0	**0**
Sustained response to treatment	0	7	4	**11**
Relapsed	2	1	6	**9**
TOTAL	**2**	**8**	**10**	**20**

ANN Prediction Accuracy = 65%, $\kappa = 0.3694$, CI = 0.0289 <> 0.7099 ($p = 0.0167$)

(c)

	Actual Outcome			
ANN Predicted Outcome	**No response to treatment**	**Sustained response to treatment**	**Relapsed**	**TOTAL**
No response to treatment	1	0	1	**2**
Sustained response to treatment	0	8	6	**14**
Relapsed	1	0	3	**4**
TOTAL	**2**	**8**	**10**	**20**

ANN Prediction Accuracy = 60%, $\kappa = 0.3443$, CI = 0.0560 <> 0.6325 ($p = 0.0096$)

(d)

C. COMPARISON OF ANNs WITH STATISTICAL ANALYSIS

Multiple discriminant analysis was used for each of the four combinations of data examined by ANNs. In all the cases investigated, except for the case where both p53 and bcl-2 were omitted from the analysis and conventional criteria were used alone, the ANN performance in predicting outcome was superior by a value of 5% to that of MDA as shown in

Table 11.2. Although this may not have reached statistical significance in the cases where p53 and bcl-2 were alternately omitted, statistical significance was attained for the case where all markers were considered (McNemar's test: $p = 0.0096$).

Table 11.2 Comparison of ANNs with conventional statistics.

	All markers	**p53 omitted**	**bcl-2 omitted**	**p53 / bcl-2 omitted**
MDA* accuracy	75%	65%	60%	65%
ANN accuracy	80%	70%	65%	60%
McNemar's 2-tail probability test	0.0192	0.1671	0.3593	0.3833

*MDA = Multiple Discriminant Analysis.

V. SUMMARY

At present, the most commonly used criteria influencing clinical decision-making in treating prostate cancer are a combination of: patient's age and life expectancy, tumour stage and grade, and serum PSA levels. In addition to these conventional criteria, novel prognostic markers are emerging continuously and are being assessed as additional information to improve management. These markers, in combination with conventional parameters, are traditionally evaluated in large observational studies of patients with long term follow-up periods using statistical analysis.

Several statistical methods such as Cox's proportional hazards [4] and logistic regression [5] have been employed to study survival patterns in different cohorts of cancer patients. Such approaches are valuable, but suffer from a number of limitations including: (1) the degree of impact of any prognostic marker on the analysis has to be assessed *a priori*, and (2) any outcome produced by the analysis cannot always apply to individual cases. ANNs, on the other hand, have the ability to predict outcome for individual patients through a thorough and generalised analysis of previous patients trends and, perhaps more importantly, patterns of tumour-associated parameters can be examined in ways that conventional statistics do not consider.

In prostate cancer, recent studies have evaluated the use of ANNs in diagnosis and the prediction of recurrence following radical surgery [6-8]. The results showed high sensitivity and specificity rates in predicting biopsy results in men with suspected prostate cancer, and recurrence following radical prostatectomy. The analysis, however, was based on variables consisting of well-established and conventional clinical and biochemical criteria. Other studies involved the use of hybrid neural and statistical classifier systems for the histopathologic grading of prostatic lesions [9] and the identification of predictors of general quality of life in patients with benign prostate hyperplasia or prostate cancer [10].

In the present study, we have evaluated the ability of ANNs to assess novel prognostic markers, in addition to established clinical and biochemical parameters. These experimental markers (p53 and bcl-2 immunopositivity) have been studied extensively by a multiplicity of workers including our own group. In the current series of patients, results of immunostaining confirmed the previously shown correlation between hormone refractory disease and the combination of p53 and bcl-2 positivity. In order to evaluate the performance of ANNs, we have compared the results of the analyses with conventional statistical methods. This comparison has demonstrated the superiority of ANNs over statistics using MDA and McNemar's tests, in three of the four investigations performed. It is worth noting that of these three investigations, in the case where both conventional and experimental markers were considered, improvement in accuracy of prediction by ANNs was statistically significant (p = 0.0096). In addition, when Fisher's exact test was used to assess ANNs in the same situation, when both bcl-2 and p53 were included, 80% accuracy of prediction was achieved compared to 60% accuracy when they were both omitted (p = 0.0032). When p53 or bcl-2 were omitted individually, although accuracy was reduced, this did not reach statistical significance. Despite the small number of patients included in this pilot study, we have demonstrated the ability of ANNs to assess prognostic markers objectively in prostate cancer.

REFERENCES

1. **Apakama I., Robinson M.C., Walter N.M., Charlton R.G., Royds J.A., Fuller C.E., Neal D.E., Hamdy F.C.,** bcl-2 overexpression combined with p53 protein accumulation correlates with hormone-refractory prostate cancer, *Br. J. Cancer,* 74, 1258-1262, 1996.
2 **Byrne R.L., Horne C.H.W., Robinson M.C., Autzen P., Apakama I., Bishop R.I., Neal D.E., Hamdy F.C.,** The expression of WAF-1, p53 and bcl-2 in prostatic adenocarcinoma, *Br. J. Urol.,* 79, 190-195, 1997.
3. **Schroeder F.H., Hermanek P., Denis L., Fair W.R., Gospodarowick M.K., Pavone-Macaluso M.,** The TNM classification of prostate cancer, *Prostate,* 4, 129-138, 1992.
4. **Cox D.R.,** Regression models and life-tables, *J. Roy. Stat. Soc. [B],* 34, 187-200.
5. **Lilford R.J., Braunholtz D.,** The statistical basis of public policy: a paradigm shift is overdue, *Br. Med. J.,* 313, 603-607, 1996.
6. **Snow P.B., Smith D.S., Catalona W.J.,** Artificial neural networks in the diagnosis and prognosis of prostate cancer: a pilot study, *J. Urol.*, 152, 1923-1926, 1994.
7. **Stamey T.A., Barnhill S.D., Zhang Z., Madyastha K.R., Zhang H.,** A neural network (ProstAsure™) with high sensitivity and specificity for diagnosing prostate cancer in men with a PSA < 4.0 ng/ml, *J. Urol.*, 157, 1425A, 1997.
8. **Barnhill S.D., Stamey T.A., Zhang Z., Zhang H., Madyastha K.R.,** The ability of the ProstAsure™ index to identify prostate cancer patients with low cancer volumes and a high potential for cure, *J. Urol.*, 157, 241A, 1997.
9. **Stotzka R., Männer R., Bartels P.H., Thompson D.,** A hybrid neural and statistical classifier system for histopathologic grading of prostatic lesions, *Analy. Quant. Cytol. Histol.*, 17, 204-218, 1995.
10. **Krongrad A., Granville L.J., Burke M.A., Golden R.M., Lai S., Cho L., Niederberger C.S.,** Predictors of general quality of life in patients with benign prostate hyperplasia or prostate cancer, *J. Urol.*, 157, 534-538, 1997.

Chapter 12

COMPARISON BETWEEN UROLOGISTS AND ARTIFICIAL NEURAL NETWORKS IN BLADDER CANCER OUTCOME PREDICTION[§]

K.N. Qureshi and J.K. Mellon

I. INTRODUCTION

Bladder cancer is the fourth most common malignancy in the western male population. Currently in England and Wales, 12,900 new cases are diagnosed each year and 5,400 patients die from the disease [1]. The American Cancer Society estimated that for 1998, bladder cancer registrations in the United States approximated 54,400 and those dying from the disease amounted to 12,500. Of newly diagnosed transitional cell carcinomas (TCC), 70% present as nonmuscle-infiltrative (pTa/pT1) tumours, 25% as muscle-invasive (T2-T4) tumours, and 5% as carcinoma *in situ* types (*cis*). Tumour recurrence following initial treatment is seen in 50-70% of patients with Ta/T1 tumours and approximately 10-25% of patients with Ta/T1 tumours progress to develop muscle-invasive or metastatic disease. Patients with organ-confined disease (T2), either arising *de-novo* or resulting from stage progression, have a 5-year survival of 50-60%, whereas patients with tumours that have penetrated beyond the detrusor muscle (T3/T4) and/or have loco-regional nodal metastasis have a 5-year survival of 15-20% [2].

In managing patients with bladder cancer, the principal problems for the clinician centre on the prompt diagnosis of bladder cancer, predicting which patients are at highest risk of tumour recurrence and stage progression in the Ta/T1 group and the relatively poor cancer-specific survival in the muscle-invasive group.

Urine cytology is a well-documented, noninvasive method for diagnosing patients with urothelial malignancy. Exfoliated cells from both normal and neoplastic urothelium can be readily identified in voided urine. Examination of cytological specimens allows for tumour detection at the time of initial presentation or during surveillance. However, the detection rates vary depending on the adequacy of the specimen, the grade and volume of the tumour and the experience of the cytologist. Presently, methods are being developed to increase the diagnostic accuracy of voided urine testing.

§ Many sections in this chapter have been extracted from our paper: Qureshi, K.N., Hamdy, F.C., Neal, D.E., and Mellon, J.K., Neural network analysis of clinicopathological and molecular markers in bladder cancer, *J. Urol.*, 163, 630-633, 2000.

0-8493-9692-1/01/$0.00+$1.50

Currently, a number of conventional clinicopathological factors are of use in predicting survival, with the greatest predictor being clinical stage followed by histological grade [3, 4]. Other informative factors include tumour type (papillary vs. solid), tumour size, the presence of concomitant *cis,* patient age, and tumour location [5]. In Ta/T1 bladder cancer, an increased recurrence rate is associated with lamina propria invasion or poorly differentiated tumours [6]. Using multivariate analysis, two additional factors have been shown to significantly influence the recurrence rate of newly diagnosed Ta/T1 bladder cancer: (1) a positive check cystoscopy at 3 months after initial resection and (2) the presence of multiple tumours at diagnosis, which when apparent either individually or in combination can be used to stratify patients into three prognostic groups with different risks of tumour recurrence [7]. A further risk factor for recurrence is tumour size. Abnormal mucosal biopsies have been demonstrated to be of significant prognostic value in predicting future tumour recurrence in cases of Ta/T1 bladder cancer [8], however, a recent study using decision analysis did not show any difference in the recurrence rate or risk of progression in patients in whom random urothelial biopsies were taken when compared to the control group [9]. Progression to muscle-invasive disease is highest in the T1G3 subgroup of bladder tumours. Additional prognostic factors for progression are number of tumours (≥4) and tumour size (≥5cm) [6]. The identification of *cis* and/or atypia in normal, incidentally resected mucosa adjacent to the tumour has also been reported to be a positive predictor for subsequent muscle-invasion [10].

Recently, a variety of molecular markers have been assessed for their ability to predict the outcome in patients with bladder cancer, although only a few give truly independent prognostic information. The epidermal growth factor receptor (EGFR) is the product of the c-*erb*B-1 gene (located on chromosome 7q22) [11] and is found in the plasma membrane of many cells. Previously, we have demonstrated that using immunohisto-chemistry of frozen tumour sections, strong staining for EGFR is associated with recurrence, progression, and reduced survival [12]. Upon extension of this study, EGFR status was confirmed to be an independent predictor of stage progression in Ta/T1 bladder cancer and survival in the group as a whole [13].

The c-*erb*B-2 proto-oncogene, located on chromosome 17q21, encodes a 185 kDa transmembrane phosphoglycoprotein with significant sequence homology to the EGFR. In primary bladder tumours, we have previously reported that strong immunoreactivity is apparent in 21% (20/95) of tumours with weak staining in a further 14% (13/95). This study also reported a weak association between expression of c-*erb*B-2 and tumour stage but none with tumour grade [14]. In a further study of 236 bladder tumours from 89 patients, c-*erb*B-2 gene amplification and protein overexpression were demonstrated to be of value in predicting death due to bladder cancer using multivariate analysis, although tumour stage and grade remained the most significant variables [15]. Similarly, in a series of 88 patients with TCC of the bladder, the immunohistochemical detection of c-*erb*B-2 was associated with reduced survival when compared to patients whose tumours did not express the c-*erb*B-2 gene product [16].

The tumour-suppressor gene, p53 (located on chromosome 17p) has been reported to be mutated in over half of all human tumours [17]. The detection of the p53 onco-protein has been related to outcome in bladder cancer. In a series of 243 patients treated with radical cystectomy, nuclear p53 status was demonstrated to be a predictor of recurrence and reduced survival, independent of stage, grade, and lymph node status in cancer confined to the bladder [18].

Artificial neural networks (ANNs) are algorithms that can be trained to recognise complex patterns in data sets. They have an advantage over conventional statistics in that they are not constrained by predefined mathematical relationships between dependent and independent variables; thus they are able to model complex nonlinear parameters. In previously published urological studies, ANNs have been used to predict the risk of prostate cancer in men with a PSA ≤ 4.0 ng/ml [19], to predict tumour recurrence following radical prostatectomy [20], to predict outcome in prostate cancer [21,22], and to predict sperm function using data derived from semen analysis [23]. However neural network technology remains in its infancy with regards to bladder cancer. Previous studies have investigated the power of ANNs to discriminate benign from malignant lower urinary tract lesions [24]. Images of routinely processed voided urine smears stained by the Giemsa technique from 470 patients with benign and malignant urothelial lesions were analysed using a neural network custom image based system. The back-propagation ANN correctly classified 100% of those with benign and 94.51% of those with malignant disease with an overall accuracy of 96.96%. However, more importantly the overall accuracy of the ANN predictions were significantly better than conventional cytological examinations. When a learning vector quantiser (LVQ)-type of ANN was employed similar results were obtained when compared with urine cytology [25], although there was no significant difference with the predictions between the two different types of ANN [26]. These results illustrate the value of a neural net-based image analysis of voided urine specimens which may complement cytologists' predictions with regards to achieving more accurate diagnoses.

The following work is based on the prediction of clinical outcome for patients with bladder cancer utilising prognostic markers identified at initial presentation [27]. In this study, we sought to assess the ability of an ANN to predict bladder cancer recurrence and stage progression in a group of patients with newly diagnosed Ta/T1 bladder cancer, and 12-month cancer-specific survival in a group of patients with primary T2-T4 bladder cancer using clinicopathological and molecular prognostic indicators. In addition, the network's predictions were compared with those of four consultant urologists supplied with the same data.

II. MATERIALS AND METHODS

A comprehensive database which included clinicopathological and molecular markers formed the basis for the study. A total of 212 patients with newly diagnosed bladder cancer were initially recruited although for 11 of these patients, complete data were unavailable. The remaining 201 patients had follow-up ranging from 1 to 96 (mean 26.5) months in the final analysis [13]. Patients were recruited from the practices of five consultant urologists, thus there were minor variations in clinical management. Standard immunohistochemical techniques had been used to detect EGFR, c-*erb*B-2 and p53 as previously described [13,18].

For the prediction of stage progression in Ta/T1 bladder cancers, the input neural data included tumour stage (Ta/T1), grade (1/2/3), tumour size (<5 cm, ≥5 cm), tumour number (single/multiple), gender (male/female), and EGFR status (+/-). For the prediction of tumour recurrence within 6 months for Ta/T1 tumours and 12-month cancer-specific survival for T2-T4 tumours, additional inputs were employed: smoking habit (yes/no), histology of mucosal biopsies (mild, moderate, severe dysplasia), presence of concomitant *cis* (yes/no), tumour metaplasia (yes/no), tumour architecture (papillary/solid), tumour site (lateral, anterior, posterior bladder wall, trigone, dome, ureteric orifice, widespread disease), c-*erb*B2 (+/-), and p53 (+/-) status.

The analysis presented was simulated on the NeuralWorks Professional II/Plus software package (NeuralWare, Pittsburgh, PA, USA) and was based on self-organising maps and the radial basis function algorithm [29]. The patient cohort was divided randomly into two sets, for the learning and testing phases of the neural simulation (Table 12.1). Before training, the network was assigned a randomised set of initial weights and a bias neuron. As training progressed, those weights and bias were modified and converged toward values representing a solution to the prediction problem. The rate of convergence was determined by a threshold set upon the root mean square (RMS) of the error between the desired and actual outputs. The weights were constantly updated to reflect this gradual convergence and to further contribute to the overall reduction in the RMS error. No retraining of the network was permitted after validation using the test data. The same input neural data used to validate the network were presented to four consultant urologists who were asked to predict recurrence within 6 months and stage progression in the Ta/T1 group of patients and 12-month cancer-specific survival in the patients with invasive disease. The data were coded and supplied in tabulated form only and the clinicians were not able to interview or examine the patients, or confer with the hospital notes before making their predictions. These results were then compared with the performance of the ANN.

Table 12.1 Number of patients in the learning and the validation/test set for each of the analyses performed.

	Number of patients		
Subset	**Learning Set**	**Test Set**	**Total**
Stage progression (Ta/T1)	45	60	105
Recurrence within 6 months (Ta/T1)	36	20	56
12-month cancer-specific survival (T2-T4)	25	15	40

The outcomes of the data analysis by the ANN and the clinicians were expressed in terms of mean accuracy (sum of correct predictions divided by total number of predictions), sensitivity, specificity, and positive/negative predictive values. The McNemar test [30] was used to analyse the relative accuracy of the predictions from clinicians and the ANN in relation to actual patient outcomes; whereas to compare their predictions with each other, Fisher's exact test was used [31]. p-values of < 0.05 were considered statistically significant. All statistical analyses were performed using UNISTAT® Statistical Package Version 4.5.01.

III. RESULTS

A. CLINICAL OUTCOME: RECURRENCE, PROGRESSION, AND SURVIVAL

During the study period, stage progression was noted in 17/105 (16%) Ta/T1 tumours. In the test set, 10/60 (17%) tumours underwent stage progression and, from within this, 4/19 (21%) T1G3 tumours progressed to muscle-invasive disease. Recurrence within 6 months of diagnosis in primary Ta bladder cancer occurred in 12/33 (36%) tumours; whereas 16/23 (70%) T1 tumours recurred within the same period ($p = 0.03$, Fisher's exact test). In the test set, 10/20 (50%) Ta/T1 tumours recurred within the 6-month-period following diagnosis. In the muscle-invasive group, 12-month cancer-specific survival was noted in 27/40 (68%) patients in the entire cohort, a similar proportion survived in the test set 10/15 (67%).

B. PREDICTIONS BY THE ANN AND CLINICIANS

The performance of the ANN and clinicians is shown in Table 12.2; the comparisons of both with actual outcomes are illustrated in Table 12.3. There was no significant difference between the ANN and the clinicians' predictions of stage progression and tumour recurrence in Ta/T1 tumours, or 12-month cancer-specific survival in the muscle-invasive group ($p = 0.33$, $p = 0.5$, and $p = 0.12$, respectively, Fisher's exact test).

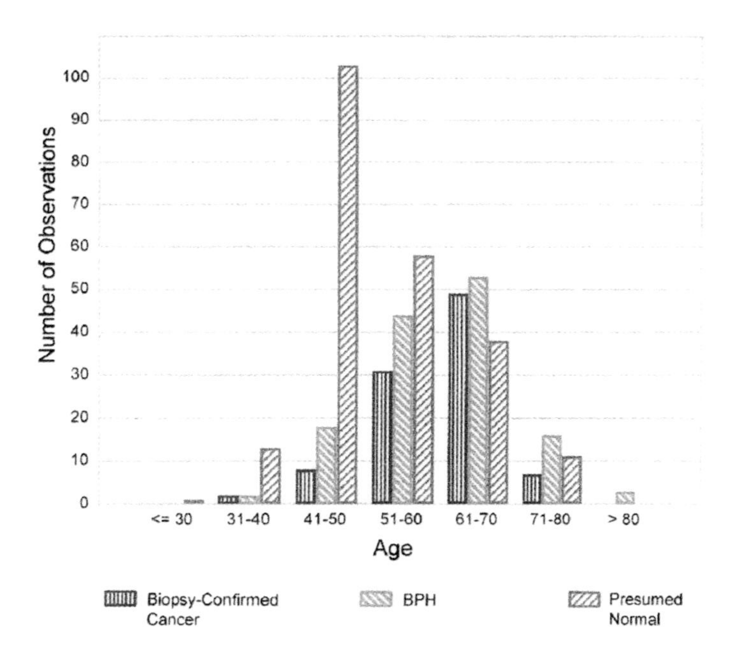

Chapter 10, Colour Figure 1
Age distribution of 457 test cases with a PSA < 4.0 ng/mL.

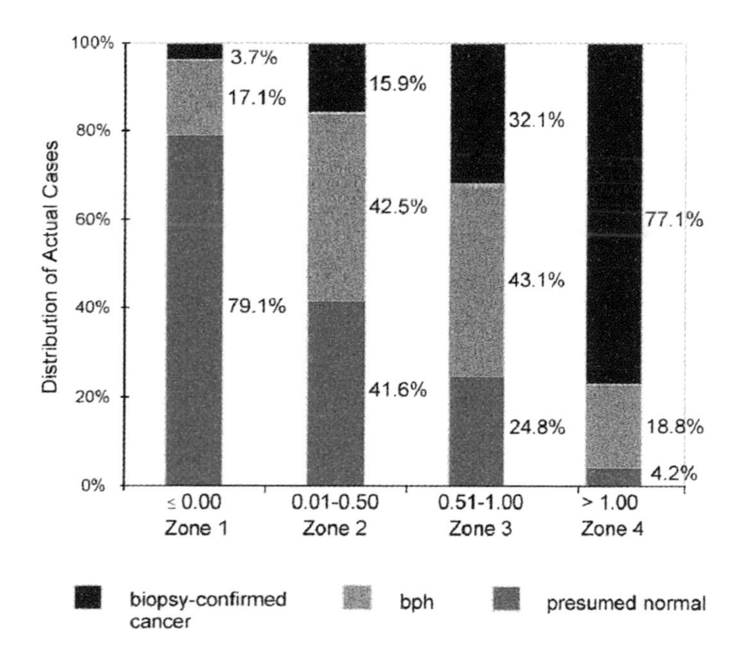

Chapter 10, Colour Figure 2
Distribution of ProstAsure™ index zones and diagnostic groups of 457 test cases with a PSA < 4.0 ng/mL.

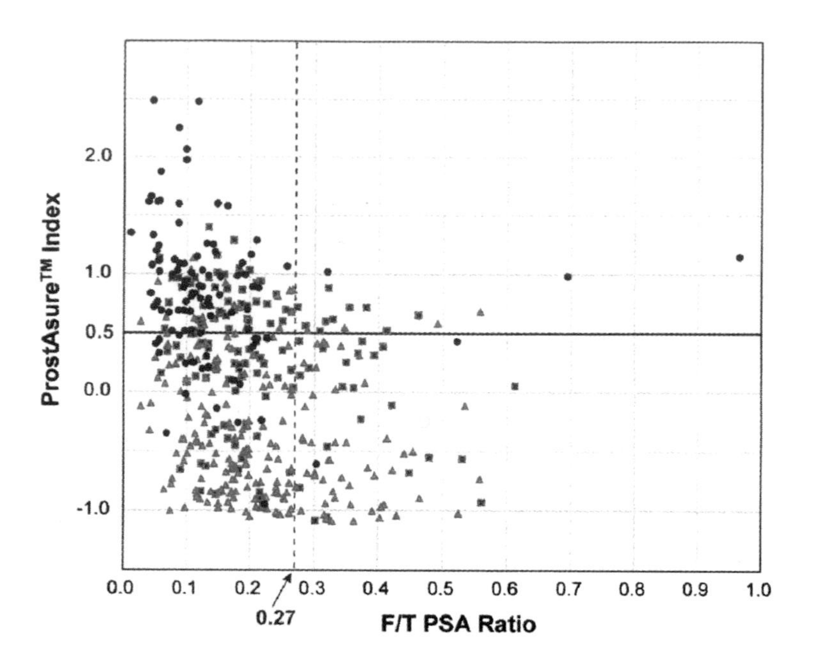

Chapter 10, Colour Figure 3
Scatterplot of 457 patients with a PSA < 4.0 ng/mL, comparing ProstAsure™ index against free/total PSA ratio.

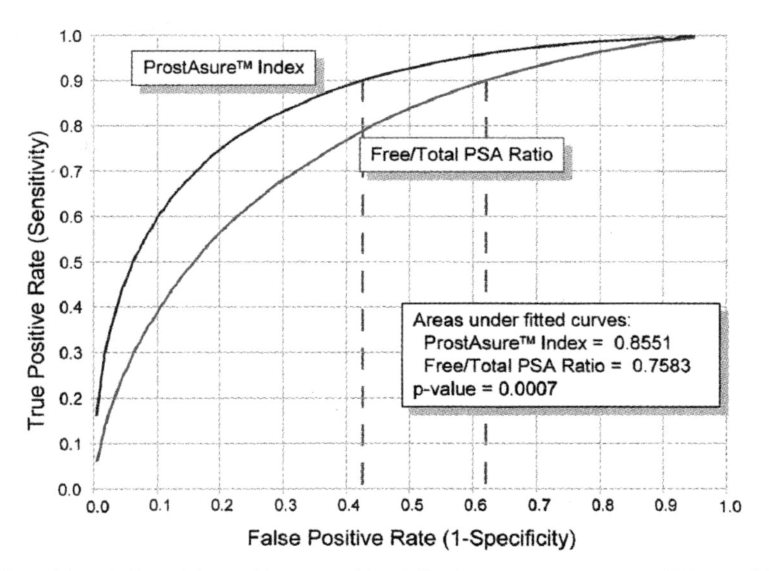

Chapter 10, Colour Figure 4
ROC curves estimated using 457 patients with PSA < 4.0 ng/mL for comparing ProstAsure™ index against free/total PSA ratio.

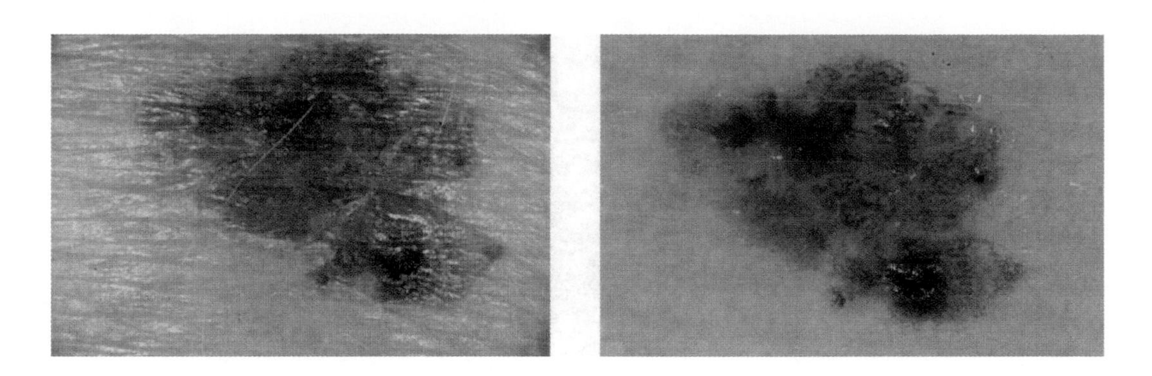

Chapter 13, Colour Figure 1
Example of pigmented skin lesion. Left: Traditional imaging technique. Right: Dermatoscopy imaging technique.

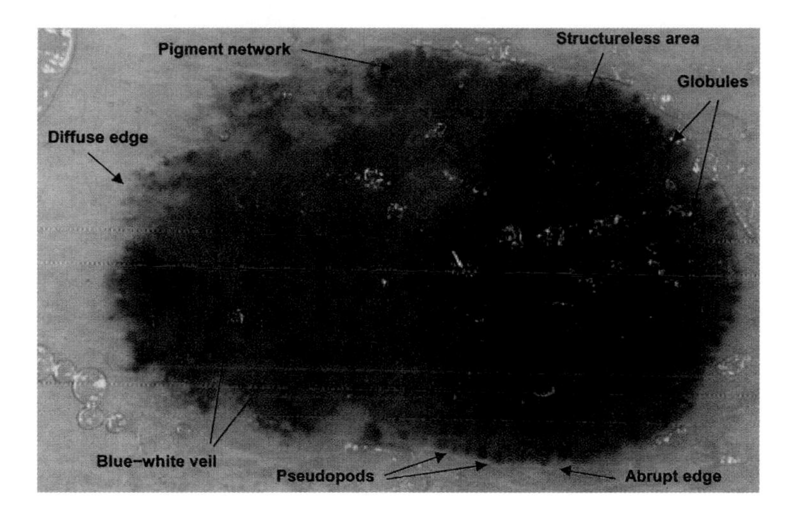

Chapter 13, Colour Figure 2
Pigmented skin lesion with several dermatoscopic features.

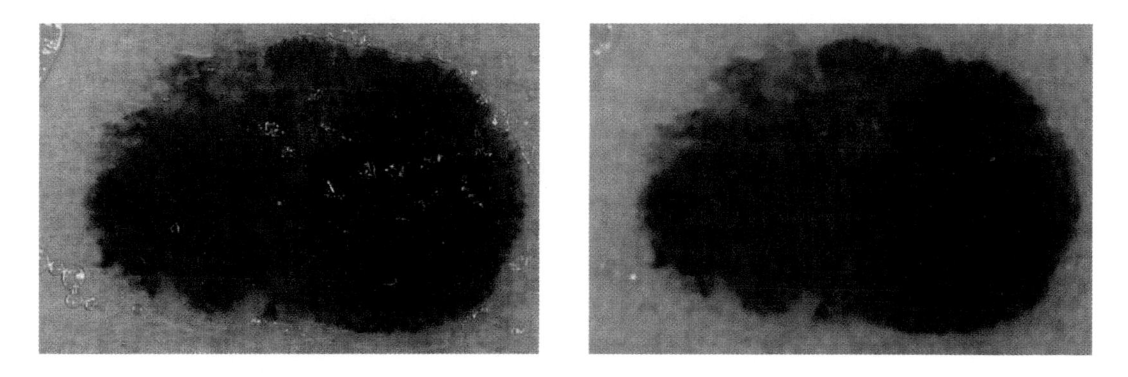

Chapter 13, Colour Figure 4
The effect of filtering an 885 × 590 dermatoscopic image with an 11 × 11 median filter. Left: Original image. Right: Filtered image. Notice how the air bubble artefacts have been reduced, especially around the lesion edge in the upper right hand corner.

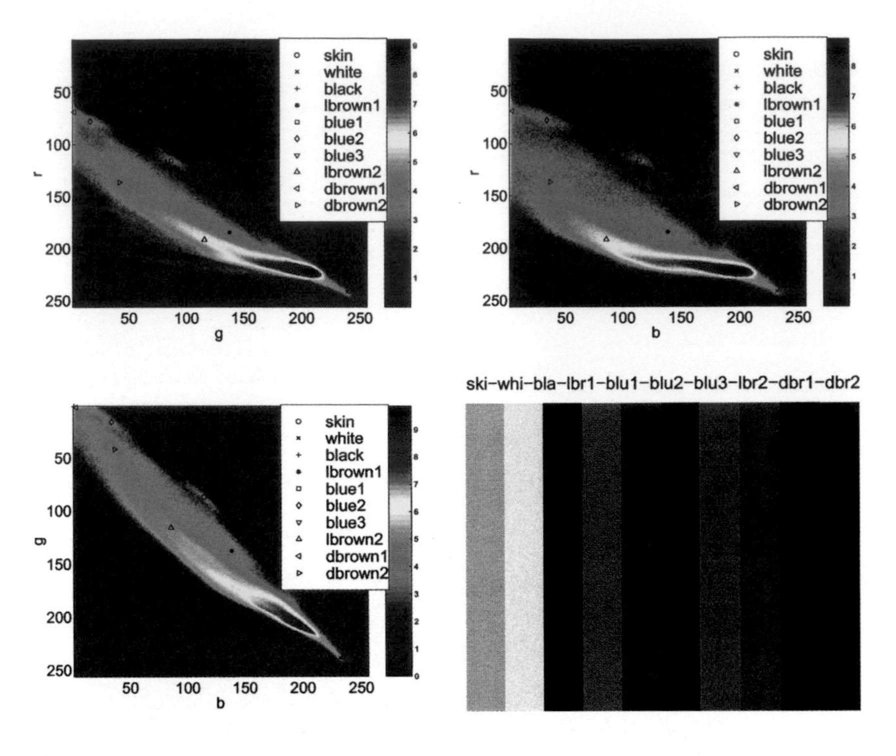

Chapter 13, Colour Figure 8

Colour prototypes have been found manually by inspecting the combined 2-D histograms of 18 randomly selected images. The perceived cluster centres are chosen as prototypes. Upper left: Red-green 2-D histogram. The histogram values, $h(r,g)$, have been compressed by the transformation, $h_C(r,g) = \log(1 + h(r,g))$, in order to enhance the visual quality. Upper right: Red-blue 2-D histogram (log-transformed). Lower left: Green-blue 2-D histogram (log-transformed). Lower right: The determined colour prototypes. The *skin* colour prototype is left out since it is eliminated by the segmentation process. Only colours inside the lesion are of interest in this work.

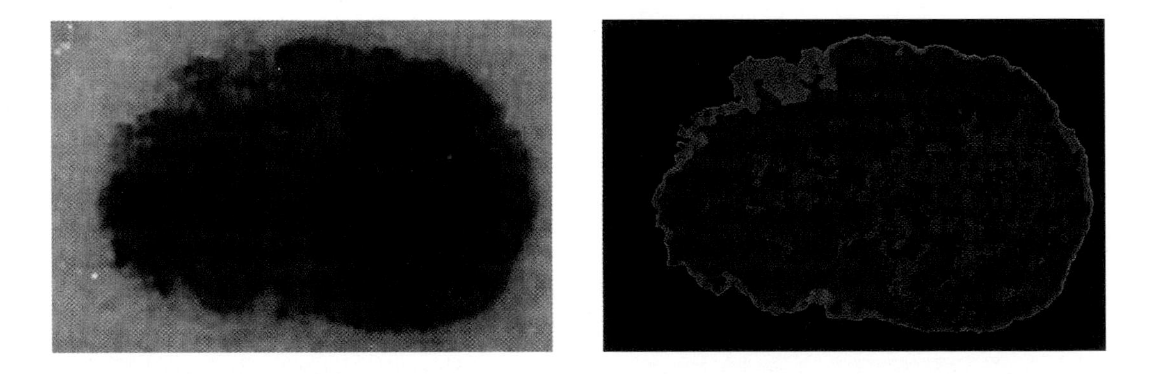

Chapter 13, Colour Figure 9

Examples of colour detection in a dermatoscopic image. Left: Original median filtered image. Right: Results of comparing the skin lesion image in the left panel with colour prototypes in the RGB colour-space using the Euclidean difference measure. Note that all shades of blue are represented by the *blue 1* prototype seen in Figure 8, all shades of dark-brown by *dbrown2* and all shades of light-brown by *lbrown2*.

Table 12.2 Performance of the ANN vs. clinicians.

	Sensitivity (%)	**Specificity (%)**	**Positive Predictive Value (%)**	**Negative Predictive Value (%)**	**Overall Accuracy (%)**
Stage Progression in Ta/T1 Tumours					
Clinicians	55	78	33	90	74
Network	70	82	44	93	80
Recurrence within 6 Months in Ta/T1 Tumours					
Clinicians	75	83	81	77	79
Network	70	80	78	73	75
12-Month Cancer-Specific Survival in Invasive Tumours					
Clinicians	60	68	48	77	65
Network	100	80	63	100	82

Table 12.3 The performance of the ANN and clinicians compared with actual events (McNemar test for difference between the predicted and the actual population). The overall accuracy of the ANN and the mean accuracy for the clinicians are given in parentheses.

	***p* Values of McNemar Test Results**			
Analysis	**Stage Progression in Ta/T1 Tumours**	**Stage Progression in T1G3 Tumours**	**Recurrence within 6 Months in Ta/T1 Tumours**	**12-Month Cancer-Specific Survival in T2-T4 Tumours**
ANN	0.07 *(80%)*	0.25 *(82%)*	0.50 *(75%)*	0.12 *(82%)*
Clinicians	0.26 *(74%)*	0.008 *(41%)*	0.16 *(79%)*	0.28 *(65%)*

On restricting the validation set for stage progression to T1G3 tumours, the ANN analysis became 100% sensitive and 78% specific with an overall accuracy of 82%. For the same high risk group, the predictions of the clinicians showed a sensitivity of 100%, specificity of 28%, and overall accuracy of 41%. The performance of the ANN in predicting stage progression in T1G3 tumours was significantly better than that of the four clinicians (McNemar test, $p = 0.25$

for the ANN and $p = 0.008$ for clinicians) (Table 12.3). Correspondingly, there was a significant difference when the ANN and clinicians' predictions for T1G3 stage progression were compared with each other ($p = 0.04$, Fisher's exact test).

IV. DISCUSSION

When confronted with a patient who specifically enquires about prognosis, most clinicians reply with an empirical answer based on past experience. This common problem relates to the shortcomings of conventional statistical methods based on population studies in providing prognostic information for individual patients.

Currently for bladder cancer, we lack accurate methods of diagnosing urothelial malignancy and of predicting stage progression and recurrence in Ta/T1 tumours and cancer-specific survival in patients with invasive disease. Using ANNs, we have demonstrated that using standard clinico-pathological factors at diagnosis combined with molecular markers of mixed prognostic significance, one can predict tumour behaviour accurately.

Traditionally, statistical techniques such as Cox's proportional hazards and logistic regression are employed when analysing prognostic information. However, in this situation, where markers interact in a complex fashion, the processing rules or mathematical equations are often very difficult to determine. ANNs can accommodate large numbers of prognostic variables and can analyse their varying degrees of impact on the outcome which is not possible using conventional statistical techniques. This is important as recent studies have shown that molecular markers used in combination can predict overall survival in patients with bladder cancer [32,33]. Therefore, as more prognostic indicators are discovered, their effect could be assessed by incorporation into a neural model. Thus it would be possible to distinguish those indicators or combination of markers that may have a more pronounced impact on outcome.

We have demonstrated in this study that an ANN is significantly more accurate at predicting stage progression in T1G3 tumours than clinicians, however when analysing the entire Ta/T1 cohort, no significant difference was shown. We have shown previously using multivariate analysis that EGFR is an independent prognostic indicator for stage progression in Ta/T1 bladder tumours. More importantly, EGFR status was found to be 90% accurate, 80% sensitive, and 93% specific in predicting stage progression in T1G3 bladder cancer [13]. When employing EGFR status as the sole predictor of stage progression for T1G3 tumours in the validation set for the ANN, the overall accuracy was 91%, this compares with 82% for the ANN analysis utilising the various inputs mentioned. Although the accuracy of the ANN in predicting T1G3 stage progression was less than when EGFR status was used as the sole parameter, there was no significant difference between these two methods of prediction ($p = 0.50$, Fisher's exact test). These findings are important, as of the tumours which are noninfiltrative at diagnosis, the T1G3 group of tumours has the greatest propensity to progress to muscle-invasive disease. Thus, the prediction at diagnosis of future stage progression in patients with T1G3 disease may indicate the need for adjuvant treatment to be instigated in order to improve clinical outcome.

Future large scale prospective studies investigating the application of ANNs utilising large numbers of variables may help clinicians in improving accuracy of diagnosis and predicting prognosis. Scientists will also be guided in their quest to determine those important molecular markers affecting tumour behaviour. We are not advocating ANNs should replace expert decision-making in clinical practice, but suggest they may have a role in complementing traditional methods to produce a more accurate prediction of clinical outcome.

REFERENCES

1. **Walker L., (Ed.),** The challenge we face, fighting cancer on all fronts: Cancer Research Campaign scientific yearbook, Park Communication Ltd, London, 2, 1997-98.
2. **Pagano F., Bassi P., Galetti T.P., Meneghini A., Milani C., Artibani W., Garbeglio A.,** Results of contemporary radical cystectomy for invasive bladder cancer: a clinicopathological study with an emphasis on the inadequacy of the tumour, nodes and metastasis classification, *J. Urol.*, 145, 45, 1991.
3. **Anderstrφm C., Johansson S., Nilsson, S.,** The significance of lamina propria invasion on the prognosis of patients with bladder tumours, *J. Urol.*, 124, 23, 1980.
4. **Cummings K.B.,** Carcinoma of the bladder: predictors, *Cancer*, 45, 1849, 1980.
5. **Liebert M., Seigne, J.,** Characteristics of invasive bladder cancers: histological and molecular markers, *Sem. Urol. Oncol.*, 14, 62, 1996.
6. **Heney N.M., Ahmed S., Flanagan M.J., Frable W., Corder M.P., Hafermann M.D., Hawkins I.R.,** Superficial bladder cancer: progression and recurrence, *J. Urol.*, 130, 1083, 1983.
7. **Parmar M.K.B., Freedman L.S., Hargreave T.B., Tolley, D.A.,** Prognostic factors for recurrence and follow-up policies in the treatment of Ta/T1 bladder cancer: report from the British medical research council subgroup on Ta/T1 bladder cancer (urological cancer working party), *J. Urol.*, 142, 284, 1989.
8. **Smith G., Elton R.A., Beynon L.L., Newsam J.E., Chisholm G.D., Hargreave T.B.,** Prognostic significance of biopsy results of normal-looking mucosa in cases of Ta/T1 bladder cancer, *Br. J. Urol.*, 55, 665, 1983.
9. **Kiemeney L.A.L.M., Witjes J.A., Heijbroek R.P., Koper N.P., Verbeek A.L.M., Debruyne F.M.J. and the Members of the Dutch South-East Co-operative Urological Group,** Should random urothelial biopsies be taken from patients with primary superficial bladder cancer? A decision analysis, *Br. J. Urol.*, 73, 164, 1994.
10. **Althausen A.F., Prout G.R., Daly J.J.,** Non-invasive papillary carcinoma of the bladder associated with carcinoma *in situ*, *J. Urol.*, 116, 575, 1976.
11. **Kondo I., Schimizu N.,** Mapping of the human gene for epidermal growth factor receptor (EGFR) on the p13 leads to q22 region of chromosome 7, *Cytogenet. Cell Genet.*, 35, 9, 1983.
12. **Neal D.E., Sharples L., Smith K., Fennelly J., Hall R.R., Harris, A.L.,** The epidermal growth factor receptor and the prognosis of bladder cancer, *Cancer*, 65, 1619, 1990.
13. **Mellon J.K., Wright C., Kelly P., Horne C.H.W., Neal, D.E.,** Long-term outcome related to epidermal growth factor receptor status in bladder cancer, *J. Urol.*, 153, 919, 1995.
14. **Mellon J.K., Lunec J., Wright C., Horne C.H.W., Kelly P., Neal, D.E.,** c-*erb*B-2 in bladder cancer: molecular biology, correlation with epidermal growth factor receptors and prognostic value, *J. Urol.*, 155, 321, 1996.
15. **Underwood M., Bartlett J., Reeves J., Gardiner D.S., Scott R., Cooke, T.,** c-*erb*B-2 gene amplification: a novel marker in recurrent bladder tumors? *Cancer Res.*, 55, 2422, 1995.
16. **Sato K., Moriyama M., Mori S., Saito M., Watanuki T., Terada K., Okuhara E., Akiyama T., Toyoshima K., Yamamoto T., Kato, T.,** An immunohistologic evaluation of c-*erb*B-2 gene product in patients with urinary bladder carcinoma, *Cancer*, 70, 2493, 1992.
17. **Hollstein T., Sidransky D., Vogelstein B., Harris C.C.,** p53 mutations in human cancers, *Science*, 253, 49, 1991.

18. **Esrig D., Elmajian D., Groshen S., Freeman J.A., Stein J.P., Chen S.C., Nichols P.W., Skinner D.G., Jones P.A., Cote, R.J.,** Accumulation of nuclear p53 and tumour progression in bladder cancer, *N. Eng. J. Med.*, 331, 1259, 1994.
19. **Babaian R.J., Fritsche H.A., Zhang Z., Zhang K.H., Madyastha K.R., Barnhill S.D.,** Evaluation of ProstAsure index in the detection of prostate cancer: a preliminary report, *Urology*, 51, 132, 1998.
20. **Snow P.B., Smith D.S., Catalona, W.J.,** Artificial neural networks in the diagnosis of prostate cancer: a pilot study, *J. Urol.*, 152, 1923, 1994.
21. **Naguib R.N.G., Robinson M.C., Apakama I., Neal D.E., Hamdy, F.C.,** Neural network analysis of prognostic markers in prostate cancer, *Br. J. Urol.*, 77, 50, 1996.
22. **Naguib R.N.G., Robinson M.C., Neal D.E., Hamdy F.C.,** Neural network analysis of combined conventional and experimental prognostic markers in prostate cancer: a pilot study, *Br. J. Cancer*, 78, 246, 1998.
23. **Niederberger C.S., Lipshultz L.I., Lamb D.J.,** A neural network to analyse fertility data, *Fertil. Steril.*, 60, 324, 1993.
24. **Pantazopoulos D., Karakitsos P., Iokim-Liossi A., Pouliakis A., Botsoli-Stergiou E., Dimopoulos, C.,** Back propagation neural network in the discrimination of benign from malignant lower urinary tract lesions, *J. Urol.*, 159, 1619, 1998.
25. **Pantazopoulos D., Karakitsos P., Pouliakis A., Iokim-Liossi A., Dimopoulos, M.,** Static cytometry and neural networks in the discrimination of lower urinary system lesions, *Urology*, 51, 946, 1998.
26. **Pantazopoulos D., Karakitsos P., Iokim-Liossi A., Pouliakis A., Dimopoulos K.,** Comparing neural networks in the discrimination of benign from malignant lower urinary tract lesions, *Br. J. Urol.*, 81, 574, 1998.
27. **Qureshi K.N., Naguib R.N.G., Mellon J.K., Neal D.E.,** Neural network analysis of clinicopathological and molecular prognostic factors in bladder cancer, *Proc. Br. Assoc. Urol. Surg.*, 1998.
28. **Wright C., Mellon K., Johnston P., Lane D.P., Harris A.L., Horne C.H.W., Neal, D.E.,** Expression of mutant p53, c-*erb*B2 and the epidermal growth factor receptor in transitional cell carcinoma of the urinary bladder, *Br. J. Cancer*, 63, 967, 1991.
29. NeuralWorks Professional II/Plus Reference Guide, NeuralWare Inc., Pittsburgh, PA, USA, 1995.
30. **McNemar Q.,** Note on the sampling error of the difference between correlated proportions or percentages, *Psychometrica*, 12, 153, 1947.
31. **Fisher, R.A., (Ed.),** *Statistical Methods for Research Workers, 13th Ed.,* Hafner, New York, 365.
32. **Grossman H.B., Liebert M., Antelo M., Dinney C.P.N., Hu S., Palmer J.L., Benedict W.F.,** p53 and RB expression predict progression in T1 bladder cancer, *Clin. Cancer Res.*, 4, 829, 1998.
33. **Cote R.J., Dunn M.D., Chatterjee S.J., Stein J.P., Shi S., Tran Q., Hu S., Xu H.J., Groshen S., Taylor C.R., Skinner D.G., Benedict W.F.,** Elevated and absent pRb expression is associated with bladder cancer progression and has co-operative effects with p53, *Cancer Res.*, 58, 1090, 1998.

Chapter 13

A PROBABILISTIC NEURAL NETWORK FRAMEWORK FOR THE DETECTION OF MALIGNANT MELANOMA

M. Hintz-Madsen, L.K. Hansen, J. Larsen, and K.T. Drzewiecki

I. INTRODUCTION

The work reported in this chapter concerns the classification of dermatoscopic images of skin lesions. The overarching goals of the work are

To develop an objective and cost-efficient tool for classification of skin lesions

This involves extracting relevant information from dermatoscopic images in the form of dermatoscopic features and designing reliable classifiers.

To gain insight into the importance of dermatoscopic features

The importance of dermatoscopic features is still very much a matter of research. Any additional insight into this area is desirable.

To develop a probabilistic neural classifier design framework

In order to obtain reliable classification systems based on neural networks, a principled probabilistic approach will be followed.

Hence, the work should be of interest to both the dermatological and engineering communities.

A. MALIGNANT MELANOMA

Malignant melanoma is the deadliest form of skin cancer and arises from cancerous growth in pigmented skin lesions. The cancer can be removed by a fairly simple surgical incision if it has not entered the blood stream. It is thus vital that the cancer is detected at an early stage in order to increase the probability of a complete recovery. Skin lesions may in this context be grouped into three classes:

- *Benign nevi* is a common name for all healthy skin lesions. These have no increased risk of developing cancer.
- *Atypical nevi* are also healthy skin lesions but have an increased risk of developing into cancerous lesions. The special type of atypical nevi, called *dysplastic nevi,* has the highest risk and is, thus, often referred to as the precursor of malignant melanoma.
- *Malignant melanoma* are as already mentioned cancerous skin lesions.

Upon inspection and suspicion of a skin lesion, the dermatologist will remove the lesion and a biopsy is performed in order to determine the exact type of skin lesion. If the lesion is found to be malignant, a larger part of the surrounding skin will be removed depending on the

0-8493-9692-1/01/$0.00+$1.50

degree of malignancy. If a lesion is not considered to be suspicious, it is not usually removed unless there is some cosmetic reason to do so.

It is not an easy task for dermatologists to visually determine whether a skin lesion is, or might be, malignant. A study at Karolinske Hospital, Stockholm, Sweden, has shown that dermatologists with less than 1 year of experience of detect 31% of the melanoma cases they are presented with, while dermatologists with more than 10 years of experience are able to detect 63% [1]. Another study shows that experienced dermatologists are capable of detecting 75% of cancerous skin lesions [2].

Malignant melanoma is usually only seen in Caucasians.

B. EVOLUTION OF MALIGNANT MELANOMA

The incidence of malignant melanoma in Denmark has increased five- to sixfold from 1942 to 1982, while the mortality rate has doubled from 1955 to 1982 [3]. Currently, approximately 800 cases of malignant melanoma are reported in Denmark every year. In Germany 9,000–10,000 new cases are expected every year with an annual increase of 5–10% [4].

Due to the rather steep increase in the number of reported malignant melanoma cases, it is becoming increasingly important to develop simple, objective and preferably non-invasive methods that are capable of diagnosing malignant melanoma. Today, the only accurate diagnostic technique is a biopsy and a histological analysis of the skin tissue sample. This is an expensive procedure as well as an uncomfortable experience for the patient. For patients with many skin lesions or *dysplastic nevus syndrome* (patients with *dysplastic nevus syndrome* have multiple dysplastic nevi – often in the dozens or even hundreds), this is clearly not a feasible diagnostic technique. The problem is further complicated due to the increasing awareness of skin cancer among the general population. People are consulting dermatologists more often, which again calls for a simple and accurate diagnostic technique.

C. IMAGE ACQUISITION TECHNIQUES

1. Traditional imaging

In larger dermatological clinics, records of patients' skin lesions are kept in form of a diagnosis and one or more traditional photographs of the lesion. Some patients may be predisposed to melanoma due, for example, to cancer in the family or dysplastic nevus syndrome. These patients will often be regularly checked in order to detect any changes in their skin lesions. Photographs taken at each checkup are compared and any change is an indication of a possible malignancy. In this case, the lesion is removed and a biopsy performed.

It is mainly due to this monitoring over time that traditional imaging is used today. An example of a traditional photograph is shown in Figure 13.1.

2. Dermatoscopic imaging

Since traditional imaging is just a recording of what the human eye sees, it does not reveal any information unavailable to the eye. *Dermatoscopy,* also known as *epiluminescence microscopy*, on the other hand, is an imaging technique that provides a more direct link between biology and distinct visual characteristics.

Dermatoscopy is a noninvasive imaging technique that renders the *stratum corneum* (top layer of the skin) translucent and makes subsurface structures of the skin visible. The technique is fairly simple and involves removing reflections from the skin surface. This is done by applying immersion oil onto the skin lesion and pressing a glass plate with the same reflection index as the stratum corneum onto the lesion. The oil ensures that small cavities between the skin and the glass plate are filled in order to reduce reflections. With a strong light source, usually a halogen lamp, it is now possible to see skin structures below the skin surface. Usually the glass plate and light source are integrated into devices like a *dermatoscope* or a *dermatoscopic camera.* Both of these have lenses allowing a 10×

magnification of pigmented skin lesions. In Figure 13.1* an example of a skin lesion, recorded by the dermatoscopic imaging technique, is shown.

Although this imaging technique is not new, it is only in the last decade that it has been thoroughly investigated, especially in Western Europe [5]. However, it is still not a widely used technique primarily due to the lack of formal training in evaluating and understanding the visual characteristics in the images. Some of these characteristics will be briefly described in the next section.

A few studies concerning processing and analysis of digital dermatoscopic images have been published. In references [6] and [7], results of colour segmentation techniques based on fuzzy *c*-means clustering are shown. Preliminary results using a minimum-distance classifier for discriminating between benign nevi, dysplastic nevi, and malignant melanoma are presented in reference [8]. Based on features describing various properties including shape and colour, researchers were able to classify 56% of skin lesions in a test set correctly.

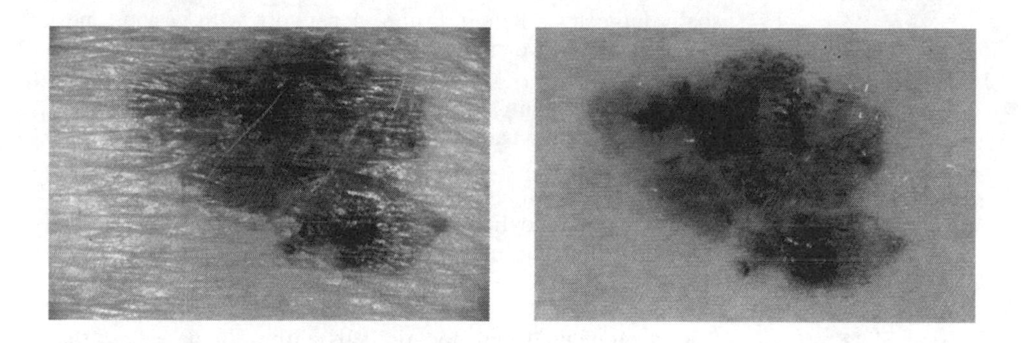

Figure 13.1 Example of pigmented skin lesion. Left: Traditional imaging technique. Right: Dermatoscopy imaging technique.

D. DERMATOSCOPIC FEATURES

The dermatoscopic imaging technique produces images that are quire different from traditional images. Several visual characteristics have been defined and analysed in recent studies, e.g., references [9-11]. These visual characteristics will be called *dermatoscopic features* or just *features* for short.

Table 13.1 lists the most important dermatoscopic features together with a short description. The features all describe specific biological behaviour (refer to reference [10] for a more detailed description). In Figure 13.2* several dermatoscopic features are shown on a pigmented skin lesion.

* Chapter 13, Colour Figures 1 and 2 follow page 136.

Table 13.1 Definition of dermatoscopic features.

Features	Description
Asymmetry	An asymmetric shape is the result of different local growth rates. This indicates malignancy. Asymmetry may be defined in numerous ways though. In Section II, one such definition is presented.
Edge abruptness	A sharp abrupt edge suggests melanoma while a gradual fading of the pigmentation indicates a benign lesion.
Colour distribution	Six different colours may be observed: light-brown, dark-brown, white, red, blue, and black. A large number of colours present indicates melanoma.
Pigment network	Area with honeycomb-like pigmentation. A regular network usually indicates a benign lesion. A network with varying mesh size suggests an atypical/dysplastic nevus or a melanoma.
Structureless area	Area with pigmentation but without any visible network. Unevenly distributed areas indicate melanoma.
Globules	Nests with a diameter of more than 0.1 mm of heavily pigmented melanocytic cells. These may be brown or black. If evenly distributed, it indicates a benign lesion.
Black dots	Heavily pigmented melanocytic cells with a diameter less than 0.1 mm. If located close to the perimeter, it suggests an atypical lesion or a melanoma.
Pseudopods	Large "rain-drop" shaped melanoma nests located at the edge of the lesion. A very strong indicator of malignant melanoma.
Radial streaming	Radial growth of melanoma. Looks like streaks. Very indicative of malignant melanoma.
Blue-white veil	Areas with a blue-white shade of colour. Indicates melanocytic cells located deep in the skin. An indictor of melanoma.
Depigmentation	Loss of pigmentation. An indicator of melanoma.

As can be seen in Figure 13.2, there is one prominent artefact due to the use of immersion oil. Small air bubbles occur in the oil layer and appear as small white circles or ellipses. This artefact can be avoided if the oil is carefully applied. Usually the area occupied by air bubbles is very small, but important features such as black dots or *pseudopods* may be obscured by air bubbles.

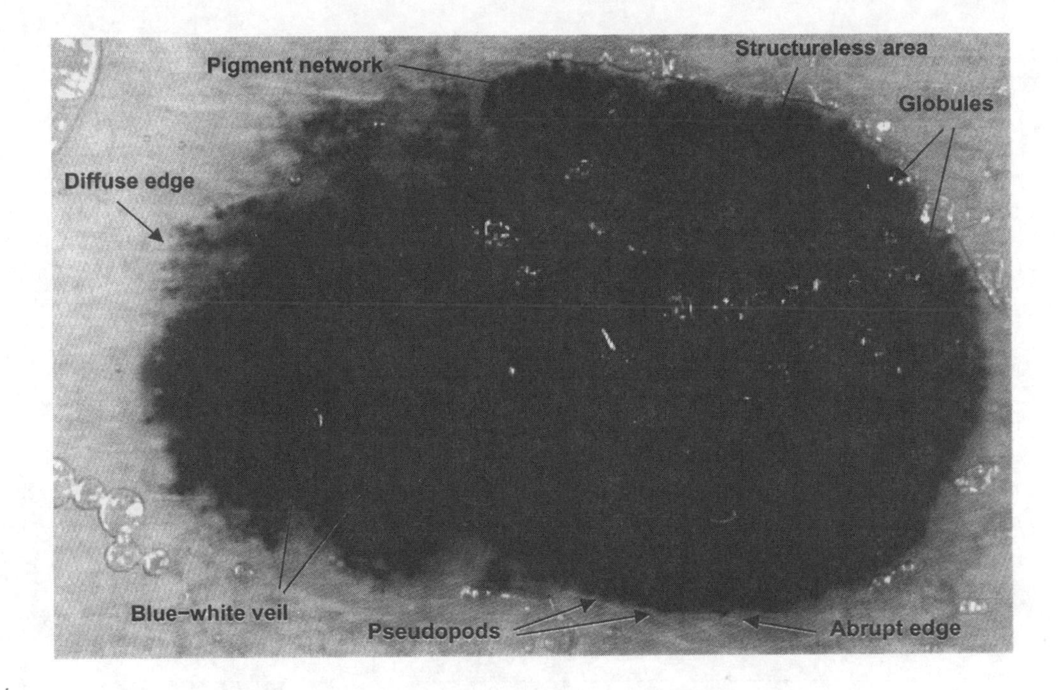

Figure 13.2 Pigmented skin lesion with several dermatoscopic features.

II. FEATURE EXTRACTION IN DERMATOSCOPIC IMAGES

In the previous section, dermatoscopic images and features were introduced. In this section, we will describe the image processing techniques used in order to extract and describe dermatoscopic features.

In Figure 13.3*, a flowchart describing the feature extracting process is shown. The four main blocks, image acquisition, preprocessing, segmentation, and dermatoscopic feature description are presented in the following sections.

A. IMAGE ACQUISITION

All dermatoscopic images used in this work have been acquired at Rigshospitalet, Copenhagen, Denmark, using a *Dermaphot* camera (*Heine Optotechnik*).

The images are developed as slides and digitised with a resolution of 1270 dots per inch and 24 bit colour (8 bits for each of the colour channels: red, green, and blue) using an *Eskoscan 2540* colour scanner (*Eskofot*). The image resolution has subsequently been digitally reduced by a factor 2 in order to limit the computational resources needed for processing the images, thus reducing the size of each image to 885×590.

* Chapter 13, Colour Figure 3 follows page 136.

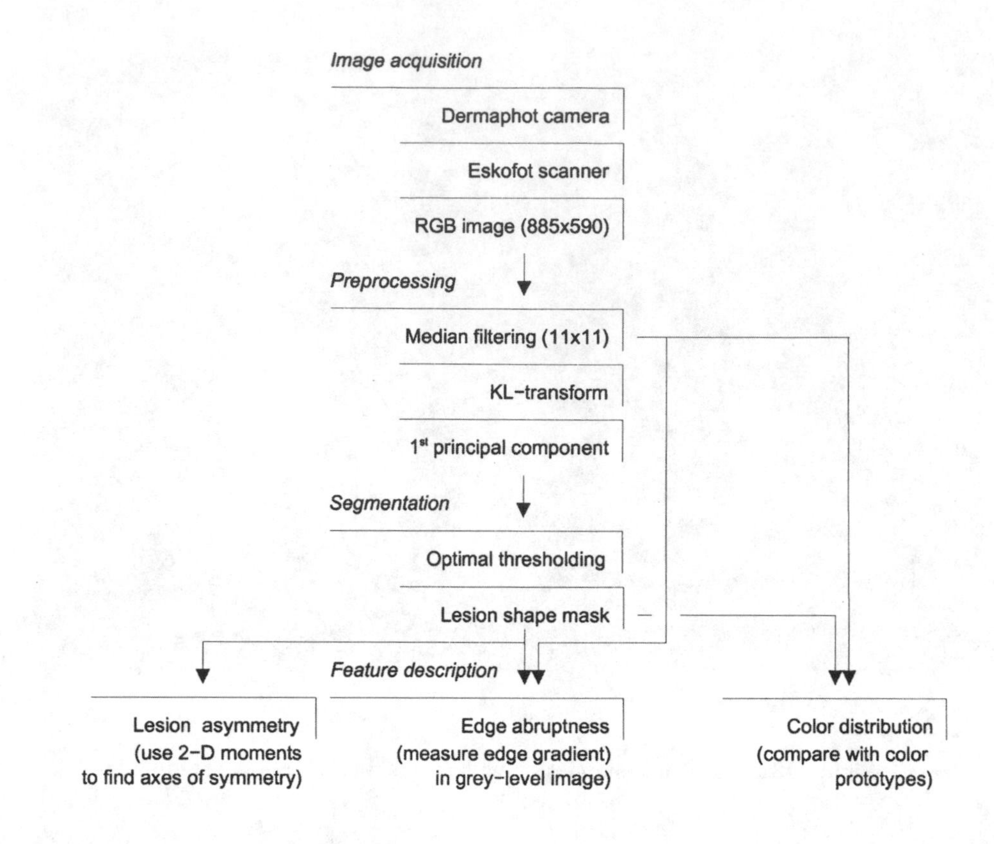

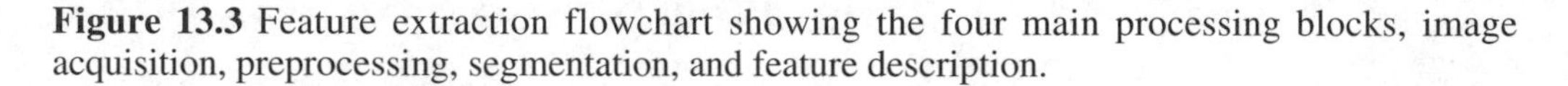

Figure 13.3 Feature extraction flowchart showing the four main processing blocks, image acquisition, preprocessing, segmentation, and feature description.

B. IMAGE PREPROCESSING

The first step in the feature extraction process is the preprocessing of images with the purpose of reducing noise and facilitating image segmentation by using median filtering and the Karhunen-Loève transform.

Now, let us first define a grey-level image of size $M \times N$ as a sequence of numbers,

$$z(m,n) \qquad 1 \le m \le M,\ 1 \le n \le N \tag{1}$$

where $z(m,n)$ is the luminance of pixel (m,n). If dealing with an 8-bit grey-level image, then each element, $z(m,n)$, will be an integer in the interval [0; 255]. In any processing of 8-bit images, we will abandon the integer restriction and process the image in a floating point representation in order to minimise quantisation effects.

Next, we define a colour image of size $M \times N$ as 3 sequences, $r(m,n)$, $g(m,n)$ and $b(m,n)$, with $r(m,n)$ representing the red, $g(m,n)$ the green, and $b(m,n)$ the blue colour components, respectively. The individual colour components are typically represented by 8 bits, but again any processing will be done using floating point precision.

1. Median filtering

As noted in Section I.D., the immersion oil used in the dermatoscopic imaging technique may produce small air bubbles manifesting themselves as small white ellipses, lines or dots. This artefact can be considered as impulsive noise and may thus be reduced using a median filter given by

$$z_{med}(m,n) = median\left\{ z(m-k,n-l) \middle| -\frac{N_{med}-1}{2} \leq k,l \leq \frac{N_{med}-1}{2} \wedge 1 \leq m-k \leq M \wedge 1 \leq n-l \leq N \right\} \quad (2)$$

where N_{med} is odd (if the median kernel size is even, there will be two middle values. One could then define the median as the mean of these two values) and indicates the size of the two-dimensional median filter. Note that we only consider a square median filter kernel. We may in fact consider any shape of filter kernel if desirable. Equation (2) is valid for a grey-level image. When working with colour images, one should apply the same median filter to all 3-colour components.

Skin Lesion Specific Comments

The main purpose of filtering dermatoscopic images is to reduce localised reflection artefacts while at the same time preserving edges. In Figure 13.4*, the results of applying a 11×11 median filter to a dermatoscopic image is shown. This kernel size is used for all median filtering in this work.

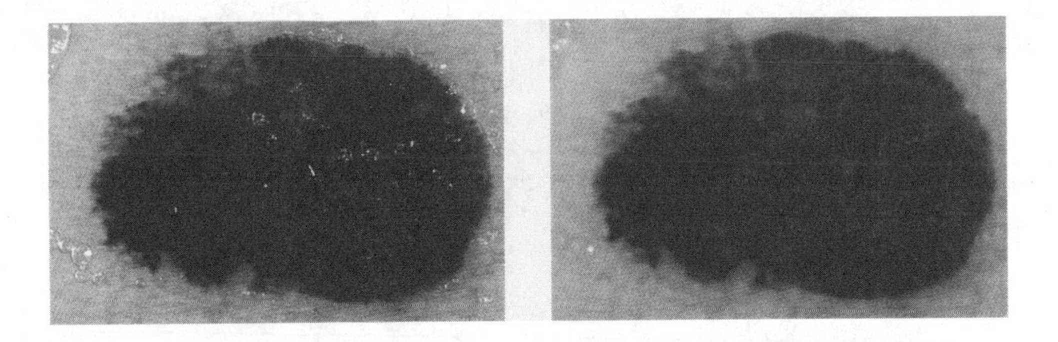

Figure 13.4 The effect of filtering a 885×590 dermatoscopic image with an 11×11 median filter. Left: Original image. Right: Filtered image. Notice how the air bubble artefacts have been reduced, especially around the lesion edge in the upper right hand corner.

* Chapter 13, Colour Figure 4 follows page 136.

2. Karhunen-Loève transform

The next preprocessing stage aims at facilitating the segmentation process by enhancing the edges in the image. For this purpose the *Karhunen-Loève* (KL) transform, also known as the *Hotelling* transform or the method of principal components [12,13], is used.

The KL transform is a linear transformation that uncorrelates the input variables by employing an orthonormal basis found by an eigenvalue decomposition of the sample covariance matrix for the input variables.

In image processing applications, the KL transformation is often applied to the 2-D image domain. Here, we will apply the transformation to the 3-D colour space spanned by $r(m,n)$, $g(m,n)$, and $b(m,n)$.

Now, let us define the following $3 \times MN$ matrix containing all pixels from the 3 colour channels,

$$\mathbf{V} = \begin{bmatrix} r(1,1) & r(1,2) & \cdots & r(1,N) & r(2,1) & \cdots & r(M,N) \\ g(1,1) & g(1,2) & \cdots & g(1,N) & g(2,1) & \cdots & g(M,N) \\ b(1,1) & b(1,2) & \cdots & b(1,N) & b(2,1) & \cdots & b(M,N) \end{bmatrix} \tag{3}$$

where we view $[r(m, n)\ g(m, n)\ b(m, n)]^T$ as a sample of a stochastic variable.

Let $\bar{\mathbf{v}}$ contain the sample mean of the 3 colour components,

$$\bar{\mathbf{v}} = \frac{1}{MN} \sum_{m=1}^{M} \sum_{n=1}^{N} \begin{bmatrix} r(m,n) \\ g(m,n) \\ b(m,n) \end{bmatrix} \tag{4}$$

The sample covariance matrix is now given by

$$\mathbf{C} = \frac{1}{MN} \mathbf{V}\mathbf{V}^T - \bar{\mathbf{v}}\bar{\mathbf{v}}^T \tag{5}$$

which can be eigenvalue decomposed, so that

$$\mathbf{C} = \mathbf{E}\Lambda\mathbf{E}^T \tag{6}$$

where $\mathbf{E} = [e_1 \quad e_2 \quad e_3]$ is a matrix containing the eigenvectors of $\mathbf{C}$, and $\mathbf{\Lambda}$ is a diagonal matrix containing the corresponding eigenvalues of $\mathbf{C}$ in decreasing order: $\lambda_1 \geq \lambda_2 \geq \lambda_3 \geq 0$.

The KL transformation is now defined as

$$\mathbf{z} = \mathbf{E}^T (\mathbf{v} - \bar{\mathbf{v}}) \tag{7}$$

where $\mathbf{v}$ is a column vector in $\mathbf{V}$ and $\mathbf{z}$ contains what is known as the *principal components*.

Due to the decreasing ordering of the eigenvalues and the corresponding eigenvectors, the first principal component will contain the maximum variance. In fact, no other linear transformation using unit length basis vectors can produce components with a variance larger than λ_1 [14].

Skin Lesion Specific Comments

For median filtered dermatoscopic images, the first principal component will typically account for more than 95% of the total variance. Since most variation occurs at edges between regions with similar luminance levels, the first principal component is a natural choice for segmentation. Another study also shows that the Karhunen-Loève transform is appropriate for segmenting dermatoscopic images [6].

C. IMAGE SEGMENTATION

The next step in the feature extraction process is *image segmentation*. The main goal is to divide an image into regions of interest from which appropriate features can be extracted. Here, we will consider a complete segmentation that divides the entire image into disjoint regions. Denoting the image, R, and the N regions, R_i, $i = 1, 2, \ldots, N$, this may be formalised as

$$R = \bigcup_{i=1}^{N} R_i, \qquad R_i \cap R_j = 0, \quad i \neq j \tag{8}$$

The regions are usually constructed so that they are homogeneous with respect to some chosen property such as luminance, colour, or context. We will now consider the case where the objective is to group pixels containing the same approximate luminance level.

1. Optimal thresholding

Thresholding is a very simple segmentation method based on using thresholds on the luminance level of pixels in order to determine what region a pixel belongs to. Denoting the non-negative luminance of a pixel, $z(m,n)$, a thresholding process using N–1 thresholds to divide an image into N regions may be written as

$$z(m,n) \in \begin{cases} R_1 & \text{if } z(m,n) < T_1 \\ R_2 & \text{if } T_1 \leq z(m,n) < T_2 \\ \cdot & \ldots \\ R_i & \text{if } T_{i-1} \leq z(m,n) < T_i \\ \cdot & \ldots \\ R_N & \text{if } T_{N-1} \leq z(m,n) \end{cases} \tag{9}$$

where T_i is the threshold separating pixels in region R_i from pixels in region R_{i+1}.

Let us consider the luminance level, $z(m,n)$, to be a sample of a stochastic variable, z, and let the conditional luminance probability distribution be denoted by $p(z|R_i)$ and the prior region probability by $P(R_i)$. Assuming we know $p(z|R_i)$ and $P(R_i)$, we may view the problem of selecting the thresholds as a classification problem and use Bayesian decision theory to minimise the probability of misclassifying a pixel.

Let us now assume that the conditional luminance probability distributions, $p(z|R_i)$, are Gaussian with mean $\mu_{R'}$ and equal variance $\sigma_{R_i}^2 = \sigma^2$. We thus obtain the following closed-form solution for the optimal thresholds,

$$T_i = \frac{\mu_{R_i} + \mu_{R_{i+1}}}{2} + \frac{\sigma^2}{\mu_{R_i} - \mu_{R_{i+1}}} \log \frac{P(R_{i+1})}{P(R_i)} \tag{10}$$

where $i = 1, 2, \ldots, N - 1$. Assuming the prior probabilities, $P(R_i)$, are equal, equation (10) reduces to

$$T_i = \frac{\mu_{R_i} + \mu_{R_{i+1}}}{2} \tag{11}$$

A simple iterative scheme based on equation (11) for estimating the $N - 1$ optimal thresholds and the N luminance means is [15]

1. Initialise thresholds, so that $T_1 < T_2 < \ldots < T_{N-1}$.

2. At time step t, compute the luminance region means

$$\mu_{R_i}^{(t)} = \frac{\sum_{(m,n)\in R_i^{(t)}} z(m,n)}{N_{R_i}^{(t)}} \quad (12)$$

where $N_{R_i}^{(t)}$ is the number of pixels in region R_i at time step t and $i = 1, 2, \ldots, N$.

3. The thresholds at time step $t + 1$ are now computed as

$$T_i^{(i+1)} = \frac{\mu_{R_i}^{(t)} + \mu_{R_{i+1}}^{(t)}}{2} \quad (13)$$

where $i = 1, 2, \ldots, N - 1$.

4. If $T_i^{(t+1)} = T_i^{(t)}$ for all $i = 1, 2, \ldots, N - 1$, then stop; otherwise return to step 2.

Skin Lesion Specific Comments

All dermatoscopic images in this work have been segmented by the optimal thresholding algorithm using 2 thresholds. A typical first principal component of a median filtered dermatoscopic image consists of a very light background and a dark skin lesion with even darker areas inside. These 3 regions are usually fairly homogeneous making the assumption of Gaussian luminance probability distributions a sound one. The assumptions of equal variances, $\sigma_{R_i}^2$, and equal priors, $P(R_i)$, are usually not warranted. Nevertheless, the algorithm provides good results using dermatoscopic images.

Note that the main purpose of segmentation in this application is to find a lesion shape mask defining the edge location of the lesion. Thus, we are only interested in the threshold separating the light skin background and the darker skin lesion. In some cases the segmentation produces several skin lesion candidates due to other small nonlesion objects. Usually the largest object is the skin lesion and is thus selected for further processing.

In Figure 13.5, the results of using the optimal thresholding algorithm on a dermatoscopic image using 2 thresholds to separate 3 regions are shown. Note the similar shape of the sample histogram and the estimated histogram indicating the usability of the optimal thresholding algorithm in the context of dermatoscopic images.

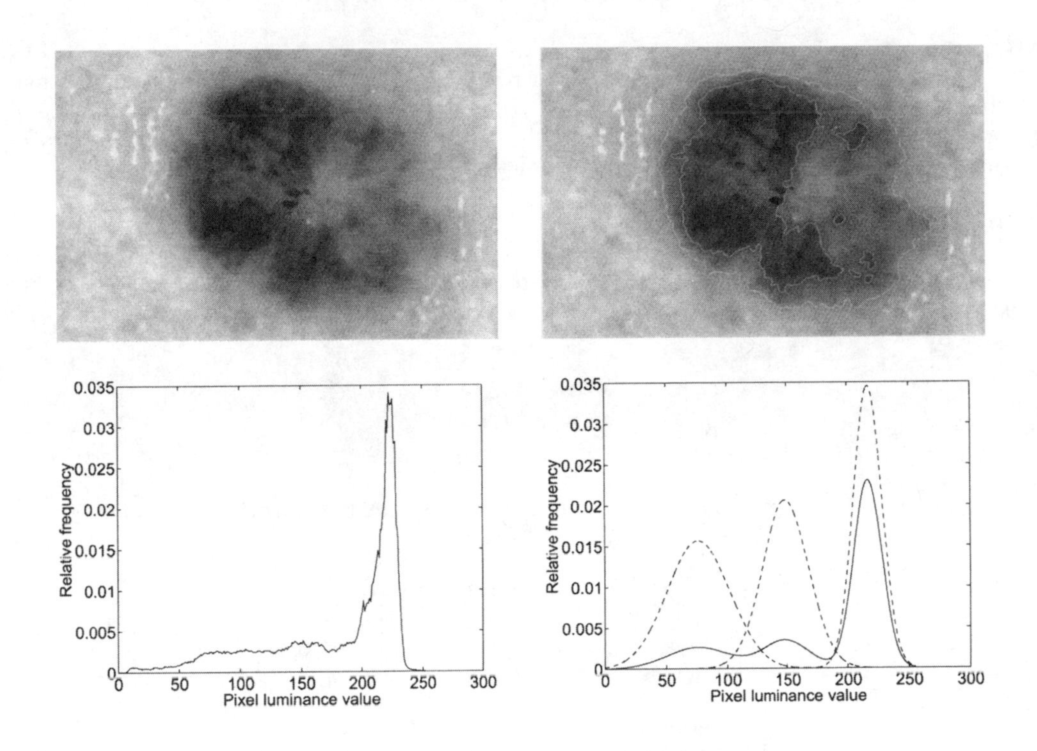

Figure 13.5 Example of results using the optimal thresholding algorithm on the first principal component of a median filtered dermatoscopic image. Upper left: Median filtered first principal component. Upper right: The segmentation result using 2 thresholds to separate 3 regions. The solid white lines indicate region borders. Lower left: The sample histogram of the upper left image. Lower right: Estimated histogram. The dashed lines show the luminance probability densities, $p(z \mid R_i)$, estimated by the optimal thresholding algorithm. The solid line shows the estimated histogram computed by assuming that the prior probabilities of the 3 regions are 1/6, 1/6, and 4/6 from left to right. Note that the overall shape of the estimated histogram matches the sample histogram fairly well.

D. DERMATOSCOPIC FEATURE DESCRIPTION

The final step in the feature extraction process is the actual extraction and description of features. In this section we will present methods for describing the following skin lesion properties:

- Asymmetry of the lesion border.
- Transition of the pigmentation from the skin lesion to the surrounding skin.
- Colour distribution of the skin lesion including the blue-white veil.

1. Asymmetry

An asymmetric skin lesion shape is the result of different local growth rates and may indicate malignancy.

In order to measure asymmetry, we will first look at 2-D moments and how these may be used for describing certain geometrical properties of an object or a region in an image.

Moments

Moment representations interpret a normalised grey-level image function, $z(x,y)$, as a probability density function of a 2-D stochastic variable. Properties of this variable may thus be described by 2-D moments [16]. For a digital image, $z(m,n)$, the moment of order $(p + q)$ is given by

$$m_{pq} = \sum_{m=1}^{M} \sum_{n=1}^{N} m^p n^q z(m,n) \tag{14}$$

Translation invariant moments are obtained by considering the *centralised moments*

$$m_{pq}^{c} = \sum_{m=1}^{M} \sum_{n=1}^{N} (m - m_c)^p (n - n_c)^q z(m,n) \tag{15}$$

where (m_c,n_c) is the *centre of mass* given by $m_c = \dfrac{m_{10}}{m_{00}}$, $n_c = \dfrac{m_{01}}{m_{00}}$.

We will now consider the case where $z(m,n)$ is binary and represents a region, R, so that $z(m,n) = 1$ if $(m,n) \in R$, otherwise $z(m,n) = 0$. This could, for instance, be the result of a segmentation process.

The moment of inertia for a binary object or region R, w.r.t. an axis through the centre of mass with an angle θ as shown in Figure 13.6 is defined as [17]

$$I(\theta) = \sum_{(m,n) \in R} \sum D_{\theta}^{2}(m,n) \tag{16}$$

$$= \sum_{(m,n) \in R} \sum \left[-(m - m_c)\sin\theta + (n - n_c)\cos\theta\right]^2 \tag{17}$$

where $D_\theta(m,n)$ is found by translating the object so that its centre of mass coincides with the centre of origin of the coordinate system, and by rotating the object otherwise by the angle θ so that the n-coordinate of the translated and rotated point (m,n) equals the desired distance $D_\theta(m,n)$. (Rotation of a point (m,n) clockwise by the angle θ is given by: $(m_r,n_r) = (m \cos \theta + n \sin \theta, -m \sin \theta + n \cos \theta)$.)

The orientation of an object is defined as the angle of the axis through the centre of mass that results in the least moment of inertia [17]. To obtain this angle, we compute the derivative of equation (17) and set it to zero,

$$\frac{\partial I(\theta)}{\partial \theta} = 0 \Rightarrow \theta_o = \frac{1}{2}\tan^{-1}\left[\frac{2m_{11}^c}{m_{20}^c - m_{02}^c}\right] \tag{18}$$

The axis through the centre of mass defined by θ_O is also known as a *principal axis*. We will refer to this as the *major axis*. All objects have two principal axes where the second principal axis is defined by the angle yielding the largest moment of inertia (note that a circle has an infinite number of principal axes due to its rotational symmetry). This will be referred to as the *minor axis*. The principal axes are orthogonal and will in the next section be used for calculating asymmetry.

In Figure 13.6, an example of a skin lesion and its two principal axes are shown.

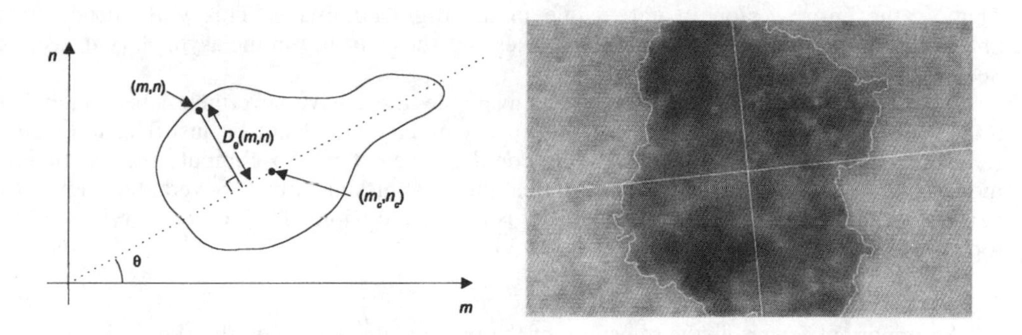

Figure 13.6 Left: The orientation angle, θ_O, of an object is defined as the angle of the axis through the centre of mass, (m_C, n_C), that minimises the moment of inertia, $I(\theta) = \sum_{m=1}^{M}\sum_{n=1}^{N} D_\theta^2(m,n)z(m,n)$. Right: Skin lesion showing the edge of the lesion and the two principal axes used for calculating asymmetry. These axes define directions of least and largest moments of inertia. The two asymmetry indexes for this lesion are 0.14, respectively. Note that this lesion is larger than the field of view of the camera. Only very large lesions, where the calculation of asymmetry cannot be justified, have been omitted from the data set.

Measuring Asymmetry

The principal axes found in the previous section will now be used as axes of symmetry. That is, we will measure how asymmetric the object is with respect to these two axes. This can be done by folding the object about its principal axes and measuring the area of the non-overlapping regions relative to the entire object area. Thus, for each principal axis, we define a measure of asymmetry as

$$S_i = \frac{\Delta A_i}{A} \tag{19}$$

where $i = 1, 2$ indicates the principal axis, ΔA_i is the corresponding nonoverlapping area of the folded object and A is the area of the entire region. For an object completely symmetric about the *i'th* principal axis, S_i' is zero while complete asymmetry yields an asymmetry measure of 1.

Skin Lesion Specific Comments

Several skin lesions included in this work are larger than the field of view of the camera. That is, the entire lesion in not visible in the digitised image. This will introduce an uncertainty in the location of the principal axes and subsequently in the asymmetry measures. See the example in Figure 13.6.

Due to the rather limited amount of data available, these have nevertheless been included. Some severe cases, where the calculation of asymmetry could not be justified, have been removed from the data set, though. One could also elect not to compute the asymmetry measures in these cases and subsequently treat them as missing values. Several techniques for dealing with missing values exist. The reader is referred to Ripley [18] for an overview on this topic.

2. Edge abruptness

An important feature is the transition of the pigmentation between the skin lesion and the surrounding skin. A sharp abrupt edge suggests malignancy while a gradual fading of the pigmentation indicates a benign lesion.

In order to measure the edge abruptness, let us first estimate the gradient of a grey-level image.

Image Gradient Estimation

In a digital image, $z(m,n)$, the gradient magnitude, $g(m,n)$ and gradient direction, $\theta_g(m,n)$, are defined by [16]:

$$g(m,n) = \sqrt{g_1^2(m,n) + g_2^2(m,n)}, \qquad \theta_g(m,n) = \tan^{-1}\left(\frac{g_2(m,n)}{g_1(m,n)}\right) \tag{20}$$

where $g_1(m,n)$ and $g_2(m,n)$ are the difference approximations to the partial derivatives in the m and n direction, respectively,

$$g_1(m,n) = \sum_i \sum_j h_1(-i,-j)z(m+i,m+j) \tag{21}$$

$$g_2(m,n) = \sum_i \sum_j h_2(-i,-j)z(m+i,m+j) \tag{22}$$

$g_1(m,n)$ and $g_2(m,n)$ are expressed as convolutions between the image and *gradient operators* denoted by $h_1(i, j)$ and $h_2(i, j)$, $-(N_h - 1)/2 \leq i, j \leq (N_h - 1)/2$, where N_h is odd and indicates the size of the gradient operators.

Several gradient operators have been suggested [17]. Here we will use the Sobel gradient operator defined by

$$\mathbf{H_1} = \begin{bmatrix} -1 & 0 & 1 \\ -2 & 0 & 2 \\ -1 & 0 & 1 \end{bmatrix}, \quad \mathbf{H_2} = \begin{bmatrix} 1 & 2 & 1 \\ 0 & 0 & 0 \\ -1 & -2 & -1 \end{bmatrix} \tag{23}$$

In the following, we will denote the gradient magnitude estimation of a grey-level digital image, $z(m,n)$, using the Sobel gradient operators by $g(m,n) = \text{grad}[z(m,n)]$.

Measuring Edge Abruptness

Let us consider the luminance component of a colour image given by

$$z(m,n) = \frac{1}{3}\left[r(m,n) + g(m,n) + b(m,n)\right] \tag{24}$$

which is just an equally weighted sum of the three colour components.

We may now estimate the gradient magnitude of the intensity component by computing $g(m,n) = \text{grad}[z(m,n)]$.

If we sample the gradient magnitude, $g(m,n)$, along the edge of the skin lesion, we obtain a set of gradient magnitude values,

$$e(k) = g(m(k), n(k)), \qquad k = 0, 1, \ldots, K-1 \tag{25}$$

where K is the total number of edge samples and $(m(k),n(k))$ are the coordinates of the k'th edge pixel.

This set of values describes the transition between the lesion and the skin background in each edge point. In order to describe the general transition or abruptness, we use the sample mean and variance of the gradient magnitude values $e(k)$,

$$m_e = \frac{1}{K}\sum_{k=0}^{K-1} e(k), \qquad v_e = \frac{1}{K}\sum_{k=0}^{K-1} e^2(k) - m_e^2 \tag{26}$$

where the sample mean, m_e, describes the general abruptness level and the sample variance, v_e, describes the variation of the abruptness along the skin lesion edge.

In Figure 13.7, an example of measuring the abruptness in a dermatoscopic image is shown.

Skin Lesion Specific Comments

As mentioned previously, several skin lesions larger than the field of view of the camera are included in this work. For these lesions the gradient magnitude has not been sampled along false edges. These occur at the boundaries of the image where the skin lesion crosses the image border (see the sample in Figure 13.6). Thus we assume that each edge information is available from the visible part of the skin lesion in order to describe the characteristics of the lesion edge, and that we can neglect the contributions outside the field of view.

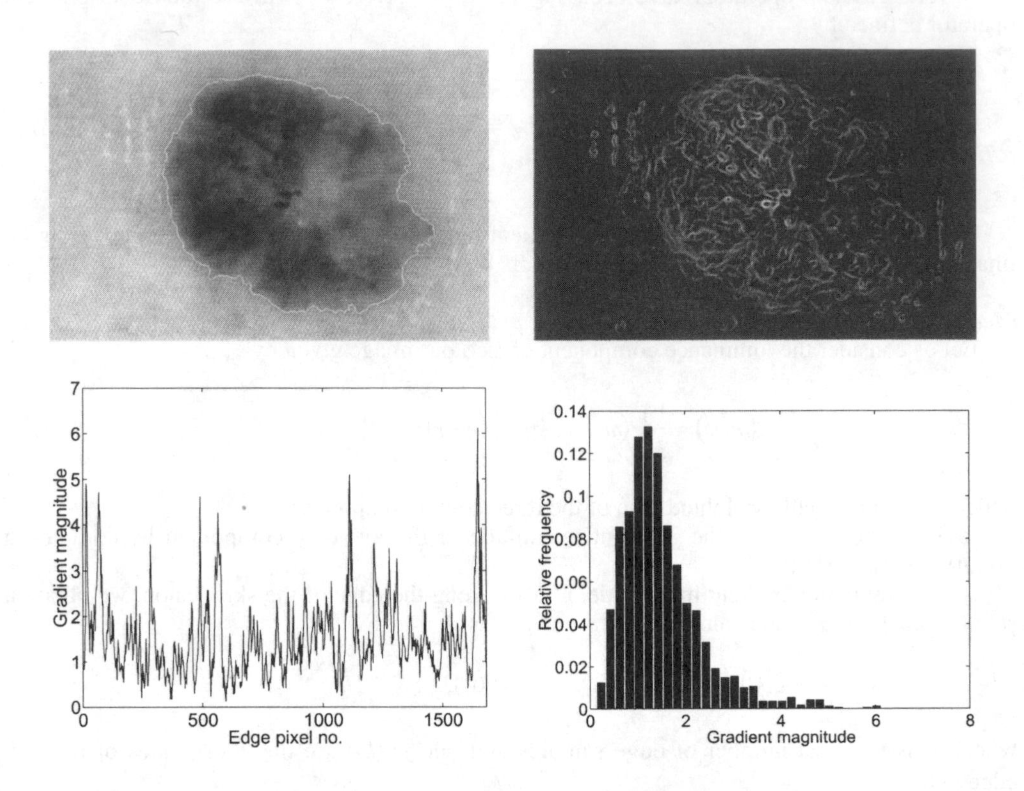

Figure 13.7 Example of measuring edge abruptness in a dermatoscopic image. Upper left: Intensity image showing the lesion edge obtained from the segmentation process. Upper right: Gradient magnitude image. *Lower left:* The gradient magnitude sampled among the lesion edge. *Lower right:* Histogram of gradient magnitude measured along the lesion edge. Note: The gradient magnitude range has been compressed by the transformation, $g_C(m,n) = \log(1 + g(m,n))$, in order to enhance the visual quality.

3. Colour

The colour distribution of a skin lesion is another important aspect that may contribute to an accurate diagnosis. Dermatologists have identified 6 shades of colour that may be present in skin lesions examined with the dermatoscopic imaging technique. These colours arise due to several biological processes [10]. The colours are *light-brown, dark-brown, white, red, blue,* and *black* [10]. This is a rather vague colour description that is likely to cause some discrepancies between how different individuals perceive skin lesion colours. Especially, there are problems with separating light-brown from dark-brown, but problems also occur with red and dark-brown due to a rather reddish glow of the dark-brown colour in skin lesions.

We will nevertheless try to define a consistent method of measuring skin lesion colours that matches the dermatologists' intuitive perception of colours. This is achieved by defining colour prototypes that are in close correspondence with the colour perception of dermatologists and using these prototypes to determine the colour contents of skin lesions. As a guideline, a large number of colours is considered to be an indicator of malignancy.

Colour Prototype Determination

The colour prototypes have been determined from three 2-D histograms (red-green, red-blue, and green-blue) of 18 randomly selected skin lesion images combined into one large image. By inspecting the histograms, several clusters matching the colour perception of dermatologists are defined and the perceived cluster centres are used as prototypes. This is shown in Figure 13.8. Note that several shades of light-brown, dark-brown and blue have been identified. No reliable prototype for red distinguishing it from dark-brown could be determined. This is a problem that is also found amongst dermatologists. One may consider a part of a lesion to be red while another may suggest dark-brown. Due to these difficulties, a red prototype has not been defined.

It is clear that this way of determining prototypes is a very subjective process, yet great care has been taken in order for the prototypes to match the colour perception of dermatologists. (The authors have spent numerous sessions with dermatologists viewing and discussing skin lesions in order to gain insight into their colour perception).

A standard *k-means* clustering algorithm using the Euclidean distance measure in the RGB colour space has also been employed but did not yield acceptable colour prototypes. It is obvious, through inspection of the 2-D histograms, that the Euclidean distance measure is not the most appropriate choice due to the varying shape of the different clusters. It would be beneficial to allow the distance measure to vary between clusters, acknowledging that different probability distributions generate the individual clusters. Often these distributions may be considered Gaussian [19].

Another contributing factor to the failure of the standard *k-means* algorithm is the number of pixels in each cluster. The histograms in Figure 13.8* are log-transformed, that is the dynamic range has been compressed in order to enhance the visual quality. Thus the number of pixels close to the centre of some of the clusters seems relatively large compared to, for example, the dominant *skin* colour cluster even though the number of pixels in these clusters is in fact rather small. In the standard *k-means* algorithm, these clusters are likely to be suppressed by the higher populated dominant clusters resulting in unacceptable results.

Thus in order to overcome these problems and to incorporate the colour perception of dermatologists, the manually selected prototypes are used in this work. Note that 10 colour clusters have been defined but only 9 prototypes are used. The *skin* prototype is left out as this colour is eliminated by the segmentation process and normally only found outside the lesion. The 9 colour prototypes thus correspond to *white*, *black*, *light-brown 1*, *light-brown 2*, *dark-brown 1*, *dark-brown 2*, *blue 1*, *blue 2,* and *blue 3* representing 5 different colours.

---

* Chapter 13, Colour Figure 8 follows page 136.

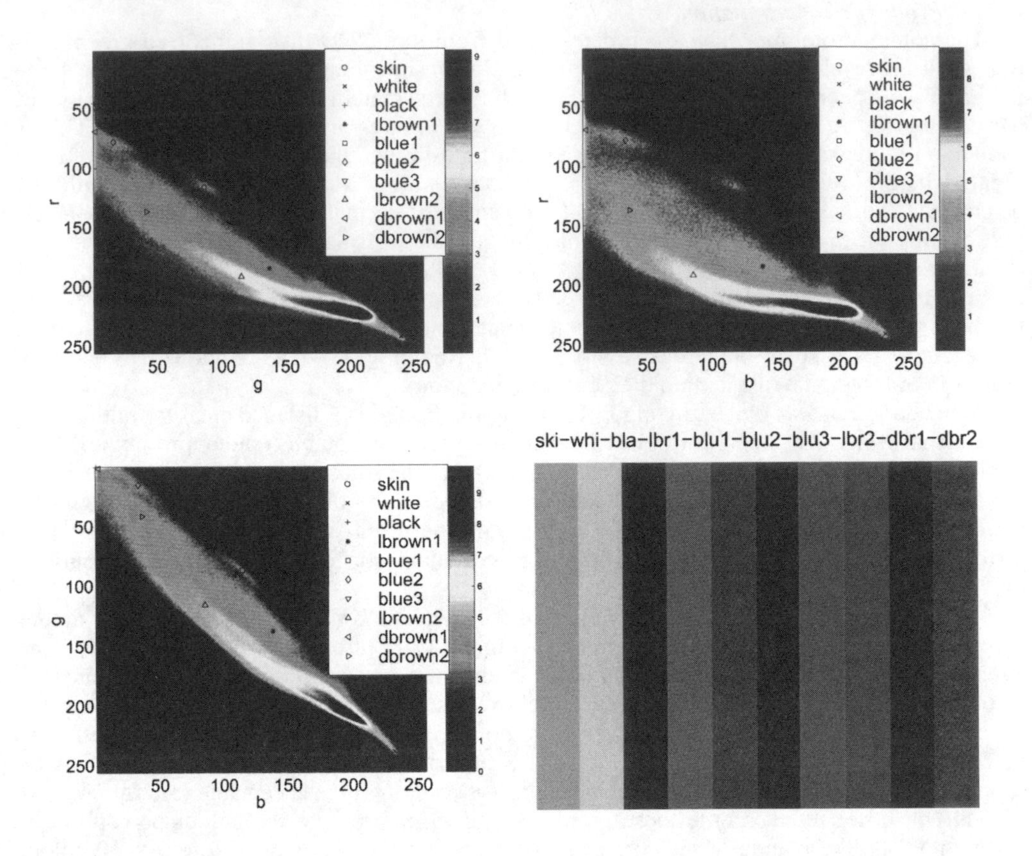

Figure 13.8 Colour prototypes have been found manually by inspecting the combined 2-D histograms of 18 randomly selected images. The perceived cluster centres are chosen as prototypes. Upper left: Red-green 2-D histogram. The histogram values, $h(r,g)$, have been compressed by the transformation, $h_C(r,g) = \log(1 + h(r,g))$, in order to enhance the visual quality. Upper right: Red-blue 2-D histogram (log-transformed). Lower left: Green-blue 2-D histogram (log-transformed). Lower right: The determined colour prototypes. The *skin* colour prototype is left out since it is eliminated by the segmentation process. Only colours inside the lesion are of interest in this work.

Measuring Colour

The colour contents of a skin lesion may be determined by comparing the skin lesion pixels with colour prototypes. Here we will use the Euclidean distance measure for comparing colours,

$$d_i^2(m,n) = [r(m,n) - r_i]^2 + [g(m,n) - g_i]^2 + [b(m,n) - b_i]^2, \quad i = 1,2,...,9 \qquad (27)$$

where $d_i(m,n)$ is the distance in RGB "colour-space" from pixel (m,n) to the *i'th* colour prototype defined by $cp_i = [r_i, g_i\, b_i]^T$.

Every skin lesion pixel can now be assigned a prototype colour by selecting the shortest distance. That is, the pixel *(m,n)* should be assigned the prototype colour cp_i if

$$d_i(m,n) < d_j(m,n) \qquad \text{for all } i \neq j \tag{28}$$

We may now describe the colour contents of a skin lesion as a set of relative areas – one for each colour prototype. This may be written as:

$$a_i = \frac{A_{cp_i}}{A} \tag{29}$$

where A is the area of the skin lesion, A_{cp_i} the area inside the skin lesion occupied by pixels close to prototype colour cp_i as defined by equation (28), and a_i the relative measure of the colour content of the prototype colour cp_i. Since we do not wish to distinguish between different shades of the same colour, the colour content of light-brown is defined as the sum of a_i for the two light-brown colour shades. The same applies to the blue and dark-brown colour shades.

As mentioned in the previous section, the choice of distance measure is not trivial. The most appropriate distance measure in this context would be one that takes the colour perception of dermatologists into account. The international committee on colour standards, CIE (Commission Internationale de L'Eclairage), has proposed the perceptually uniform colour-spaces, CIE-Lab and CIE-Luv, in which the Euclidean distance measure matches the average human perception of colour differences [20]. In order to transform pixels in RGB colour-space to either CIE-Luv or CIE-Lab colour-space, one must first empirically determine a linear 3×3 transformation matrix for the complete imaging system (the imaging system in this application consists of camera, film, development process, and image scanning) that transforms the RGB colour-space of the imaging system to the standardised CIE-RGB colour-space [21]. The CIE-RGB values may then be converted through a non-linear transformation into either CIE-Luv or CIE-Lab values [17]. Using the Euclidean distance measure in either of these colour-spaces for comparing colours may yield results corresponding better with the colour perception of dermatologists.

An example of skin lesion comparison with the colour prototypes is shown in Figure 13.9*.

Skin Lesion Specific Comments

Note that the use of colour prototypes requires that the conditions of the imaging system are very controlled in order to achieve colour consistency. This involves camera, lighting conditions, film type, film development process, and scanner.

---

* Chapter 13, Colour Figure 9 follows page 136.

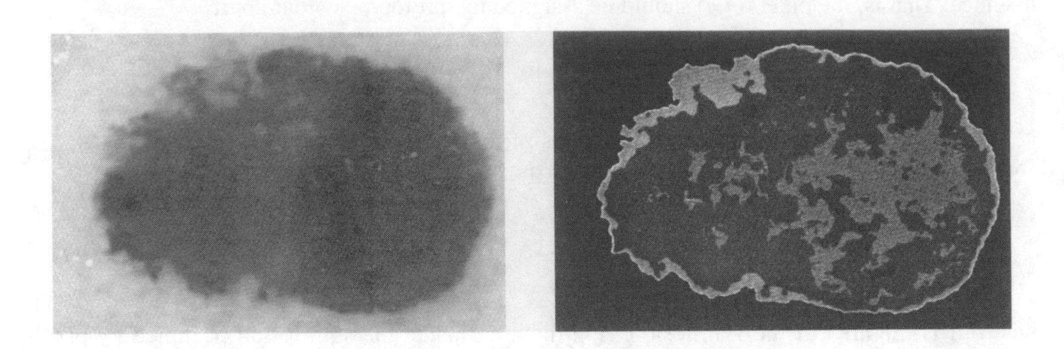

Figure 13.9 Examples of colour detection in a dermatoscopic image. Left: Original median filtered image. Right: Results of comparing the skin lesion image in the left panel with colour prototypes in the RGB colour-space using the Euclidean difference measure. Note that all shades of blue are represented by the *blue 1* prototype seen in Figure 13.8, all shades of dark-brown by *dbrown2* and all shades of light-brown by *lbrown2*.

III. A PROBABILISTIC FRAMEWORK FOR CLASSIFICATION

A. BAYES' DECISION THEORY

Bayes' decision theory is based on the assumption that the classification problem at hand can be expressed in probabilistic terms and that these terms are either known or can be estimated.

Suppose the classification problem is to map an input pattern $\mathbf{x}$ into a class C_l out of n_c classes where $l = 1, 2, \ldots, n_c$. We can now define several probabilistic terms that are related through *Bayes' theorem* [22],

$$P(C_l \mid \mathbf{x}) = \frac{p(\mathbf{x} \mid C_l)P(C_l)}{p(\mathbf{x})} \tag{30}$$

$P(C_l)$ is the class *prior* and reflects our prior belief of an unobserved pattern $\mathbf{x}$ belonging to class C_l. $p(\mathbf{x} \mid C_l)$ is the *class-conditional probability density function* and describes the probability characteristics of $\mathbf{x}$ once we know it belongs to class C_l. The *posterior* probability is denoted by $P(C_l \mid \mathbf{x})$ and is the probability of an observed pattern $\mathbf{x}$ belonging to class C_l. The unconditional probability density function, $p(\mathbf{x})$, describing the density function for $\mathbf{x}$ regardless of the class, is given by

$$p(\mathbf{x}) = \sum_{l=1}^{n_c} p(\mathbf{x} \mid C_l)P(C_l) \tag{31}$$

In short, Bayes' theorem shows how the observation of a pattern $\mathbf{x}$ changes the prior probability $P(C_l)$ into a posterior probability $P(C_l \mid \mathbf{x})$.

A classification system usually divides the input space into a set of n_c decision regions, R_1, R_2, ..., R_{n_c}, so that a pattern, $\mathbf{x}$, located in R_l is assigned to class C_l. The boundaries between the regions are called *decision boundaries*. Often the aim of a classifier is to minimise the probability of error, that is, to minimise the probability of classifying a pattern **x** belonging to class C_l as a different class due to **x** not being in decision region R_l. This leads to *Bayes' minimum-error decision rule* saying that a pattern should be assigned to class C_l if [22]

$$P(C_l \mid \mathbf{x}) > P(C_m \mid \mathbf{x}) \qquad \text{for all } l \neq m \tag{32}$$

As already mentioned, Bayes' minimum-error decision rule assumes that the aim is to minimise the probability of error. This makes sense if every possible error is associated with the same cost. If this is not the case, one could adopt a *risk-based approach* [23]. It may also be appropriate not to divide the entire input space into n_c decision regions. If a pattern has a low posterior probability for all classes, it may be beneficial to reject the pattern, rather than assigning it to a class. This is called *error-reject trade-off* [22,24,25].

B. MEASURING MODEL PERFORMANCE

Up till now we have assumed that we know the true posterior probabilities for the classes or that we have some estimate of the posterior probabilities. We will now introduce the notion of a model producing estimates of the posterior probabilities.

Assume we have a data set, D, which we shall call a *training set*, consisting of q_D input–output pairs drawn from the joint probability distribution $p(\mathbf{x},\mathbf{y})$

$$D = \left\{ \left(\mathbf{x}^{\mu}, \mathbf{y}^{\mu}\right) \mid \mu = 1,\ 2,\ \ldots,\ q_D \right\} \tag{33}$$

where **x** is an input pattern vector and **y** is an output vector containing the corresponding class label: $\mathbf{y}^{\mathrm{T}} = (y_1, y_2, \ldots, y_{n_c})$ with $y_l = 1$, if $\mathbf{x} \in C_l$, otherwise $y_l = 0$. This class labelling scheme is known as 1-*of*-n_c coding.

Let us also assume we have a model, M, parameterised by a vector, **u**, that is estimated on the basis of the training set, D, and let the model be capable of producing estimates of the posterior probabilities for the classes

$$M(\mathbf{u}) : \mathbf{x} \rightarrow \hat{\mathbf{y}} \tag{34}$$

where $\hat{\mathbf{y}}^{T} = \left(\hat{y}_1, \hat{y}_2, \ldots, \hat{y}_{n_c}\right)$ contains estimates of the true posterior probabilities, i.e., $\hat{y}_l = \hat{P}(C_l \mid \mathbf{x})$. We can now use Bayes' theorem to define several probabilistic terms for the model M:

$$p(\mathbf{u} \mid D) = \frac{p(D \mid \mathbf{u})\, p(\mathbf{u})}{p(D)} \tag{35}$$

$p(\mathbf{u})$ is the *prior parameter* and reflects our prior knowledge of the model parameters before observing any data. $p(D \mid \mathbf{u})$ is the *likelihood of the model* and describes how probable it is that the data, D, is generated by the model parameterised by **u**. The *posterior parameter distribution* is denoted by $p(\mathbf{u} \mid D)$ and quantifies the probability distribution of the model parameters once the data has been observed. The unconditional probability distribution, $p(D)$, is a normalisation factor given by $p(D) = \int p(D \mid \mathbf{u}) p(\mathbf{u}) d\mathbf{u}$.

Now, in order to design a model as close to the true underlying model as possible, we may find the parameters that maximise the posterior parameter distribution

$$\hat{\mathbf{u}}^{\mathrm{MAP}} = \arg\max_{\mathbf{u}} \left[p(D \mid \mathbf{u})\, p(\mathbf{u}) \right] \tag{36}$$

This is known as *maximum a posteriori* (MAP) estimation.

If we have a uniform parameter prior, $p(\mathbf{u})$, the MAP estimate reduces to the *maximum likelihood* (ML) estimate,

$$\hat{\mathbf{u}}^{\mathrm{ML}} = \arg\max_{\mathbf{u}}\left[p(D \mid \mathbf{u})\right] \tag{37}$$

The MAP and ML estimates are based on the assumption that there is one near-optimal model matching the true model the best. Bayesians argue that one should use the entire posterior parameter distribution as a description of the model when performing output predictions. Examples of Bayesian approaches include David MacKay's *Bayesian framework for classification* based on approximating the posterior weight distribution [26-28] and *Markov Chain Monte Carlo* schemes based on sampling the posterior weight distribution [29,30]. We will pursue the ML principle.

Assuming that the individual samples in D are drawn independently, the likelihood of the model can be written as

$$p(D \mid \mathbf{u}) = \prod_{\mu=1}^{q_D} p\left(\mathbf{y}^{\mu} \mid \mathbf{x}^{\mu}, \mathbf{u}\right) p\left(\mathbf{x}^{\mu}\right) \tag{38}$$

Instead of maximising the likelihood, we may choose to minimise the negative logarithm of the likelihood (since the logarithm is a monotonic function, the two approaches lead to the same results):

$$-\log p(D \mid \mathbf{u}) = -\sum_{\mu=1}^{q_D}\left[\log p\left(\mathbf{y}^{\mu} \mid \mathbf{x}^{\mu}, \mathbf{u}\right) + \log p\left(\mathbf{x}^{\mu}\right)\right] \tag{39}$$

Since $p(\mathbf{x})$ is independent of the parameter vector, $\mathbf{u}$, we can discard this term from equation (39) and minimise the following function instead,

$$E_D(\mathbf{u}) = -\frac{1}{q_D}\sum_{\mu=1}^{q_D} \log p\left(\mathbf{y}^{\mu} \mid \mathbf{x}^{\mu}, \mathbf{u}\right) \tag{40}$$

$$= \frac{1}{q_D}\sum_{\mu=1}^{q_D} e\left(\mathbf{x}^{\mu}, \mathbf{y}^{\mu}, \mathbf{u}\right) \tag{41}$$

where $E_D(\mathbf{u})$ is called an *error function* and $e(\mathbf{x}, \mathbf{y}, \mathbf{u})$ a *loss function*. Note that the negative log-likelihood has been normalised with the number of samples in the training set D, thus making $E_D(\mathbf{u})$ an expression of the average pattern error.

Now let us return to the MAP technique. As with the ML estimate, instead of maximising the posterior parameter distribution, we can choose to minimise the negative logarithm of the posterior parameter distribution.

$$-\log p(D \mid \mathbf{u}) - \log p(\mathbf{u}) = -\frac{1}{q_D}\sum_{\mu=1}^{q_D}\left[\log p\left(\mathbf{y}^{\mu} \mid \mathbf{x}^{\mu}, \mathbf{u}\right) + \log p\left(\mathbf{x}^{\mu}\right)\right] - \log p(\mathbf{u}) \tag{42}$$

Again we note that $p(\mathbf{x})$ is independent of $\mathbf{u}$, so we may discard this term and minimise the following function instead,

$$-\frac{1}{q_D}\sum_{\mu=1}^{q_D} \log p\left(\mathbf{y}^{\mu} \mid \mathbf{x}^{\mu}, \mathbf{u}\right) - \frac{1}{q_D}\log p(\mathbf{u}) \tag{43}$$

This function that we wish to minimise can now be written as

$$C(\mathbf{u}) = E_D(\mathbf{u}) + R(\mathbf{u}) \tag{44}$$

where $C(\mathbf{u})$ is called a *cost function* and $R(\mathbf{u}) \propto -\frac{1}{q_D}\log p(\mathbf{u})$ is a *regularisation function.* The latter is determined by the prior parameter and we shall return to this subject later in this chapter.

In the next section, we will derive a loss function for multiple-class problems based on the ML principle.

1. Cross-entropy error function for multiple classes

We will now consider the case where we have multiple exclusive classes, i.e., a pattern belongs to only one class. As per our previous analysis, we assume that we have a model capable of producing estimates of the true posterior probabilities for the classes $\hat{y}_l = \hat{P}(C_l \mid \mathbf{x})$. We use a 1-of-$n_c$ coding scheme for the class labelling and the distributions of the different class labels y_l are independent. The probability of observing a class label, $\mathbf{y}$, given a pattern, $\mathbf{x}$, is $\hat{P}(C_l \mid \mathbf{x})$ if the true class is C_l, which can be written as

$$p(\mathbf{y} \mid \mathbf{x}, \mathbf{u}) = \prod_{l=1}^{n_c} (\hat{y}_l)^{y_l} \tag{45}$$

Inserting equation (45) in equation (40), we obtain the following error function,

$$E_D(\mathbf{u}) = -\frac{1}{q_D} \sum_{\mu=1}^{q_D} \sum_{l=1}^{n_c} y_l^\mu \log \hat{y}_l^\mu \tag{46}$$

which is known as the *cross-entropy* error function [23].

C. MEASURING GENERALISATION PERFORMANCE

When modelling, we would like our model to be as close as possible to the true model described by $p(\mathbf{x},\mathbf{y})$. In order to measure this, we define the *generalisation ability* of a model as its ability to predict the output of the true model. Thus, the *generalisation error* of a model can be defined as

$$G(\mathbf{u}) = \langle e(\mathbf{x}, \mathbf{y}, \mathbf{u}) \rangle_{p(\mathbf{x},\mathbf{y})} \tag{47}$$

$$= \int e(\mathbf{x}, \mathbf{y}, \mathbf{u}) p(\mathbf{x}, \mathbf{y})\, d\mathbf{x} d\mathbf{y} \tag{48}$$

where the loss function, $e(\mathbf{x}, \mathbf{y}, \mathbf{u})$, could be, for example, the cross-entropy error. The lower bound of $G(\mathbf{u})$ is $G(\mathbf{u}^*)$, where $\mathbf{u}^*$ denotes the parameters of the true model.

In the limit of an infinite training set, D, the training error converges to the generalisation error,

$$\lim_{q_D \to \infty} E_D(\mathbf{u}) = \lim_{q_D \to \infty} \frac{1}{q_D} \sum_{\mu=1}^{q_D} e(\mathbf{x}, \mathbf{y}, \mathbf{u}) \tag{49}$$

$$= \int e(\mathbf{x}, \mathbf{y}, \mathbf{u}) p(\mathbf{x}, \mathbf{y})\, d\mathbf{x} d\mathbf{y} \tag{50}$$

Note that $G(\mathbf{u})$ is dependent on the training set through the model parameters $\mathbf{u}$. We may remove this dependency by defining the *expected generalisation error* as the average generalisation error w.r.t. all possible training sets of size q_D,

$$\overline{G} = \langle G(\mathbf{u}) \rangle_{p_D} \tag{51}$$

$$= \int G(\mathbf{u}) p(D) dD \tag{52}$$

Here we have acknowledged that the generalisation error itself is a stochastic variable and defined the expected or average generalisation error. We could equally well have defined other interesting measures such as, for example, the median. Refer to Larsen and Hansen [31] for a discussion of different generalisation error statistics.

Usually, we do not know the true joint input-output distribution, $p(\mathbf{x},\mathbf{y})$, and thus cannot determine neither $G(\mathbf{u})$ nor $\overline{G}$. Instead, we can compute either empirical or algebraic estimates of these quantities which we shall discuss in the next two sections.

1. Empirical estimates

Since we usually cannot assess the true joint input-output distribution, $p(\mathbf{x},\mathbf{y})$, we may resolve to using empirical estimates of this distribution.

One such estimator is obtained by employing a data set that is independent of the training set but drawn from the same true distribution, $p(\mathbf{x},\mathbf{y})$. We call this a *test set*,

$$T = \{(\mathbf{x}^\mu, \mathbf{y}^\mu \mid \mu = 1,\ 2,\ \ldots,\ q_T)\} \tag{53}$$

If we use the empirical joint input-output distribution, $\hat{p}_T(\mathbf{x}, \mathbf{y})$, based on the test set, we may now use the *test error* as an estimate of the generalisation error,

$$\hat{G}_T(\mathbf{u}) = \frac{1}{q_T} \sum_{\mu=1}^{q_T} e(\mathbf{x}^\mu, \mathbf{y}^\mu, \mathbf{u}) \tag{54}$$

As with the training error, $\hat{G}_T(\mathbf{u})$ converges to the generalisation error, $G(\mathbf{u})$, when the test set, T, is infinite.

Now, we would like the training set to be as large as possible in order to create an accurate model. At the same time, the test set should be large in order to get a reliable estimate of the generalisation ability of the model. Unfortunately, the available data is usually rather limited, so we have to deal with a trade-off between having a large training set and a large test set. A method trying to overcome this trade-off is called *cross-validation* [32,33]. The idea of cross-validation is based on training and testing on disjunct subsets of data resampled from the available database. If we split the database up into K disjunct data sets, we may estimate a model using $K - 1$ sets and evaluate its performance on the remaining set. This can be done K times resulting in K different models with K measures of the generalisation performance. The cross-validation error is then defined as

$$\hat{G}_{\text{CV}} = \frac{1}{K}\sum_{i=1}^{K}\hat{G}_{T^{(i)}}\left(\mathbf{u}^{(i)}\right) \tag{55}$$

where $\hat{G}_{T^{(i)}}\left(\mathbf{u}^{(i)}\right)$ is the test error defined by equation (54) and i the split label. This provides us with an estimate of the expected generalisation error defined by equation (51).

If each of the K disjunct data sets only contains one pattern, we obtain the special case called *leave-one-out cross-validation*.

Cross-validation has one major drawback, though, and that is the high computational costs involved. K models have to be estimated which for leave-one-out cross-validation corresponds to estimating as many models as there are available patterns in the data set. A scheme trying to remedy this based on linear unlearning of patterns has been proposed in Hansen and Larsen [34]. An application using this technique is presented in Sørensen et al. [35].

2. Algebraic estimates

Empirical generalisation error estimates require a fraction of the available data to be set aside thus reducing the amount of data available for the training set. And as stated previously, we would prefer a large training set in order to model the true model as accurately as possible.

In order to maximise the size of the training set, we will now consider an algebraic estimate of the average generalisation error based only on the data in the training set. We will assume the following:

- Independence of input and error on output.
- There exists a set of parameters, $\mathbf{u}^*$, that implements the true model, i.e., the chosen model architecture should be capable of implementing the true model.
- The number of patterns in the training set is large.

Under these assumptions, the following estimate of the average generalisation error can be derived [36-38]:

$$\langle G(\mathbf{u})\rangle_{p(D)} \approx E_D(\mathbf{u}) + \frac{1}{q_v}\left[\mathbf{J}^{-1}\mathbf{H}\right]^T \tag{56}$$

where $\mathbf{H}$ and $\mathbf{J}$ are the Hessian matrices for the unregularised and regularised cost functions, respectively.

This estimate may be used to select an optimal model among a hierarchy of models with decreasing complexity, i.e., every model should be a sub-model of the previous model in the hierarchy [38].

For other texts on algebraic generalisation error estimates, refer to references [39-42].

D. CONTROLLING MODEL COMPLEXITY

When estimating models, we face the problem of choosing a model that has an appropriate complexity. That is, the model should be flexible enough to adequately model the underlying function of the true model. At the same time, we should ensure that the model is not too flexible in order not to capture the noise in the data. The latter case is known as *overfitting* [23,43].

In brief, the purpose of controlling the model complexity is to maximise the generalisation performance of the model. We will in the next two sections consider two such techniques based on parameter regularisation and parameter pruning, respectively. Both methods are based on the assumption that the model is too complex.

1. Weight decay regularisation

As we saw in previous sections, the MAP technique involves a prior for the model parameters, and the cost function could thus be written as

$$C(\mathbf{u}) = E_D(\mathbf{u}) + R(\mathbf{u}) \tag{57}$$

where $R(\mathbf{u}) \propto \frac{1}{q_D} \log p(\mathbf{u})$ is called a *regularisation function.*

In order to avoid overfitting, we should consider a prior that has the potential of limiting the model complexity by ensuring that the decision boundaries are smooth. One such prior that favours small parameters is a zero mean Gaussian prior parameter with the individual parameters being independent. (Here we assume that small parameters lead to very constrained models while large parameters allow very flexible models, which will be the case for the neural network models considered in Section IV).

$$p(u_k) = \frac{1}{\sqrt{(2\pi)/\alpha_k}} \exp\left[-\frac{1}{2}\alpha_k u_k^2\right] \tag{58}$$

where α_k is the inverse prior parameter variance that can be used for controlling the range of u_k. We can now write the normalised negative logarithm of the prior parameter as

$$-\frac{1}{q_D} \log p(\mathbf{u}) = -\frac{1}{q_D} \sum_{k=1}^{n_u} \log p(u_k) \tag{59}$$

$$= -\frac{1}{q_D} \sum \left[-\frac{1}{2}\alpha_k u_k^2 - \log \frac{2\pi}{\alpha_k}\right] \tag{60}$$

where n_u is the total number of parameters.

We have seen from the MAP estimate that $R(\mathbf{u})$ should really equal $-\frac{1}{q_D} \log p(\mathbf{u})$, but since the second term in equation (60), $\log \frac{2\pi}{\alpha_k}$ does not depend on $\mathbf{u}$, and we wish to minimise $C(\mathbf{u}) = E_D(\mathbf{u}) + R(\mathbf{u})$ with respect to $\mathbf{u}$, we may discard this term and define the regularisation function as

$$R(\mathbf{u}) = \frac{1}{2q_D} \sum_{k=1}^{n_u} \alpha_k u_k^2 = \frac{1}{2} \mathbf{u}^T \mathbf{R} \mathbf{u} \tag{61}$$

where $\mathbf{R}$ is a diagonal positive semi-definite matrix with elements α_k / q_D in the diagonal. This particular form of the regularisation function is called *weight decay* in the neural network community since it penalises large parameters or weights, whereas, for regression problems in traditional statistics, it is known as *ridge regression* when all α_k's are equal [44]. The regularisation parameters, α_k, are also known as *hyperparameters* since they control other parameters, in this case, the model parameters.

2. Optimal brain damage pruning

As we saw previously, we could limit the effect of a parameter or implicitly remove it by setting its regularisation parameter, i.e., the inverse parameter variance, to a very large value. We could instead explicitly remove a parameter using one of several pruning techniques.

These methods are often based on computing the importance of each parameter by estimating the increase in an error measure that the removal of a parameter causes. All parameters are then ranked according to their importance – denoted as *saliency* — and a percentage of the parameters with the lowest saliencies can be removed. The model is then reestimated and the procedure is repeated until no parameters remain. This results in a family of models with decreasing complexity. For each model, an estimate of the generalisation error may be computed and used for selecting the optimal model.

We will consider a pruning technique, called *optimal brain damage* (OBD) [45], that is based on the following assumptions:

- The regularised cost function is at a minimum.
- The terms of third and higher orders in a Taylor expansion of the error and regularised cost function can be neglected.
- The off-diagonal elements in the Hessian matrix can be neglected if more than one parameter is removed.

Under these assumptions the OBD saliency for a weight, $\hat{u}_k$, is

$$s_k^{\mathrm{OBD}} = \left(\frac{\alpha_k}{q_D} + \frac{1}{2}\mathbf{H}_{kk} \right) \hat{u}_k^2 \tag{62}$$

where $\mathbf{H}_{kk}$ is the *k'th* diagonal element of the Hessian matrix.

IV. NEURAL CLASSIFIER MODELLING

The traditional approach to classification is statistical and concerns the modelling of stationary class-conditional probability distributions by a set of basis functions, e.g., Parzen windows or Gaussian mixtures [18,22,23].

Neural networks have, in the last decade, been employed extensively for classification applications. The two most common neural network architectures for supervised classification are the multilayer perceptron and the radial basis function network with two layers of weights. We will consider the multilayer perceptron architecture in greater detail in the next section.

Both classes of neural networks possess the important *universal approximation* capability, i.e., they may approximate any given function with arbitrary precision as long as the number of hidden units is large enough [18,46]. (If the network output function imposes bounds on the output values, it can of course only approximate equally bounded functions). Since neural networks "learn by example", they are particularly effective in situations where no suitable traditional statistical model may be identified, i.e., knowledge about the true data-generating system is poor.

Radial basis function networks will not be discussed any further. For a more thorough introduction, the reader is referred to Bishop [23].

A. MULTILAYER PERCEPTRON ARCHITECTURE

We will now focus on two-layer perceptrons and define a particular model architecture that is used throughout the rest of this chapter.

The hidden unit activation function used is the hyperbolic tangent function. Thus, the output of the hidden units for a pattern, $\mathbf{x}^\mu$ may be written as

$$h_j(\mathbf{x}^\mu) = \tanh\left(\sum_{k=1}^{n_I} w_{jk}^I x_k^\mu + w_{j0}^I \right), \qquad j = 1,\ 2,\ \ldots,\ n_H \tag{63}$$

where w_{jk}^I is the weight connecting input *k* and hidden unit *j*, w_{j0}^I is the threshold for hidden unit *j*, n_I is the number of inputs, and n_H is the number of hidden units.

The hidden unit outputs are weighted and summed, yielding the following unbounded network outputs:

$$\phi_i\left(\mathbf{x}^\mu\right) = \sum_{j=1}^{n_H} w_{ij}^H h_j\left(\mathbf{x}^\mu\right) + w_{i0}^H, \qquad i = 1,\ 2,\ \ldots,\ n_O \tag{64}$$

where w_{ij}^H is the weight connecting hidden unit j and the unbounded output unit i, w_{i0}^H is the threshold for the unbounded output unit i and n_O is the number of unbounded output units.

In order to employ the probabilistic framework derived in Section III, the neural classifier outputs must be normalised so that the classifier may be used for estimating posterior probabilities. We will now consider two slightly different normalisation schemes and discuss their properties.

1. Softmax normalisation

The standard way of ensuring that network outputs may be interpreted as probabilities is by using the normalised exponential transformation known as *softmax* [47],

$$\hat{y}_i^\mu = \hat{P}\left(C_i \mid \mathbf{x}^\mu\right) = \frac{\exp\left[\phi_i\left(\mathbf{x}^\mu\right)\right]}{\sum_{i'=1}^{n_O} \exp\left[\phi_{i'}\left(\mathbf{x}^\mu\right)\right]} \tag{65}$$

where $\hat{y}_i^\mu$ represents the estimated posterior probability that the pattern $\mathbf{x}^\mu$ belongs to class C_i. We thus have the following properties: $0 \le \hat{y}_i^\mu \le 1$, $\sum_{i=1}^{n_O} \hat{y}_i^\mu = 1$. As can be seen, the softmax normalisation introduces a redundancy in the output representation due to the property that the posterior probability estimates for a pattern sum to one.

An effect of this is that the unregularised Hessian matrix for a well-trained network will be singular due to the output redundancy, resulting in a dependency between the weights going to one output unit and the weights going to the other output units. This effectively reduces the rank of the unregularised Hessian matrix by the number of hidden units plus one (threshold unit). It will also affect any computations involving the inverse Hessian matrix. Employing regularisation reduces the problem, since this usually reestablishes the full rank of the regularised Hessian.

The standard softmax network is shown in Figure 13.10.

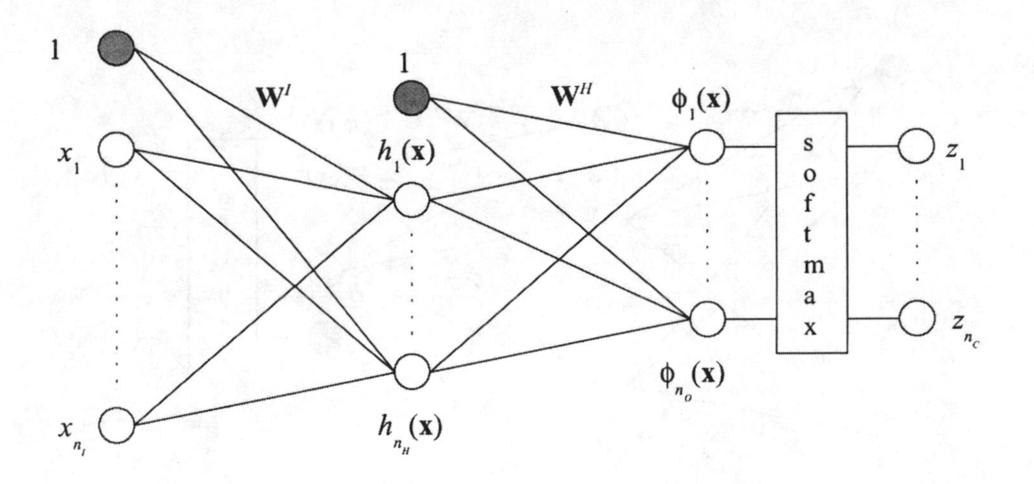

Figure 13.10 The standard two-layer softmax network. This has an inherent output redundancy yielding the unregularised Hessian singular for a well-trained network.

2. Modified softmax normalisation

In order to remove the output redundancy introduced by the standard softmax normalisation, we may remove one of the unbounded outputs. This yields the following *modified softmax* normalisation

$$\hat{y}_i^{\mu} = \begin{cases} \dfrac{\exp\left[\phi_i\left(\mathbf{x}^{\mu}\right)\right]}{1 + \sum_{i'=1}^{n_C - 1} \exp\left[\phi_{i'}\left(\mathbf{x}^{\mu}\right)\right]}, & \text{for } i = 1,\ 2,\ \ldots,\ n_C - 1 \\ 1 - \sum_{i'=1}^{n_C - 1} \hat{y}_{i'}^{\mu}, & \text{for } i = n_C \end{cases} \tag{66}$$

where n_C is the number of classes.

Another way of obtaining this modification is by removing all input connections to the unbounded output $\phi_{n_C}(.)$ and setting $\phi_{n_C}(.)$ to zero for all input patterns. Using the standard softmax normalisation (65), we now effectively obtain the modified softmax normalisation. This is illustrated in Figure 13.11.

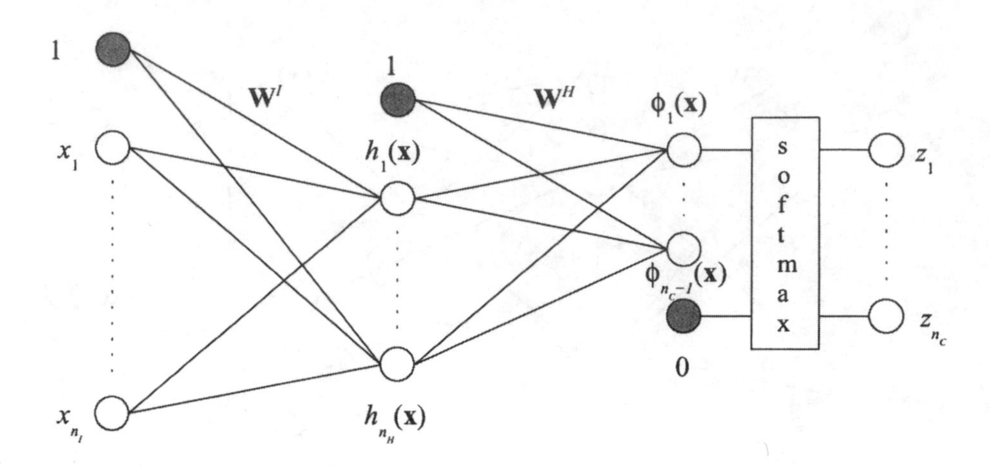

Figure 13.11 The modified two-layer softmax network. This does not have the inherent output redundancy.

The modified softmax normalisation has several benefits compared to the standard softmax normalisation. With a certain number of hidden units, the modified softmax normalisation reduces the network complexity, i.e., the number of weight parameters is reduced by the number of hidden units plus one. This improves the number of training patterns per weight relationship. The dependency between weights is removed, thus improving the performance of algorithms based on the computation of the inverse Hessian, e.g., the Newton scheme of updating weights which will be discussed later. Another example where the modified softmax normalisation may be beneficial is in MacKay's Bayesian framework for classification [26,27]. This framework approximates the posterior probability distribution of the weights by a Gaussian distribution centred on the MAP solution of the weights and with the inverse Hessian as covariance matrix. The posterior class probabilities are then found by using the entire posterior weight distribution. Any inaccuracies in the Hessian may affect the results considerably in this framework.

The modified softmax scheme is recommended for output normalisation.

B. ESTIMATING MODEL PARAMETERS

With the neural classifier architecture in place, we now need to address the task of estimating the model parameters. We will pursue the MAP approach with a Gaussian prior weight. As we recall from Section III, this yields the following cost function:

$$C(\mathbf{u}) = E_D(\mathbf{u}) + R(\mathbf{u}) \tag{67}$$

where $\mathbf{u}$ is a column vector containing all n_u network weights and thresholds, $E_D(\mathbf{u})$ is the cross-entropy error function (46), and $R(\mathbf{u})$ is a regularisation function proportional to the log prior weight.

The MAP solution for the network weights and thresholds will be found by using a training set, D, of size q_D and by using optimisation methods based on gradient and curvature information.

Common for these approaches is an iterative weight updating scheme that may be formulated as

$$\mathbf{u}^{(t+1)} = \mathbf{u}^{(t)} + \Delta\mathbf{u}^{(t)} \tag{68}$$

where t indicates the iteration time-step and $\Delta\mathbf{u}^{(t)}$ is the weight parameter change.

In the following sections, we will need the first and second derivatives of the cross-entropy error function w.r.t. the weights. Note, if the modified softmax normalisation is used then $\phi_{n_C}\left(\mathbf{x}^{\mu}\right) = 0$ in the following.

The gradient is

$$\frac{\partial E_D(\mathbf{u})}{\partial u_j} = -\frac{1}{q_D} \sum_{\mu=1}^{q_D} \sum_{i=1}^{n_C} \frac{y_i^{\mu}}{\hat{y}_i^{\mu}} \frac{\partial \hat{y}_i^{\mu}}{\partial u_j} \tag{69}$$

and the Hessian,

$$\frac{\partial^2 E_D(\mathbf{u})}{\partial u_j \partial u_k} = -\frac{1}{q_D} \sum_{\mu=1}^{q_D} \sum_{i=1}^{n_C} \frac{y_i^{\mu}}{\hat{y}_i^{\mu}} \left[-\frac{1}{\hat{y}_i^{\mu}} \frac{\partial \hat{y}_i^{\mu}}{\partial u_k} \frac{\partial \hat{y}_i^{\mu}}{\partial u_j} + \frac{\partial^2 \hat{y}_i^{\mu}}{\partial u_j \partial u_k} \right] \tag{70}$$

where the derivative of the posterior probability w.r.t. the weights is given by

$$\frac{\partial \hat{y}_i^{\mu}}{\partial u_j} = \hat{y}_i^{\mu} \sum_{i'=1}^{n_C} \left(\delta_{i,i'} - \hat{y}_{i'}^{\mu} \right) \frac{\partial \phi_{i'}\left(\mathbf{x}^{\mu}\right)}{\partial u_j} \tag{71}$$

and the second derivative is given by

$$\frac{\partial^2 \hat{y}_i^{\mu}}{\partial u_j \partial u_k} = \sum_{i'=1}^{n_C} \left[\left(\left(\delta_{i,i'} - \hat{y}_{i'}^{\mu} \right) \frac{\partial \hat{y}_i^{\mu}}{\partial u_k} - \hat{y}_i^{\mu} \frac{\partial \hat{y}_{i'}^{\mu}}{\partial u_k} \right) \frac{\partial \phi_{i'}\left(\mathbf{x}^{\mu}\right)}{\partial u_j} + \hat{y}_i^{\mu} \left(\delta_{i,i'} - \hat{y}_{i'}^{\mu} \right) \frac{\partial^2 \phi_{i'}\left(\mathbf{x}^{\mu}\right)}{\partial u_j \partial u_k} \right] \tag{72}$$

Note that we have expressed the derivatives as a function of the derivatives for a standard neural network with linear outputs: $\frac{\partial \phi_{i'}\left(\mathbf{x}^{\mu}\right)}{\partial u_j}$ and $\frac{\partial^2 \phi_{i'}\left(\mathbf{x}^{\mu}\right)}{\partial u_j \partial u_k}$.

It is often desirable for computational reasons to use the Gauss-Newton approximation of the Hessian instead,

$$\frac{\partial^2 E_D(\mathbf{u})}{\partial u_j \partial u_k} \approx \frac{1}{q_D} \sum_{\mu=1}^{q_D} \sum_{i=1}^{n_C} \frac{1}{\hat{y}_i^{\mu}} \frac{\partial \hat{y}_i^{\mu}}{\partial u_k} \frac{\partial \hat{y}_i^{\mu}}{\partial u_j} \tag{73}$$

This is motivated by Fisher's property [48],

$$\left\langle \frac{\partial^2 e(\mathbf{x},\mathbf{y},\mathbf{u})}{\partial \mathbf{u} \partial \mathbf{u}^T} \right\rangle_{p(D)} = \left\langle \frac{\partial e(\mathbf{x},\mathbf{y},\mathbf{u})}{\partial \mathbf{u}} \frac{\partial e(\mathbf{x},\mathbf{y},\mathbf{u})}{\partial \mathbf{u}^T} \right\rangle_{p(D)}$$

and is valid when using a log-likelihood cost function. An important property of this approximation is that the Hessian is guaranteed to be positive semi-definite, thus ensuring that a Newton step is in a descent direction. The Newton algorithm will be described shortly.

The detailed derivations of equations (69) through (73) may be found in Hintz-Madsen [49].

1. Gradient descent optimisation

One of the simplest optimisation algorithms is *gradient descent*, also known as *steepest descent*, derived from a first-order Taylor approximation to the regularised cost function. It is based on iteratively updating the weight vector so that we move in the direction of the largest rate of decrease of the cost function, i.e., in the direction of the negative gradient of the cost function evaluated at time-step t. This may be written as

$$\Delta\mathbf{u}^{(t)} = -\eta\frac{\partial C\left(\mathbf{u}^{(t)}\right)}{\partial\mathbf{u}} = -\eta\left(\frac{\partial E_D\left(\mathbf{u}^{(t)}\right)}{\partial\mathbf{u}} + \frac{\partial R\left(\mathbf{u}^{(t)}\right)}{\partial\mathbf{u}}\right) \tag{74}$$

where η is called a *learning rate* that ensures that the cost error decreases for each iteration when η is sufficiently small.

It is clear that too small a learning rate will result in slow convergence, while a too large learning rate will yield an inadequate first order approximation, which may result in an error increase. A simple approach for iteratively adapting the learning rate is described in the following first-order optimisation scheme with fixed regularisation parameters:

1. Initialise weights, e.g., uniformly over [–0.5; 0.5].
2. Compute $C(\mathbf{u}^{(t)})$, initialise the learning rate, η, (through initial experiments, a suitable value may be found), and compute the weight parameter change $\Delta\mathbf{u}^{(t)} = -\eta\partial C(\mathbf{u}^{(t)})/\partial\mathbf{u}^{(t)}$.
3. Update the weights, $\mathbf{u}^{(t+1)} = \mathbf{u}^{(t)} + \Delta\mathbf{u}^{(t)}$, and compute $C(\mathbf{u}^{(t+1)})$.
4. If $C(\mathbf{u}^{(t+1)}) > C(\mathbf{u}^{(t)})$, then set $\eta = \eta/2$ and go to step 3.
5. If the convergence criterion is not met (e.g., when the 2-norm of the gradient is below some small value), then set $t = 1$ and go to step 2.

This simple gradient descent scheme is not very efficient but it may be employed when more sophisticated optimisation schemes are not applicable. For example, this could be the case in the start-up phase for optimisation algorithms based on a second-order Taylor expansion where the quadratic approximation may be poor initially. That is, the gradient descent algorithm may be applied as initialisation for more advanced optimisation schemes.

2. Newton optimisation

There are several optimisation algorithms based on a second-order Taylor expansion of the cost function. One of these is the *Newton optimisation* method [43].

Using a second-order Taylor expansion of the regularised cost function, the weights are updated by

$$\Delta\mathbf{u}^{(t+1)} = \mathbf{u}^{(t)} - \eta\left(\frac{\partial^2 E_D\left(\mathbf{u}^{(t)}\right)}{\partial\mathbf{u}\partial\mathbf{u}^T} + \frac{\partial^2 R\left(\mathbf{u}^{(t)}\right)}{\partial\mathbf{u}\partial\mathbf{u}^T}\right)^{-1}\left(\frac{\partial E_D\left(\mathbf{u}^{(t)}\right)}{\partial\mathbf{u}} + \frac{\partial R\left(\mathbf{u}^{(t)}\right)}{\partial\mathbf{u}}\right) \tag{75}$$

where η is a step-size parameter that ensures a cost error decrease when the second-order Taylor expansion is poor.

The Newton algorithm may be formulated through the following iterative scheme:

1. Initialise weights; use for example the gradient descent scheme in the previous section.
2. Compute $C(\mathbf{u}^{(t)})$ and initialise the step-size, η, to 1.
3. Update the weights according to equation (75) and compute $C(\mathbf{u}^{(t+1)})$.

4. If $C(\mathbf{u}^{(t+1)}) > C(\mathbf{u}^{(t)})$, then set $\eta = \eta/2$ and go to step 3.
5. If the convergence criterion is not met (e.g., when the 2-norm of the gradient is below some small value), then set $t = t + 1$ and go to step 2.

The Newton algorithm converges in very few iterations but may be computationally expensive due to the need for computing and inverting the regularised Hessian.

C. OVERVIEW OF DESIGN ALGORITHM

Based on the optimisation algorithms described in this section and the probabilistic framework described in Section III, we will suggest a scheme for designing neural network classifiers based on adaptive estimation of the network architecture by using the optimal brain damage pruning technique described earlier. The regularisation parameters are fixed throughout the pruning scheme. The algebraic test error estimate described in Section III is used for the selection of the optimal network architecture.

In brief, the algorithm may be described as:

1. Determine the regularisation parameters. For example, these may be found by sampling the algebraic test error estimate as a function of these parameters, and selecting those that minimise the algebraic test error estimate. An example of this is shown in Hintz-Madsen et al. [50].
2. Train/retrain the network using the Newton optimisation algorithm. After pruning a small percentage of weights, only a few retraining iterations are usually required.
3. Compute the algebraic test error estimate.
4. Compute the OBD saliencies and remove a small percentage of the weights with the smallest saliencies. Go to step 2 if any weights are left.
5. Select the network with the smallest algebraic test error estimate as the optimal network.

After designing a classifier using this algorithm, Bayes minimum-risk decision rule and rejection thresholds may be applied.

Examples of using the algorithm are shown in Hintz-Madsen et al. [51,52].

V. EXPERIMENTS

We employ the design algorithm described in Section IV.C. using fixed values of the regularisation parameters combined with network pruning. Of particular interest is the pruning of dermatoscopic input features.

A. EXPERIMENTAL SETUP

A total of 58 dermatoscopic images distributed in 3 skin lesion categories are available as follows: *benign nevi*: 25, *atypical nevi*: 11, and *malignant melanoma*: 22. For each image, 9 features have been extracted. In summary, these are: 2 asymmetry measures, 2 edge abruptness measures, and 5 colour measures (see Section II for details).

One approach for attempting to overcome the limited data problem would be to employ bootstrapping methods for increasing the training set size [53-55].

We will use the empirical leave-one-out test error estimator described in Section III.C. for evaluating the designed classifiers. This provides us with 58 training sets, each with 57 patterns, and 58 test sets with 1 pattern. Thus, in order to design a complete classifier for solving the malignant melanoma problem, we need to design 58 classifiers for the 58 training sets.

The used network architecture consists of 9 inputs, 4 hidden units, and 2 output units with 2 regularisation parameters, α_{w^I} and α_{w^H}, for the weights/biases in the input layer and the weights/biases in the output layer, respectively.

The network weights are initialised uniformly over [–0.5; 0.5] and the regularisation parameters are set to $\alpha_{w^I} = 0.5$ and $\alpha_{w^H} = 0.9$. These are chosen in order to prevent significant overfitting of the training data. A more systematic approach for determining the regularisation parameters without the use of a validation set is to sample the algebraic test error estimate as a function of the regularisation parameters and use the regularisation parameters that minimise the algebraic test error estimate. Examples of this are shown in Hintz-Madsen [50]. Thirty gradient descent iterations are performed prior to using the Newton algorithm in order to identify a minimum cost function. Training is stopped when the 2-norm of the gradient of the training error w.r.t. the weights is below 10^{-5} or the maximum number of allowed iterations is reached. Matrix inversion is done using the Moore-Penrose pseudo inverse [48] ensuring that the eigenvalue spread is less than 10^8 (the eigenvalue spread should not be larger than the square root of the machine precision [56]). This is not a problem for this application due to the rather large regularisation parameters.

Next, the network is pruned and the optimal pruned model is selected as the model with the lowest algebraic test error estimate. Recall that this is an asymptotic estimate. Thus, its use may be questionable in an application with only 57 training patterns. During pruning, the *training patterns per weight* relationship improves, thus hopefully improving the validity of the estimator.

B. RESULTS

A total of 10 classifiers each consisting of 58 pruned networks, as described in the previous section, are designed. All results reported are the averages and standard deviations for the 10 classifiers.

1. Classifier results

Table 2 lists the cross-entropy error rates for the training and test sets before and after pruning. As expected, the training error increases as a result of pruning due to the reduced network complexity while the test error decreases only slightly.

Following Bayes' minimum-error decision rule as described in Section III.A., the network output with the highest probability determines the class. One could also adopt Bayes' minimum-risk decision rule [23]. The corresponding classification results are shown in Table 3. Here we see a more noticeable decrease of the test error from 0.441 ± 0.023 to 0.400 ± 0.007 after pruning. Note that there is still some discrepancy between the training error and test error suggesting that we are still somewhat overfitting the training set.

While the cross-entropy and classification errors yield some insight into the performance of a classifier, it is of great interest to see how the classification errors are distributed in the 3 classes. This information is contained in *confusion matrices*.

Since we employ the leave-one-out empirical test error estimator for model evaluation, the full classifier consists of 58 pruned networks.

Table 13.2 Cross-entropy error for the malignant melanoma problem. The averages and standard deviations over 10 runs are reported. One run is a full leave-one-out scheme using 58 training sets.

Cross-Entropy Error	Nonpruned Neural Classifier	Pruned Neural Classifier
Training	0.689 ± 0.002	0.757 ± 0.003
Test	1.022 ± 0.016	1.007 ± 0.006

Table 13.3 Probability of misclassification for the malignant melanoma problem. The averages and standard deviations over 10 runs are reported.

Probability of Misclassification	**Nonpruned Neural Classifier**	**Pruned Neural Classifier**
Training	0.273 ± 0.004	0.306 ± 0.001
Test	0.441 ± 0.023	0.400 ± 0.007

In Tables 13.4 and 13.5, the confusion matrices for the test set before and after pruning are shown. We see that the performance for the *atypical nevi* class is rather poor before pruning and even worse after pruning. The reason that the *atypical nevi* class suffers is the lower prior class compared to the *benign nevi* and *melanoma* class (recall that only 11 of 58 lesions in the training set are atypical). Thus, the error contribution from the *atypical nevi* class is relatively small making it fairly inexpensive to ignore this class during training. A method for minimising the risk of completely ignoring a class is to weigh each error contribution from a pattern in the cross-entropy error function with the inverse prior class. This corresponds to creating equal prior classes. In order to take the real imbalanced priors into account, the network outputs should be reweighed with the real imbalanced prior classes divided by the balanced prior classes [23]. This approach has not been employed in this work. It is interesting to note that the majority of the *atypical nevi* before and after pruning are assigned to the *benign nevi* class when recalling that the *atypical nevi* are in fact healthy. 72.7% ± 0.0% are actually classified as benign for the pruned classifiers. This suggests that the information in the extracted dermatoscopic features is not adequate for distinguishing the *benign nevi* from the *atypical nevi*, but is more appropriate for separating healthy lesions, i.e., *benign nevi* and *atypical nevi*, from cancerous lesions. Acknowledging this, we might be able to obtain a higher detection of the *melanoma* lesions by considering only these two categories of lesions when designing the classifiers. This has not been attempted, though. If we compare the test set results before and after pruning, we note that pruning has improved the detection of the *benign nevi* and the *melanoma* lesions significantly. In fact, a detection rate of 75.0% ± 2.4% for the *melanoma* lesions are comparable with the detection rates of very experienced dermatologists [2].

In Figure 13.12, the results of a typical run of the design algorithm are shown. For the non-pruned networks, the cross-entropy and classification test errors exhibit only very little overfitting. Notice how the Newton optimisation sets in after 30 iterations. If smaller regularisation parameters were used, the effects would have been much more dramatic. The pruning plots show that the decrease of the cross-entropy test error and classification test error occur at the end of the pruning session, i.e., when only 12 to 20 weights remain. Notice also that the minimum of the algebraic test error estimate coincides fairly well with the region where the test error is lowest.

For comparison, a standard *k-nearest-neighbour* (*k*-NN) classification was performed. Within a *k*-NN, a pattern is classified according to a majority vote among its *k* nearest neighbours using the Euclidean metric [22]. The training error may be computed from the training set by including each training pattern in the majority vote. The *leave-one-out* test error is computed by excluding each training pattern from the vote. Figure 13.13 shows the classification error on the training and test sets as a function of *k*. We see that for a wide range of *k*-values, the *k*-NN classifier has similar classification error rates on the test set compared with the nonpruned and pruned neural classifiers, suggesting that the *k*-NN classifier and the neural classifiers perform similarly. If we inspect the confusion matrix for the test set for a 15-NN classifier, shown in Table 13.6, we see that they classify quite differently despite having approximately the same overall classification error rate. The 15-NN classifier performs much better for the *benign nevi* class at the expense of the *melanoma* class. This is very unfortunate since the cancerous lesions are our major concern. From a medical point of view, it is significantly more expensive to classify a cancerous lesion as healthy. Again, we note that a large majority of the *atypical nevi* are classified as *benign nevi* supporting our earlier statement concerning the discriminating power of the extracted dermatoscopic features.

Table 13.4 Confusion matrix for the test set using nonpruned networks. The averages and standard deviations over 10 runs are reported.

Confusion Matrix for the Test Set	Nonpruned Neural Classifier		
	Benign Nevi	**Atypical Nevi**	**Melanoma**
Benign Nevi†	0.684 ± 0.058	0.709 ± 0.038	0.273 ± 0.000
Atypical Nevi†	0.108 ± 0.033	0.018 ± 0.038	0.041 ± 0.014
Melanoma†	0.208 ± 0.041	0.273 ± 0.000	0.686 ± 0.014

†Indicates the estimated output classes.

Table 13.5 Confusion matrix for the test set using pruned networks. The averages and standard deviations over 10 runs are reported.

Confusion Matrix for the Test Set	Pruned Neural Classifier		
	Benign Nevi	**Atypical Nevi**	**Melanoma**
Benign Nevi†	0.732 ± 0.019	0.727 ± 0.000	0.241 ± 0.037
Atypical Nevi†	0.032 ± 0.017	0.000 ± 0.000	0.000 ± 0.019
Melanoma†	0.236 ± 0.013	0.273 ± 0.000	0.750 ± 0.024

†Indicates the estimated output classes.

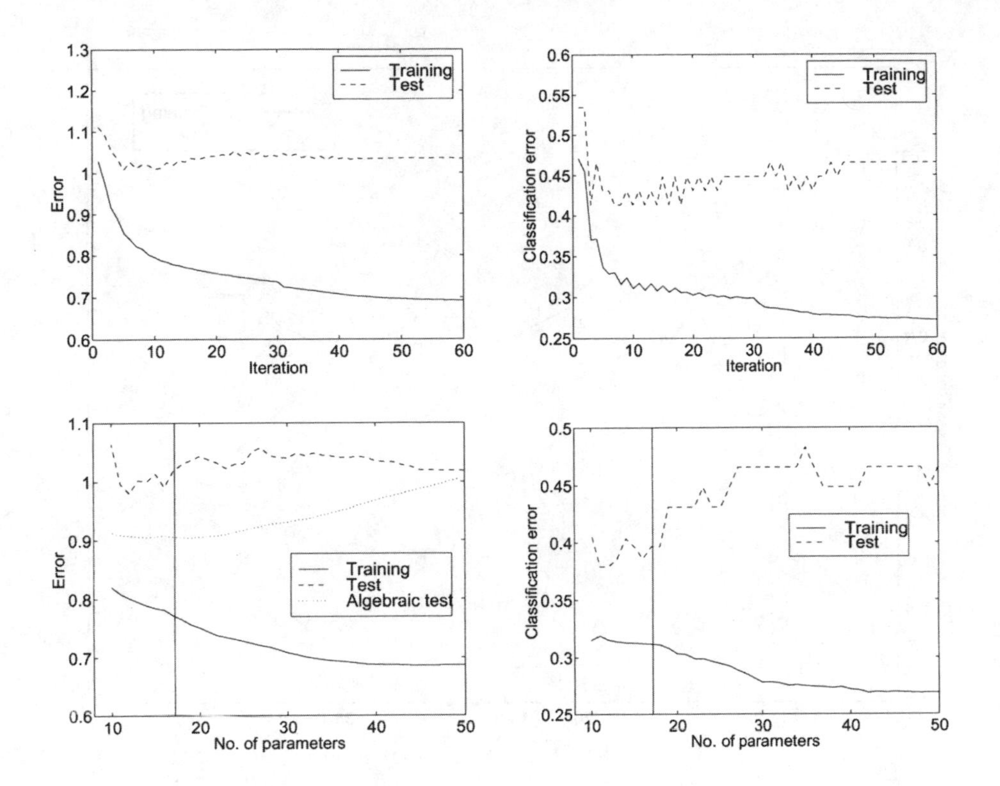

Figure 13.12 Results of a run of the design algorithm for the malignant melanoma problem. Each run consists of 58 networks. Upper left: The development of the cross-entropy error during training of the nonpruned networks. Gradient descent is used for the first 30 iterations, thereafter Newton optimisation is used. Upper right: The development of the classification error during training of the nonpruned networks. Lower left: The development of the cross-entropy error during pruning. The vertical line indicates the mean location of the minimum estimated test error. Lower right: The development of the classification error during pruning.

Table 13.6 Confusion matrix for the test set using a 15-NN classifier. Note that the classifier "favours" the *benign nevi* class, thus making costly errors in the *melanoma* class from a medical point of view.

Confusion Matrix for the Test Set	***k*-NN Classifier (*k* = 15)** Benign Nevi	Atypical Nevi	Melanoma
Benign Nevi†	0.920	0.818	0.455
Atypical Nevi†	0.000	0.000	0.000
Melanoma†	0.080	0.182	0.545

†Indicates the estimated output classes.

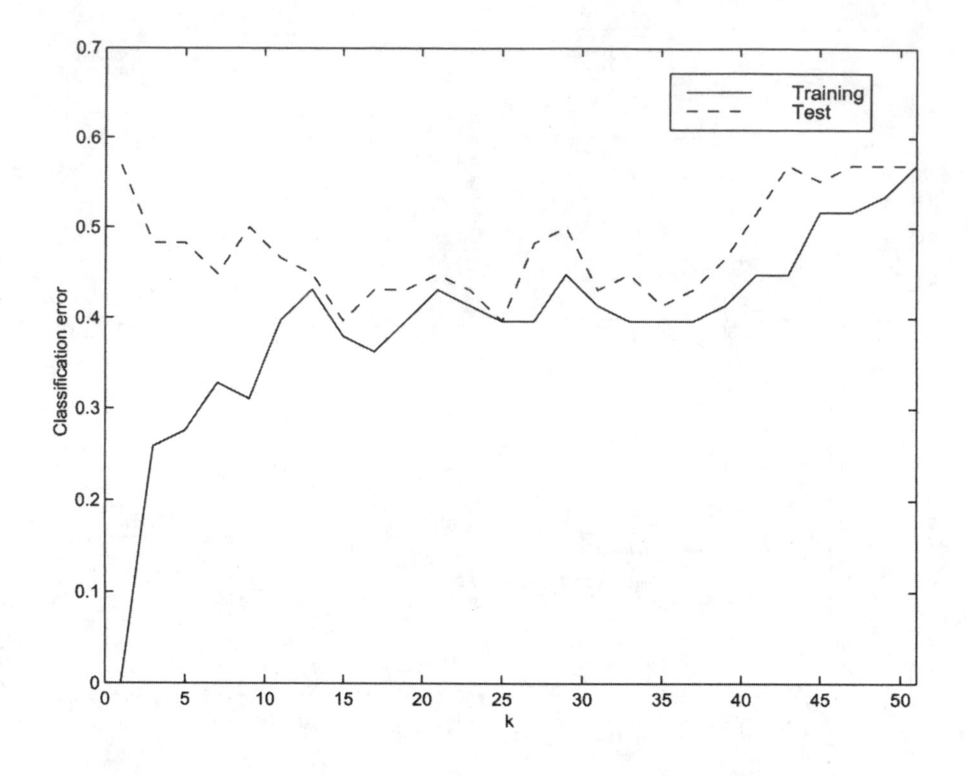

Figure 13.13 Classification results for a *k*-NN classifier as a function of *k*. Note that for a wide range of *k*-values, the *k*-NN classifier performs in a similar fashion to the nonpruned and pruned neural classifiers when comparing the classification rates.

2. Dermatoscopic feature importance

One of the most interesting effects of pruning is that it may provide information about the importance of the input variables. This is of particular interest for this application where the discriminating power of the dermatoscopic features is still rather unclear. Figure 14 shows an example of a pruned network selected by the minimum of the algebraic test error estimate. Two inputs have been completely removed by the pruning process. For this particular network, these are the *minor axis asymmetry* measure and the *dark-brown colour* measure. Those two measures are in fact the two most commonly removed dermatoscopic input features as can be seen in Table 13.7. This table also shows how often the individual dermatoscopic features have been completely removed during the runs of the design algorithm. Recall that each run results in 58 pruned networks. Thus, for each run the number of times a feature has been removed is computed relative to the maximum number of times it could have been removed (58). This enables us to compute the mean and standard deviation over 10 runs and sort the features according to their importance, assuming that the number of times a feature has been removed is inversely proportional to its importance.

It is worth noting that two features were never pruned: the *major axis asymmetry* measure and the *blue colour* measure. We know that the presence of blue colour in a lesion indicates *blue-white veil* and thus malignancy. So this is an expected result. We would also expect asymmetry to be important since this indicates different local growth rates in the lesion and thus malignancy. It is interesting to note that while the *major axis asymmetry* measure seems very important, the *minor axis asymmetry* measure is nearly always removed. The reason for this is probably that these two measures often are very similar which is also indicated by the skin lesion example in Figure 13.6. That is, they both contain the same information, thus only one asymmetry measure is needed. The *dark-brown colour* measure is the most often pruned feature. This is a bit surprising since the number of different colours present in a skin lesion is normally considered to correlate with the degree of malignancy. The removal of this feature could be due to the fact that the five colour measures sum to 1 for a skin lesion. Thus, it is possible to infer a missing colour measure from the remaining four. We also note that the *white colour* measure is often removed. This could invalidate the explanation of the inference of a missing colour measure but the amount of white colour, if present, is typically under 0.5%. That is, the *white colour* measure could easily be ignored in the inference of the missing *dark-brown colour* measure.

In summary, the three most important dermatoscopic features seem to be the *major axis asymmetry* measure and the *blue and black colour* measures, while the three least important ones are the *dark-brown* and *white colour* measures and the *minor axis asymmetry* measure.

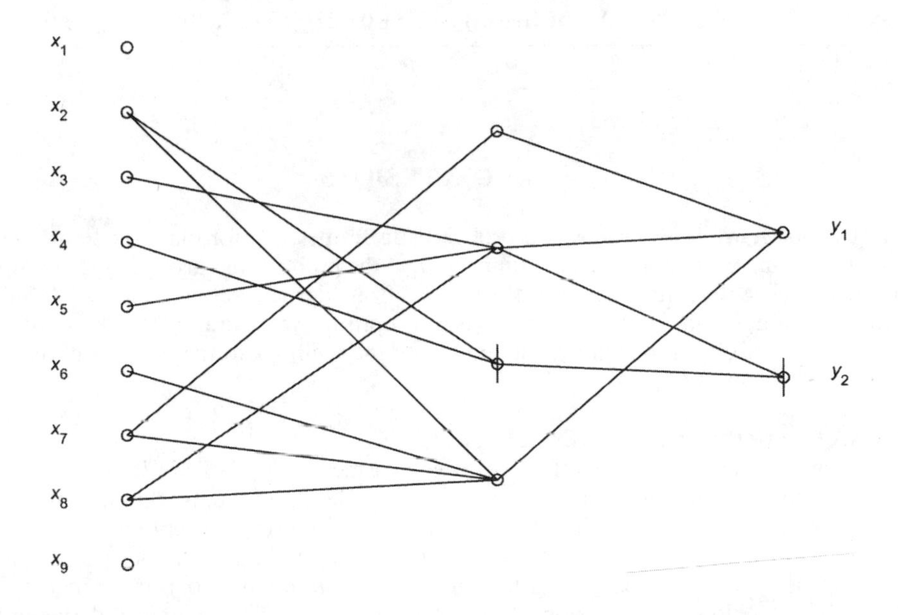

Figure 13.14 Example of a pruned malignant melanoma network with 17 weights. A vertical line through a node indicates a bias. The two pruned dermatoscopic input features are the *minor axis asymmetry* measure and the *dark-brown colour* measure. These are the two most commonly pruned input features. Recall that we only have two network outputs with weight connections due to the modified softmax normalisation.

Table 13.7 Table showing how often the individual dermatoscopic features have been completely pruned during the 10 runs. A zero pruning index for a feature indicates that it was never removed, while a pruning index of 1 indicates that the feature was always removed. The averages and standard deviations over 10 runs are reported.

Feature Importance	Pruning Index	Feature Importance	Pruning Index	Feature Importance	Pruning Index
Asymmetry: Major Axis	0.000 ± 0.000	**Edge Abrupt.: Std. Dev.**	0.053 ± 0.025	**Colour: White**	0.272 ± 0.031
Colour: Blue	0.000 ± 0.000	**Edge Abrupt.: Mean**	0.083 ± 0.021	**Asymmetry: Minor Axis**	0.772 ± 0.048
Colour: Black	0.022 ± 0.008	**Colour: Light-Brown**	0.097 ± 0.023	**Colour: Dark-Brown**	0.783 ± 0.054

VI. CONCLUSIONS

In this chapter, we have proposed a probabilistic framework for classification based on neural networks and we have applied the framework to the problem of classifying skin lesions.

This involved extracting relevant information from dermatoscopic images, defining a probabilistic framework, proposing methods for optimising neural networks capable of estimating posterior class probabilities, and applying the methods to the malignant melanoma classification problem.

A. DERMATOSCOPIC FEATURE EXTRACTION

The extraction of dermatoscopic features involved measuring the skin lesion asymmetry, the transition of pigmentation from the skin lesion to the surrounding skin and the colour distribution within the skin lesion. The latter involved determining colour prototypes by inspecting 2-D histograms and by using knowledge of dermatologists' colour perception. No reliable red prototype colour could be identified, though, partially due to a strong reddish glow of the dark-brown colour in skin lesions. It was seen that some of the extracted dermatoscopic features single-handedly showed potential for separating, in particular, the malignant from the healthy lesions.

B. PROBABILISTIC FRAMEWORK FOR CLASSIFICATION

The defined probabilistic framework for classification included optimal decision rules, derivation of error functions, model complexity control, and assessment of generalisation performance.

C. NEURAL CLASSIFIER MODELLING

The proposed schemes for designing neural network classifiers involved defining a two-layer feed-forward network architecture and evoking methods for optimising the network weights and the network architecture. Traditionally, a standard softmax output normalisation scheme is employed in order to ensure that model outputs may be interpreted as posterior probabilities. This normalisation scheme has an inherent redundancy due to the property that the posterior probability output estimates sum to one. This redundancy is generally ignored and results in weight dependencies in the output layer and, thus, a singular unregularised Hessian matrix. In order to overcome this problem, a modified softmax output normalisation scheme removing the redundancy has been suggested.

D. THE MALIGNANT MELANOMA CLASSIFICATION PROBLEM

The neural classifier framework was applied to the malignant melanoma classification problem using the extracted dermatoscopic features and results from histological analyses of skin tissue samples. The adaptive estimation of regularisation parameters and outlier probability was not employed due to the very limited amount of data available. Instead, optimal brain damage pruning and model selection using an algebraic generalisation error estimate were employed. In a leave-one-out test set, we were able to detect 73.2% ± 1.9% of benign lesions and 75.0% ± 2.4% of malignant lesions. None of the atypical lesions were classified correctly. We argued that this is probably due to the fact that the atypical lesions class has a small prior and is thus ignored during model estimation. 72.7% ± 0.9% of the atypical lesions were classified as benign lesions. Considering that atypical lesions are in fact healthy, indicates that the extracted dermatoscopic features are effective only for separating healthy lesions from cancerous lesions — i.e., the features do not possess adequate information for discriminating between benign and atypical lesions. As a result of the pruning process, it was possible to rank the dermatoscopic features according to their importance. We found that the three most important features are shape asymmetry and the amount of blue and black colour present within a skin lesion.

REFERENCES

1. **Lindelöf B., Hedblad M.A.,** Accuracy in the clinical diagnosis and pattern of malignant melanoma at a dermatologic clinic, *J. Derm.*, 21, 7, 461-464, 1994.
2. **Koh H.K., Lew R.A., Prout M.N.,** Screening for melanoma/skin cancer, *J. Am. Acad. Derm.*, 20, 2159-2172, 1989.
3. **Østerlind A.,** Malignant melanoma in Denmark, Ph.D. thesis, Danish Cancer Registry, Institute of Cancer Epidemiology, Denmark, 1990.
4. **Rassner G.,** Früherkennung des malignen melanomas der haut, *Hausartz*, 39, 396-401, 1988.
5. **Argenyi Z.B.,** Dermoscopy (epiluminescence microscopy) of pigmented skin lesions, *Derm. Clinics*, 15, 1, 79-95, 1997.
6. **Fischer S., Schmid P., Guillod J.,** Analysis of skin lesions with pigmented networks, *Proc. Int. Conf. Image Proc.*, 1, 323-326, 1996.
7. **Schmid P., Fischer S.,** Colour segmentation for the analysis of pigmented skin lesions, *Proc. Int. Conf. Image Proc. App.*, 2, 688-692, 1997.
8. **Ganster H., Gelautz M., Pinz A., Binder M., Pehamberger P., Bammer M., Krocza J.,** Initial results of automated melanoma recognition, *Proc. Scand. Conf. Image Anal.*, 209-218, 1995.
9 **Steiner A., Binder M., Schemper M., Wolff K., Pehamberger H.,** Statistical evaluation of epiluminescence microscopy criteria for melanocytic pigmented skin lesions, *J. Am. Acad. Derm.*, 29, 4, 581-588, 1993.
10 **Stolz W., Braun-Falco O., Bilek P., Landthaler M., Cognetta A.B.,** *Colour Atlas of Dermatoscopy*, Blackwell Science, Oxford, England, 1994.
11. **Stanganelli I., Burroni M., Rafanelli S., Bucchi L.,** Intraobserver agreement in interpretation of digital epiluminescence microscopy, *J. Am. Acad. Derm.*, 33, 4, 584-589, 1995.
12. **Karhunen H.,** Über lineare methoden in der wahrscheinlichkeitsrechnung, *Am. Acad. Sci.*, 37, 3-17, 1947.
13. **Loève M.,** Fonctions aleatoires de seconde ordre, *Processus Stochastiques et Mouvement Brownien*, Hermann, 1948.
14. **Mardia K.V., Kent J.T., Bibby J.M.,** *Multivariate Analysis,* Academic Press, London, 1979.
15. **Ridler T.W., Calvard S.,** Picture thresholding using an iterative selection method, *IEEE Trans. Sys. Man. Cyber.*, 8, 8, 630-632, 1978.

16. **Sonka M., Hlavac V., Boyle R.,** *Image Processing, Analysis and Machine Vision,* Chapman & Hall, London, 1993.
17. **Jain A.K.,** *Fundamentals of Digital Image Processing,* Prentice-Hall, New Jersey, 1989.
18. **Ripley B.D.,** *Pattern Recognition and Neural Networks,* Cambridge University Press, Cambridge, Massachusetts, 1996.
19. **Scott A.J., Symons M.J.,** Clustering methods based on likelihood ratio criteria, *Biometrics*, 27, 387-397, 1971.
20. **Skarbek W., Koschan A.,** Colour image segmentation – a survey, Technical Report 94–32, Institute for Technical Informatics, Technical University of Berlin, Germany, 1994.
21. **Wyszecki G., Stiles W.S.,** *Colour Science,* Wiley-Interscience, New York, 1982.
22. **Duda R.O., Hart P.E.,** *Pattern Classification and Science Analysis,* Wiley-Interscience, New York, 1973.
23. **Bishop C.M.,** *Neural Networks for Pattern Recognition,* Oxford University Press, Oxford, England, 1995.
24. **Hintz-Madsen M., Hansen L.K., Larsen J., Olesen E., Drzewiecki K.T.,** Design and evaluation of neural classifiers – application to skin lesion classification, *Proc. IEEE Work Neural Net. Sig. Proc. V*, 484-493, 1995.
25. **Hansen L.K., Liisberg C., Salamon P.,** The error-reject tradeoff, *Open Sys. Info. Dyn.*, 4, 159-184, 1997.
26. **MacKay D.J.C.,** A practical Bayesian framework for backpropagation networks, *Neural Comp.*, 4, 3, 448-472, 1992.
27. **MacKay D.J.C.,** The evidence framework applied to classification networks, *Neural Comp.*, 4, 5, 720-736, 1992.
28. **Thodberg H.H.,** Ace of Bayes: application of neural networks with pruning, Technical Report 1132E, The Danish Meat Research Institute, Denmark, 1993.
29. **Duane S., Kennedy A.D., Pendleton B.J., Roweth D.,** Hybrid Monte Carlo, *Phys. Let. B*, 2, 195, 216-222, 1987.
30. **Neal R.M.,** Bayesian learning for neural networks, Ph.D. thesis, University of Toronto, Canada, 1994.
31. **Larsen J., Hansen L.K.,** Empirical generalisation assessment of neural network models, *Proc. IEEE Work Neural Net. Sig. Proc. V*, 30-39, 1995.
32. **Stone M.,** Cross-validatory choice and assessment of statistical predictors, *J. Roy. Stat. Soc.*, 36, 2, 111-147, 1974.
33. **Toussaint G.T.,** Bibliography on estimation of misclassification, *IEEE Trans. Info. Theory*, 20, 4, 472-479, 1974.
34. **Hansen L.K., Larsen J.,** Linear unlearning for cross-validation, *Adv. Comp. Math.*, 5, 269-280, 1996.
35. **Sørensen P.H., Nørgård M., Hansen L.K., Larsen J.,** Cross-validation with LULOO, *Proc. Int. Con. Neural Info. Proc.*, 2, 1305-1310, 1996.
36. **Murata N., Yoshizawa S., Amari S.,** A criterion for determining the number of parameters in an artificial neural network model, In *Artificial Neural Networks*, 9-14, Elsevier, Amsterdam, 1991.
37. **Amari S., Murata N.,** Statistical theory of learning curves under entropic loss Criterion, *Neural Comp.*, 5, 140-153, 1993.
38. **Murata N., Yoshizawa S., Amari S.,** Network information criterion – determining the number of hidden units for an artificial neural network model, *IEEE Trans. Neural Net.*, 5, 865-872, 1994.
39. **Akaike H.,** A new look at the statistical model identification, *IEEE Trans. Auto. Cont.*, 19, 6, 716-723, 1974.
40. **Ljung L.,** *System Identification: Theory for the User,* Prentice-Hall, New Jersey, 1987.
41. **Moody J.E.,** The effective numbers of parameters: an analysis of generalisation and regularisation in nonlinear models, *Adv. Neural Info. Proc. Sys.*, 4, 847-854, 1992.
42. **Larsen J.,** Design of neural network filters, Ph.D. thesis, Electronics Institute, Technical University of Denmark, 1993.

43. **Hertz J., Krogh A., Palmer R.G.,** *Introduction to the Theory of Neural Computation,* Addison-Wesley, Reading, Massachusetts, 1991.
44. **Hoerl A.E., Kennard R.W.,** Ridge regression, *Technometrics*, 12, 55-82, 1970.
45. **Le Cun Y., Denker J., Solla S.,** Optimal brain damage, *Adv. Neural Info. Proc. Sys.*, 2, 598-605, 1990.
46. **Park J., Sandberg I.W.,** Universal approximation using radial-basis-function networks, *Neural Comp.*, 3, 246-257, 1991.
47. **Bridle J.S.,** Probabilistic interpretation of feedforward classification network outputs with relationships to statistical pattern recognition, *Neurocomputing – Algorithms, Architectures and Applications*, 6, 227-236, Springer-Verlag, Berlin, 1990.
48. **Seber G.A.F., Wild C.J.,** Nonlinear regression, John Wiley & Sons, New York, 1995.
49. **Hintz-Madsen M.,** A probabilistic framework for classification of dermatoscopic images, *Ph.D. thesis, Department of Mathematical Modelling, Technical University of Denmark*, Denmark, 1998.
50. **Hintz-Madsen M., Hansen L.K., Larsen J., Pedersen M.W., Larsen M.,** Neural classifier construction using regularisation, pruning and test error estimation, *Neural Net.*, 1998.
51. **Hintz-Madsen M., Hansen L.K., Larsen J., Olesen E., Drzewiecki K.T.,** Detection of malignant melanoma using neural classifiers, *Proc. Int. Conf. Eng. App. Neural Net.*, 395-398, 1996.
52. **Hintz-Madsen M., Pedersen M.W., Hansen L.K., Larsen J.,** Design and evaluation of neural classifiers, *Proc. IEEE Work Neural Net. Sig. Proc. VI*, 223-232, 1996.
53. **Young G.A.,** Bootstrap: more than a stab in the dark?, *Stat. Sci.*, 9, 3, 382-415, 1994.
54. **Efron B., Tibshirani R.,** Bootstrap methods for standard errors, confidence intervals, and other measures of statistical accuracy, *Stat. Sci.*, 1, 1, 54-77, 1986.
55. **Efron B., Tibshirani R.,** *An Introduction to the Bootstrap, Monographs on Statistics and Applied Probability,* Chapman & Hall, 1993.
56. **Dennis J.E., Schnabel R.B.,** *Numerical Methods for Unconstrained Optimisation and Non-linear Equations,* Prentice-Hall, Englewood Cliffs, New Jersey, 1983.

INDEX